Team-Based Oncology Care:
The Pivotal Role of Oncology Navigation

Lillie D. Shockney
Editor

Team-Based Oncology Care: The Pivotal Role of Oncology Navigation

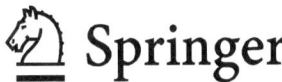 Springer

Editor
Lillie D. Shockney
Johns Hopkins University School of Medicine
Baltimore
MD, USA

ISBN 978-3-030-09861-2   ISBN 978-3-319-69038-4   (eBook)
https://doi.org/10.1007/978-3-319-69038-4

Printed on acid-free paper

This Springer imprint is published by the registered company Springer International Publishing AG part of Springer Nature
The registered company address is: Gewerbestrasse 11, 6330 Cham, Switzerland

Contents

1

Linda Burhansstipanov and Lillie D. Shockney

1.1 What Is Team-Based Oncology Care?

It takes a team of professionals to manage the diagnosis and treatment of a cancer patient today. Each brings their own skills, knowledge, and experience to the table. With the exception of multidisciplinary consultations during which time a patient will likely be seeing several providers all at once, it is more common for a cancer patient to be meeting with providers one at a time, focusing on the expertise they have that is needed by that patient at this specific juncture along their continuum of care. This can feel and look like each discipline is functioning within their own silo, and to a great degree, this is true. The challenge is continuous effective communication with one another so the patient can move smoothly from one provider to another as they continue their treatments/care. There are also members of the team who the patient will likely never personally meet; these professionals include pathologists and radiologists, for example, who have a pivotal role in diagnosing cancer, staging the cancer, and identifying other findings that may very well impact the patient's treatment going forward. At any given time, one individual may be the most important member on the team to that patient. For example, getting the results from the surgery that was performed is critically important postoperatively and rests in the hands of an experienced pathologist to determine the extent of the cancer; its prognostic factors, if all of the cancer was surgically removed; and other specifics about the cancer cells' features that will directly impact the decisions that will next be made regarding the next phase of the patient's treatment. Patients also may need to

L. Burhansstipanov, MSPH, DrPH (✉)
Native American Cancer Research Corporation, Pine, CO, USA
e-mail: lindab@natamcancer.net

L. D. Shockney, RN, BS, MAS, ONN-CG
Johns Hopkins University School of Medicine, Baltimore, MD, USA

© Springer International Publishing AG, part of Springer Nature 2018
L. D. Shockney (ed.), *Team-Based Oncology Care: The Pivotal Role of Oncology Navigation*, https://doi.org/10.1007/978-3-319-69038-4_1

1

be navigated backward along their care continuum when an unanticipated finding was learned about the cancer, which requires extending specific forms of treatment or changing the surgical plans originally made. The navigator needs to remain the constant point of contact.

In 1999 the Institute of Medicine's *Ensuring Quality Cancer Care* described the interdisciplinary cancer care team as including an oncology nurse, pathologist, radiation oncologist, medical oncologist, surgeon, nutritionist, social worker, occupational therapist, pastoral counselor, hospice volunteer, and pain management team made up of physicians, nurses, and pharmacists [1]. Of note is in the 2013 IOM report, *Delivering High-Quality Cancer Care: Charting a New Course for a System in Crisis*; patient navigators were included as team members [2]. The importance of there always being collaboration among all the team members, including the timely transfer of information among members of the team, is essential. Someone to facilitate coordination of care and undo barriers to care is a strength of the navigator professionals.

In 2011, the IOM convened the *Best Practices Innovation Collaborative of the Institute of Medicine Roundtable on Value and Science-Driven Health Care* which evolved into a discussion paper [3]. The roundtable was intended to provide common reference points to guide coordinated collaboration among health professionals, patients, and families—ultimately helping to accelerate interprofessional team-based care. This group identified five personal values that characterize the most effective members of high-functioning teams in healthcare: honesty, discipline, creativity, humility, and curiosity [3]. Additional ideals, particularly when working with underserved cancer patients, are trust, respect, patience, and the ability to truly listen to the patient as well as to other members of the healthcare team.

This IOM roundtable identified principles of team-based healthcare [3]. These are:

- Shared goals: The team, including the patient and, where appropriate, family members or other support persons, works to establish shared goals that reflect patient and family priorities and can be clearly articulated, understood, and supported by all team members.
- Clear roles: There are clear expectations for each team member's functions, responsibilities, and accountabilities, which optimize the team's efficiency and often make it possible for the team to take advantage of division of labor, thereby accomplishing more than the sum of its parts.
- Mutual trust: Team members earn each other's trust, creating strong norms of reciprocity and greater opportunities for shared achievement.
- Effective communication: The team prioritizes and continuously refines its communication skills. It has consistent channels for candid and complete communication, which are accessed and used by all team members across all settings.
- Measurable processes and outcomes: The team agrees on and implements reliable and timely feedback on successes and failures in both the functioning of the team and achievement of the team's goals. These are used to track and improve performance immediately and over time [3].

1.2   The Roles and Responsibilities of Various Oncology Team Members

The diversity of the oncology care team varies depending on the type of cancer, location of the clinical facility, and local resources. Building relationships with patients is a valued component in oncology care. These team members include support staff who frequently are ignored but are critical to making patients feel comfortable; helping making referrals; assuring timely appointments; scheduling admissions, procedures, tests, and treatments; greeting patients; answering phone calls and talking with patients politely; and assisting with financial and insurance issues [4]. As Cashavelly et al. (2008) express, "Support staff's interactions can positively impact a patient's care. A welcoming smile, a painless blood draw, or listening to a patient's fears and concerns adds value to quality care, which impacts the patient's experience and satisfaction with his or her care" [4]. They typically are the first interactions the patients and families have with the oncology team. Because the patients and families typically are stressed dealing with a life-threatening disease, it is essential that members of the oncology team are supportive of the patients and families as well as of one another who are team members. This also means that there needs to be organized and regular communication among team members about the patient so that all are "in the loop."

There has been confusion for patients as well as even oncology team members what the roles are of various individuals on the team; most commonly these professionals are navigators, nurses, physician assistants, and social workers. Their roles and responsibilities are described below.

Patients need to actually be part of their own care team too, providing accurate information about their medical history, current side effects, and compliance with taking medications as prescribed; participating in the decision-making about treatment; and also sharing their life goals as well as upcoming milestone events that should not be sacrificed to cancer and its treatment. The team should be informed, for example, about an upcoming important family event (impending birth ceremony), naming or puberty ceremony (Indigenous Peoples), or responsibilities (work retreat, firework sales in June and early July that support the family for the rest of the year, a granddaughter's wedding). This enables the oncology team member to plan treatments sooner or delay by a few weeks, avoiding the patient missing key family or work events, because patients should only need to give cancer the time it requires to get rid of it and not allow it to steal away any more of the patient's time. And for patients with advanced disease, quality of life and moments of joy are to be maximized instead of forfeited to their cancer.

1.3   Understanding the Complexity of Cancer Care

Cancer is a very complex disease and the healthcare system is overwhelming to most patients. The IOM 1999 report, *Ensuring Quality Cancer Care* [1], recognized these complexities and made a number of key recommendations to assure that all Americans receive high-quality care. These include:

Maintaining a system to measure and monitor the quality of care using a core set of quality measures and to provide quality benchmarks for use by health systems

Ensuring that key elements of quality care are provided for every person with cancer:

- Treatment by experienced professionals
  - Patients are provided an agreed-upon care plan.
- Access to the full complement of resources to implement the care plan
- Access to clinical trials
  - Policies to ensure full disclosure of information about treatment options
  - Mechanisms to coordinate services
  - Psychosocial support (p. 16) [5]

In 2005, the IOM released a landmark report, titled *From Cancer Patient to Cancer Survivor: Lost in Transition.* This report raised the awareness of cancer survivorship and clarified the toll of cancer and its treatment on the health, functioning, sense of security, and well-being of the patient [6]. This plan identified 10 key recommendations.

- Recommendation 1: Healthcare providers, patient advocates, and other stakeholders should work to raise awareness of the needs of cancer survivors, establish cancer survivorship as a distinct phase of cancer care, and act to ensure the delivery of appropriate survivorship care.
- Recommendation 2: Patients completing primary treatment should be provided with a comprehensive care summary and follow-up plan that is clearly and effectively explained. This "survivorship care plan" should be written by the principal provider(s) who coordinated oncology treatment. This service should be reimbursed by third-party payors of healthcare.
- Recommendation 3: Health-care providers should use systematically developed evidence-based clinical practice guidelines, assessment tools, and screening instruments to help identify and manage late effects of cancer and its treatment. Existing guidelines should be refined, and new evidence-based guidelines should be developed through public- and private-sector efforts.
- Recommendation 4: Quality of survivorship care measures should be developed through public/private partnerships and quality assurance programs implemented by health systems to monitor and improve the care that all survivors receive.
- Recommendation 5: The Centers for Medicare and Medicaid Services (CMS), the National Cancer Institute (NCI), the Agency for Healthcare Research and Quality (AHRQ), the Department of Veterans Affairs (VA), and other qualified organizations should support demonstration programs to test models of coordinated, interdisciplinary survivorship care in diverse communities and across systems of care.
- Recommendation 6: Congress should support Centers for Disease Control and Prevention (CDC), other collaborating institutions, and the states in developing comprehensive cancer control plans that include consideration of survivorship

care and promoting the implementation, evaluation, and refinement of existing state cancer control plans.

- Recommendation 7: The National Cancer Institute (NCI), professional associations, and voluntary organizations should expand and coordinate their efforts to provide educational opportunities to health-care providers to equip them to address the healthcare and quality of life issues facing cancer survivors.
- Recommendation 8: Employers, legal advocates, health-care providers, sponsors of support services, and government agencies should act to eliminate discrimination and minimize adverse effects of cancer on employment, while supporting cancer survivors with short-term and long-term limitations in ability to work.
- Recommendation 9: Federal and state policy makers should act to ensure that all cancer survivors have access to adequate and affordable health insurance. Insurers and payors of healthcare should recognize survivorship care as an essential part of cancer care and design benefits, payment policies, and reimbursement mechanisms to facilitate coverage for evidence-based aspects of care.
- Recommendation 10: The National Cancer Institute (NCI), Centers for Disease Control and Prevention (CDC), Agency for Healthcare Research and Quality (AHRQ), Centers for Medicare and Medicaid Services (CMS), Department of Veterans Affairs (VA), private voluntary organizations such as the American Cancer Society (ACS), and private health insurers and plans should increase their support of survivorship research and expand mechanisms for its conduct. New research initiatives focused on cancer patient follow-up are urgently needed to guide effective survivorship care [6].

Most of these recommendations were at least partially adopted by federal agencies and national organizations, positively impacting cancer care throughout the country. In particular, the recognition and potential value of patients having copies of their treatment summary and their survivorship care plan were deemed important for helping patients posttreatment to remain on track for their screenings and surveillance schedule and supporting the patient in the management of side effects from treatment as well as identification of late effects from treatment. These documents are also to assist the community providers who become responsible for the patients' long-term survivorship needs. Of note, the American College of Surgeons Commission on Cancer added standards (Standard 3.3) to their accreditation requirements for comprehensive cancer centers based on several recommendations from this 2005 IOM report.

The IOM 2013 report, *Delivering High-Quality Cancer Care* [2], again addressed and emphasized the complexity of the cancer. This report explained that the complexity of the cancer care system was "driven by the biology of cancer itself, the multiple specialists involved in the delivery of cancer care, as well as a healthcare system that is fragmented and often ill prepared to meet the individual needs, preferences, and values of patients who are anxious, symptomatic, and uncertain about where to obtain the correct diagnosis, prognosis, and treatment recommendations." The report acknowledges that receipt of high-quality cancer care is the exception rather than the rule. Many cancer patients do not have their questions answered in ways that are understandable; have no idea about information such as the stage of cancer at the time of diagnosis; and don't really understand what treatments they've received; short, long, or late effects of cancer; and what they should do next. These are all aspects that can be addressed by patient navigators through easy-to-understand communication skills and the trust relationship they hold with the patient.

The central goal of the 2013 IOM conceptual framework is delivering compre-hensive, patient-centered, evidence-based, high-quality cancer care that is accessi-ble and affordable to the entire US population, regardless of the setting where cancer care is provided [2]. The committee identified six components of high quality: (1) engaged patient; (2) an adequately staffed, trained, and coordinated workforce; (3) evidence-based cancer care; (4) a learning healthcare information technology (IT) system for cancer; (5) translation of evidence into clinical practice, quality measure-ment, and performance improvement; and (6) accessible, affordable cancer care [2].

The goals of the recommendations from the 2013 IOM report are as follows [2]:

1. Provide patients and their families with understandable information about can-cer prognosis, treatment benefits and harms, palliative care, psychosocial sup-port, and costs.
2. Provide patients with end-of-life care that meets their needs, values, and preferences.
3. Ensure coordinated and comprehensive patient-centered care.
4. Ensure that all individuals caring for cancer patients have appropriate core competencies.
5. Expand the breadth of data collected in cancer research for older adults and patients with multiple comorbid conditions.
6. Expand the depth of data collected in cancer research through a common set of data elements that capture patient-reported outcomes, relevant patient charac-teristics, and health behaviors.
7. Develop a learning healthcare information technology system for cancer that enables real-time analysis of data from cancer patients in a variety of care settings.
8. Develop a national quality reporting program for cancer care as part of a learn-ing healthcare system.
9. Implement a national strategy to reduce disparities in access to cancer care for underserved populations by leveraging community interventions.
10. Improve the affordability of cancer care by leveraging existing efforts to reform payment and eliminate waste.

Again, the patient navigator can help function as a member of the oncology team by providing consistent support and education using easy-to-understand language. They also serve as a mediator between the patient and other members of the oncol-ogy team who may have difficulty being understood by the patient.

The American College of Surgeons Commission on Cancer (CoC). The CoC is a consortium of professional organizations dedicated to improving survival and quality of life for cancer patients through standard setting, prevention, research, education, and the monitoring of comprehensive quality care. They accredit programs that meet all of their recommendations to improve their quality of patient care through various cancer-related programs. These programs are concerned with the full continuum of cancer from prevention through hospice and end-of-life care or survivorship and quality of life (p. 15) [5]. The CoC standards include patient navigation, in Standard 3.1 Patient Navigation Process. "A patient navigation process, driven by a triennial community needs assessment, is established to address health-care disparities and barriers to cancer care. Resources to address identified barriers may be provided either on-site or by referral." And patient navigators are frequently the staff to conduct Standard 3.2 Psychosocial Distress Screening. "Each calendar year, the cancer committee develops and implements a process to integrate and monitor on-site psychosocial distress screening and referral for the provision of psychosocial care" [5]. In 2015, AONN+ became the 53rd member of the Commission on Cancer. This professional organization strives to provide the training, education and mentorship, and support nurse navigators and lay patient navigators need to successfully navigate cancer patients across the continuum of care. AONN+ also measures the positive impact the navigation process has for improving patient care and delivering quality of care.

1.4   Oncology Workforce Shortage

New models of interprofessional, team-based care are an effective mechanism of responding to the existing workforce shortages and demographic changes, as well as in promoting coordinated and patient-centered care [2]. The IOM report (2013) [2] identifies several issues in the declining oncology workforce and notes that physician extenders (particularly nurse practitioners and physician assistants) will become the fastest growing medical professional group in the healthcare system. In part, this is due to the baby boomer generation of oncology specialists who are aging and retiring. The pipeline of graduating medical students is not increasing, and wooing graduates into cognitive disciplines away from more lucrative procedure-based specialties is a challenge [7]. This is all happening while the number of individuals diagnosed with a life-threatening cancer is continuing to rise.

1.5   Fragmentation of Care

The cancer patient experiences a healthcare system that is fragmented, both within a cancer center and clinical setting and between clinics in different locations. Given the diversity of the US healthcare system, such fragmentation is not unexpected, but it could be remedied through a combination of public regulation and cooperation between public- and private-sector purchasers of care [1]. Collaboration and coordination among primary care providers, oncologists, and other care providers and nonmedical members of the team are essential for patients to receive quality and timely cancer care. They need to develop and implement strategies on how to communicate with each other respectfully and to work out streamlined transitions in care [6]. The IOM 1999 report stated that the cancer care system does not ensure access to care, lacks coordination, and is inefficient in its use of resources [1]. Unfortunately, even within the IOM 2013 report, "coordination of complex cancer care, using a common electronic health record, with treating specialists who jointly discuss the patient's case and then confer with the patient about their recommendations, is the exception and not the rule" [2]. Clearly, the team needs to provide better coordination of care for all patients with cancer, but especially the growing numbers of cancer survivors [8], especially for underserved, rural, elder, and minority patients. Because most cancer patients are elders, gentle and respectful patient navigation skills are essential. Additionally, the team needs to develop efficient and coordinated ways to transition patients at low risk for cancer recurrence back to their primary care clinicians and prepare these providers and patients with plans for follow-up [8]. Patient navigators are important members of the team to help address this fragmentation.

1.6 Collaboration Between Patient Navigators and Oncology Nurse Navigators

A common saying is "it takes a village to raise a child," and similarly, it takes a team to provide quality cancer care to a patient. Oncology providers cannot work effectively in a silo and must communicate well with one another, at all levels (from the receptionist to the surgeon), for the patient to truly benefit. Kosty et al. (2015) states, "Clear communication and transparent, defined roles and responsibilities help ensure that care needs are addressed and timely decisions are made" [9]. Patients diagnosed with cancer expect that the many providers and staff with whom they interact across their care continuum will deliver a coordinated and seamless experience.

Patient navigators and oncology nurse navigators can and do collaborate with one another. Among the more common strategies is for clinical programs to have subcontracts with community patient navigation programs to access the local and cultural expertise they may need. Because they typically initiate interactions during the community outreach and education phase of the cancer continuum, their involvement with the oncology care team provides continuity. This is particularly important when considering the many different types of individuals the patient encounters during the cancer journey. Thus, the community patient navigator is a consistent source of support for the patients who are forced to cope with fragmented healthcare systems. In general, community patient navigators begin their work conducting outreach and education in the community, whereas most oncology nurse navigators are introduced to the patient once there is a suspicious finding. Domingo and Braun illustrated the relationship in Fig. 1.1 [10].

All navigators want to help patients through the cancer care continuum (from outreach and education, screening, suspicious finding, diagnosis, treatment, post-treatment, and survivorship/end of life). However, there is great benefit to the patient when community patient navigators and oncology nurse navigators collaborate. The oncology nurse navigator is an expert on medical information, identification of what

Screening	Suspicious finding	Diagnosis	Treatment	Post Treatment	Survivorship
Provide education on cancer Link clients to cancer screening	Link clients to further testing	Link clients to treatment	Support clients to complete treatment	Support clients to return to "normal life" or to hospice services	Support survivors with emotional problems and on-going screening
Links to health information, cancer care, insurance, financial assistance, transportation, housing, food, counseling, and other services.					Help family members access grief counseling, genetic testing, ongoing screening

Fig. 1.1 Cancer navigation through the cancer care continuum

resources are needed and how to access them for the patient, as well as empowering the patient. This individual also is well-versed on communication skills and can reiterate what the risks and benefits of the various treatment options are, while also addressing the patient's psychosocial needs. The community patient navigator is well-trained to translate complex medical information and terminology into easy-to-understand phrasing and language accurately, but without giving medical advice. Many community patient navigators speak the same primary and preferred language of the patient and can translate information, helping the patient avoid having to translate English into their primary language, deciding what they need and want to ask the provider in their primary language, translating that question back into English, and pronouncing the English words to phrase the question or query. The community patient navigator can also provide support, identify barriers to care, and provide resources to undo these barriers, while also arranging for referrals requested by the other oncology team members.

So each navigator has a specific focus. Depending on the medical environment, each institution needs to decide what model of navigation they will want to implement.

1.7 Navigation Includes Knowing and Distributing Information About the Patient's Life Goals

Patients had for the most part active lives before they were diagnosed and hope to resume those active lives after their treatment is completed. However, when gathering information about the patient, the focus is on their medical history and current status with less of a focus on the patient's life goals. To provide team-based oncology care, the team members must be aware of the patient's life goals are. These goals need to be acknowledged and, whenever possible and appropriate, incorporated into the decision-making process about treatment options. Patients can be too panicked to bring up any goals on their own because their focus is only on wanting to survive. Navigators can play an instrumental role by speaking with the patient specifically for this purpose. It is important to document these life goals in the medical records for the entire team to see and acknowledge so that the patient isn't sacrificing any more of himself/herself to cancer than is needed. For example, a patient may have her daughter's wedding coming up in 3 weeks. The surgeon tells that patient that she will be having a mastectomy with reconstruction performed in 2 weeks. The navigator needs to intervene with the surgeon so that the surgery can be arranged soon after the wedding rather than before so that the patient can enjoy her daughter's wedding, feel physically good that day, and have her clothes properly fit, free of drains. The navigator also can educate the patient that a slight delay in breast cancer surgery doesn't negatively impact the patient's clinical outcome.

Conclusion

This chapter summarized the importance of a comprehensive team-based care consisting of oncology specialists and a myriad of other ancillary support staff, all with specific roles and responsibilities focusing on taking care of cancer patients in the best way possible, beginning with awareness and screening in the community setting onto diagnosis, treatment, and finally survivorship or end of life. Recommendations from different organizations on how to improve collaboration within the team have been an ongoing focus and must continue to be, particularly in the fragmented healthcare delivery system we presently have across the country. The field of oncology needs more qualified and dedicated professionals and ancillary support staff entering the field to address the dwindling workforce due to retirement or of younger professionals moving into lucrative fields other than oncology. The shortage of oncology specialists simultaneous to the increasing volume of newly diagnosed cancer patients places oncology cancer care in crisis. Patient-centered care must remain the priority and focus for everyone involved today with cancer patients.

Some team members will only be involved with the patient during a finite time along their cancer journey (radiologist who performed the biopsy); others will never even meet the patient yet have a pivotal role in their care (pathologist who makes the diagnosis); and others will be alongside the patient across the continuum of care (navigators).

Navigators are essential members of the oncology team in providing continuity throughout the cancer continuum to serve as the point person for the patient as well as for the care delivery team. They also function as advocates in assuring that the patient's life goals are identified and respected by all members of the oncology team. They identify and resolve barriers to the patient's care, as well as promote patient-centered care by discussing and documenting the patient's life goals so that these future patient milestones can be preserved whenever possible.

Organizations such as the IOM and the CoC will continue to promote team-based quality cancer care and measure the ability of cancer centers to deliver such care in measurable ways.

The two members of the oncology team who are ever constant are the navigator and the patient.

References

1. Institute of Medicine. Ensuring quality cancer care. Chicago: National Academy Press; 1999. http://www.nap.edu/catalog/6467.html.
2. IOM. Delivering high-quality cancer care: charting a new course for a system in crisis. Washington, DC: National Academies Press; 2013.
3. Mitchell P, Wynia M, Golden R, McNellis B, Okun S, Webb CE, Rohrbach V, Von Kohom I. Core principles and values of effective team-based health care. Discussion Paper. Washington, DC: Institute of Medicine; 2012. www.iom.edu/tbc.
4. Cashavelly BJ, Donelan K, Binda KD, Mailhot JR, Clair-Hayes KA, Maramaldi P. The forgotten team member: meeting the needs of oncology support staff. Oncologist. 2008;13(5):530–8. https://doi.org/10.1634/theoncologist.2008-0023T.
5. American College of Surgeons, Commission on Cancer. Cancer Program Standards 2012: ensuring patient-centered care. Chicago; 2012.
6. Institute of Medicine and National Research Council. From cancer patient to cancer survivor: lost in transition. Washington, DC: National Academy of Sciences; 2005, 2006. http://www.nap.edu/catalog/11468.html.
7. Tempero M. Embracing team-based oncology care. J Natl Compr Canc Netw. 2014;12:845. https://doi.org/10.6004/jnccn.2014.0078.
8. Ganz PA. Cancer survivors: a look backward and forward. J Oncol Pract. 2014;10:289–93. https://doi.org/10.1200/JOP.2014.001552.
9. Kosty MP, Bruinooge SS, Cox JV. Intentional approach to team-based oncology care: evidence-based teamwork to improve collaboration and patient engagement. J Oncol Pract. 2015;11:247–8. https://doi.org/10.1200/JOP.2015.005058.
10. Domingo JB, Davis EL, Allison AL, Braun KL. Cancer patient navigation case studies in Hawai'i: the complimentary role of clinical and community navigators. Hawaii Med J. 2011;70(12):257–61.

History of Oncology Patient and Nurse Navigation

2

Linda Burhansstipanov, Lillie D. Shockney, and Sharon Gentry

2.1 Overview of Navigation and the Healthcare System

Over the last three decades, there have been improvements in cancer screening services as well as key developments in all types of cancer treatment [1]. During this same time, patient navigation as a health delivery support strategy has rapidly expanded and the importance of this care concept is becoming widely accepted. Interestingly, this care modality was noted in Russian culture in the 1700s as fcldshers or trained health workers to whom community members could turn for social encouragement or assistance, and later the idea was recognized in China with rural farmers who were trained to be called "barefoot doctors" [2]. The North American history started with Dr. Harold P. Freeman's patient navigation goal to improve outcomes in underserved populations by eliminating barriers to timely cancer diagnosis and treatment in a culturally sensitive manner [3]. Over time, patient navigation programs have also been shown to improve sharing of resources; enhance continuity of care, which can result in improved outcomes; improve quality of services; and increase patient satisfaction [4]. Navigation has matured across the oncology care continuum from outreach/prevention to survivorship and end of life [5].

L. Burhansstipanov, MSPH, DrPH (✉)
Native American Cancer Research Corporation, Pine, CO, USA
e-mail: lindab@natamcancer.net

L. D. Shockney, RN, BS, MAS, ONN-CG
Johns Hopkins University School of Medicine, Baltimore, MD, USA

S. Gentry, RN, MSN, ONN-CG, AOCN, CBCN
Novant Health Derrick L. Davis Cancer Center, Winston-Salem, NC, USA

© Springer International Publishing AG, part of Springer Nature 2018
L. D. Shockney (ed.), *Team-Based Oncology Care: The Pivotal Role of Oncology Navigation*, https://doi.org/10.1007/978-3-319-69038-4_2

2.2   The History of Oncology Patient Navigation

The development of the concept of patient navigation was related to the findings of the American Cancer Society (ACS) National Hearings on Cancer in the Poor that was conducted in seven American cities during 1989 [6]. The report based on the hearings revealed that the five most critical issues related to cancer and the poor were as follows:

1. Poor people endure greater pain and suffering from cancer than other Americans.
2. Poor people and their families must make extraordinary personal sacrifices to obtain and pay for care.
3. Poor people face substantial obstacles in obtaining and using health insurance and often do not seek care if they cannot pay for it.
4. Current cancer education programs are culturally insensitive and irrelevant to many poor people.
5. Fatalism about cancer is prevalent among the poor and prevents them from seeking care [7].

In 1990, as a response to this report, Dr. Freeman implemented the Harlem Cancer Education and Demonstration Project (HCEDP) to develop and pilot a patient navigation program, as well as expand community outreach and access to screening services with culturally sensitive educational programs to a predominately poor urban African American community [8]. The study compared 5-year survival rates of treated patients with breast cancer before (1964–1986) and after (1995–2000) the introduction of patient navigation, and the improvements in 5-year survival rates rose from 39% to 70% [9]. Those women who were diagnosed with cancer were supported through the entire cancer treatment process. The patient navigator movement expanded the idea that nonclinical staff members were needed to reduce health disparities.

The ACS in response to its report titled "Report to the Nation: Cancer in the Poor" was one of the first national foundations to recognize the value of patient navigation. It began supporting navigation programs in the mid-1990s by awarding grants, and by 2003, there were over 200 cancer care programs identified nationwide by the National Cancer Institute (NCI) that were providing patient navigation [10]. By 2007, the ACS funded more than 60 patient navigation programs across the United States [11]. In 2016, the Merck Foundation provided a grant of $1.58 million over 4 years to the ACS to implement a comprehensive patient navigation program in three US communities where substantial cancer care disparities exist [12]. Sites selected based on their ability to provide services to diverse, low-income, and underserved patient populations include the Queens Hospital Center in Queens, NY; the Phoenix Cancer Center/Maricopa Integrated Health System in Phoenix, AZ; and the University of New Mexico Comprehensive Cancer Center in Albuquerque, NM. This funding allowed the ACS to enhance its already substantial patient navigation program and expand its focus on access to high-quality care, patient empowerment, and care coordination.

In early 2000, Long Island College Hospital began a Breast Health Navigation Program (BHNP) to address their diverse community that was built on the HCEDP concept but incorporated an algorithm process for problem-solving and expanded the role of the navigators to enable them throughout the breast cancer trajectory. The BHNP demonstrated improved outcomes for support group attendance, patient satisfaction, follow-up appointment referrals, as well as a 1-day reduction in length of stay [13].

In 2001, a report titled "Voices of a Broken System: Real People, Real Problems" was released by the President's Cancer Panel [14]. The panel created from the 1971 National Cancer Act holds semiannual meetings in different geographic regions of the United States to gather information from government agencies, private organizations, healthcare providers, and individuals including cancer patients, to identify barriers to progress in reducing the burden of cancer [15]. Based upon the findings of these meetings, the panel generates a report for the President of the United States with high-priority topic recommendations, including actions that should be taken by relevant organizations. In 2003, they released "Facing Cancer in Indian Country," which focused on unique issues among American Indians and Alaska Natives [16]. In both the 2001 and 2003 reports, the President's Cancer Panel recommended that funding be provided to support community-based programs, such as patient navigator programs, to assist individuals in obtaining cancer information, screening, treatment, and supportive services [17].

In 2003, the US Department of Health and Human Services (HHS) Cancer Health Disparities Progress Review Group met and was assigned the task to identify strategies for the Department of Health and Human Services to address the growing cancer disparities in the United States [18]. Cancer health disparities were defined by the National Cancer Institute as "differences in the incidence, prevalence, mortality and burden of cancer and related adverse health conditions that exist among specific population groups in the United States" [19]. Nine HHS offices and agencies took part in the process, which started with 465 responses to the statement "specific actions that should be taken to eliminate cancer health disparities in the US are…" These were refined to 114 statements after removal of overlap and duplication, which then led to 29 roundtable recommendations and were finalized into 14 recommendations. These 14 recommendations were to be addressed across the three phases of "discovery" (for initiation within 1, 2, and 3 years), "development" (for initiation within 2 years), and "delivery" (for initiation within 1, 2, and 3 years) for HHS to lead the nation in eliminating cancer health disparities [20]. Throughout this process (e.g., within the original 465 responses), the need for patient navigation was emphasized for every aspect of the cancer care continuum from outreach and education through end of life.

In 2005, President George W. Bush signed the Patient Navigator Outreach and Chronic Disease Prevention Act [21]. This Act amended the Public Health Service Act to authorize the Secretary of Health and Human Services, acting through the Administrator of the Health Resources and Services Administration (HRSA), to make grants to eligible entities for the development and operation of demonstration programs to provide patient navigator services to improve healthcare outcomes.

The legislation authorized $25 million in grants through the Community Health Centers at Health Resources and Services Administration, the Office of Rural Health Policy, the National Cancer Institute (NCI), and the Indian Health Service to establish patient navigator programs by implementing a full-time navigator to empower, educate, and assist patients and families in disparate communities to journey through complex healthcare systems [22]. A key concept was that the funds supported the training and employment of patient navigators who had direct knowledge of the communities they serve so they could coordinate care and referrals, involve community organizations, facilitate enrollment in clinical trials, help assist patients with coverage by public programs or private insurance, as well as overcome barriers within the healthcare system to ensure prompt diagnosis and treatment [23].

The NCI adopted Freeman's goal for patient navigation in 2006 [24]. This 5-year cooperative agreement existed for awardees to develop operationally effective and cost-effective patient navigation interventions that would eliminate barriers to timely delivery of cancer diagnosis and treatment services [25]. Established and ongoing patient navigation programs were ineligible to apply since the grant's purpose was to initiate new, innovative navigation programs. The primary project, the Patient Navigator Research Program (PNRP), provided funding to nine sites, with a primary focus on populations that were experiencing cancer health disparities, focusing on breast, cervical, colorectal, and prostate cancers [26]. As is evident in Table 2.1, the studies were based in geographically diverse regions throughout the contiguous 48 states and the sites included both patient and nurse navigation interventions. The summary of key outcomes included:

Table 2.1 NCI patient navigation research program awardees (2005–2010)

Project titled	Principal investigator(s)	Population served
Chicago Cancer Navigation Project	Steven T. Rosen, MD Elizabeth Calhoun, PhD	African American, Hispanic/Latino
DC City-wide Patient Navigation Research Program	Steven R. Patierno, PhD	African American, Hispanic/Latino, Underserved
Improving Patient Outcomes Through System Navigation	Peter C. Raich, MD, FACP Liz Whitley, PhD	African American, Hispanic/Latino, Underserved
Moffitt Cancer Center Patient Navigator Program	Richard G. Roetzheim, MD, MSPH	Hispanic/Latino, African American, Migrant Farm Worker
Northwest Tribal Cancer Navigator Program	Victoria Warren-Mears, PhD	American Indian/Alaska Native
Ohio Patient Navigator Research Program (OPNRP)	Electra Paskett, PhD, MPH	Underserved
Patient Navigation in the Safety Net: CONNECTeDD	Karen M. Freund, MD, MPH	Racial/Ethnic Minorities and Low Income
RCT of Primary Care-based Patient Navigation-Activation	Kevin Fiscella, MD, MPH	Racial/Ethnic Minorities and Low Income
UTHSCSA Patient Navigation Research Program	Donald J. Dudley, MD	Hispanic/Latino

- Patient navigation increased rates of resolution of abnormal cancer screening findings and decreased the time it typically takes for patients to receive a diagnostic resolution.
- Patient navigation increased rates of treatment initiation among patients from a population who typically failed to begin treatment within 90 days of a cancer diagnosis.
- Navigated patients reported improved quality of life and increased satisfaction with the healthcare system/cancer care compared to non-navigated patients.
- Many patients with cancer identified financial problems and medical/mental health comorbidities as main barriers to healthcare access, and patients with abnormal screens identified language/interpreter issues as their primary barrier [27].

A previously successful NCI-funded program that supported the NCI decision to embrace navigation was the Waianae Coast Cancer Control Project that ran from 1989 to 1993 in the Pacific Islands [28]. The Native Hawaiian community-based organization, Papa Ola Lokahi, was awarded a cooperative agreement grant from the National Cancer Institute with the purpose to test the effectiveness of an integrated, community-driven cancer control intervention to increase breast and cervical cancer screening rates, as well as increase knowledge and enhance attitudinal and behavior scores among participants [28]. This intervention was designed to take advantage of Native Hawaiian social and family networks and their sense of "kokua" (Hawaiian term meaning "to help without being asked to help"). These "helpers" were called "navigators." A "navigator" was assigned to work with the community member to help them "navigate" or move successfully through the healthcare system comparable to how their ancestors navigated the waters traveling from one island to another. These navigators worked in rural native Hawaiian villages and communities to educate women and help bring them into healthcare settings for breast and cervical cancer screening. The program was very well-accepted, and the communities demanded more programs comparable to this original version [29].

In 2005–2010, the NCI Center to Reduce Cancer Health Disparities' Community Networks Program initiatives designed to reduce cancer health disparities awarded 25 programs to aid underserved populations such as racial/ethnic minorities and low-income rural residents [30]. The second initiative occurred from 2010 to 2015 and awarded 23 grants and again targeted underserved and marginalized communities. These grantees helped ensure that communities and populations experiencing a disproportionate share of the cancer burden had the resources to address cancer disparities by partnering with those communities in education, research, and training activities. Several of the programs in both rounds of grants hired, trained, and used patient navigators to carry out their respective interventions. Examples of awardees include 'Imi Hale Native Hawaiian Cancer Network, a native Hawaiian community; Mayo Clinic's Spirit of Eagles Native Navigators and the Cancer Continuum, an American Indian community; Carolina Community Network, an Appalachian and poor white community; Promoting Access to Health for Pacific Islander and Southeast Asian Women, involving Asian and Pacific Island communities; and Redes en Acción, focusing on Hispanic/Latino communities. All used patient navigation to address one or more phases of the cancer continuum from education and outreach through end of life [31].

A patient navigator is a trusted member of the local community who is employed by community organizations and trained to work directly with individuals to facilitate timely access to healthcare by eliminating or navigating barriers that may impede access to care. Community-based patient navigators begin their work by providing outreach and education but continue providing support throughout the cancer continuum. They cross the threshold of the clinic to work with the patient and other members of the healthcare team in the clinical setting.

There are other positions that serve the community and may have overlapping roles with the patient navigator. These include community health workers, promotores de salud, "kokua," peer leaders, peer health promoters, peer specialists, lay health advocates, lay health advisors, and case managers. Historically, several of these roles that are carried out by community patient navigators have a basis in cultural models and will not be covered in this chapter. The Affordable Care Act, signed into law in 2010, has patient navigation embedded within it to be "an in-person resource for Americans who want additional assistance in shopping for and enrolling in plans in the Health Insurance Marketplace" [32]. These "navigators" function primarily as insurance brokers and will not be covered in this chapter.

2.3   The Evolution of Oncology Nurse Navigation

During this same time period, the healthcare system was evolving to analytical patient-centered care [33]. It started with the utilization review prospective payment system where a patient's hospitalization had to be medically justified by an insurance-hired nurse reviewer. It set up an adversarial relationship between the physician, nurse, and hospital that escalated with the creation of concurrent chart review called utilization management (UM). UM hospital-employed nurses talked with physicians and teams to discuss more documentation to justify stay but did look at the root cause of delays in treatment and/or discharge. Then, third-party payers had their UM nurses who interacted with hospital UM nurses to encourage patient transfers to lower levels of care—more adversarial issues. The first focus on patient-centered care came about with case management where nurses experienced in chronic patient populations worked with healthcare teams to improve efficiency and adherence to care and link patients with hospital or community resources. Nursing patient navigation grew out of this focus on community outreach with emphasis on coordination of care/transitions of care [33].

Work in breast navigation was also the main patient population focus in nursing navigation as well as patient navigation. In the 1990s, the Johns Hopkins Hospital in Baltimore, Maryland, recognized the need in their community population of low-income African American women that the 40% no-show rate for screening mammograms needed to be addressed in their healthcare institution [34]. Provider and system delays were the main barriers to get follow-up care or treatment with many newly diagnosed patients presenting with stage III/IV disease and 15% showing up initially in the emergency department with pain. A focus group utilizing survivor volunteers as well as faith-based community leaders gathered personal perspectives of patients' experiences and expectations. At first, lay navigators were used to help patients access resources for care, but upon recognizing the deficit in patient education, psychosocial support, and barrier assessment, a nurse navigator role was implemented at the point of diagnosis. A key to a successful evolution of this program was the use of an operations management process map tool that allowed the care to be seen through the eyes of the patient and family [35]. The institution increased timeliness to care and most notably reduced the start time of chemotherapy by 2 weeks by using this process [36].

At the end of the 1990s, a shift from inpatient care to outpatient or ambulatory care for breast cancer treatment gave Baptist Medical Center in South Carolina an opportunity to implement a program of education and support for breast cancer patients that centered around a breast health specialist or nurse navigator who supported patients during their entire breast cancer experience [37]. In 1994, Judy Kneece began EduCare, Inc., a breast health publishing and training company to prepare nurses to successfully navigate patients in an interdisciplinary manner [38]. In 1999, Lexington Medical Center in South Carolina redesigned their breast care delivery around the concept of a breast health navigator to provide education, support, and anticipatory guidance from diagnosis through treatment, and the wait time for a diagnostic mammogram went from 2 weeks to 24 hours, with 95% of the patients receiving a breast biopsy pathology result within 24 hours [39].

In 2005, Pfizer Inc. announced the launch of a novel multimedia tool kit designed to help hospitals and health systems throughout the United States introduce patient navigation programs for cancer care [40]. Patient Navigation in Cancer Care: Guiding Patients to Quality Outcomes was aimed to equip hospitals and health systems with detailed guidance on how to establish and evaluate navigation programs and also provide resources and training information for navigators [41]. The comprehensive tool kit was developed as a cooperative effort between Pfizer and the Healthcare Association of New York State, in consultation with Dr. Harold Freeman, President and Founder of the Ralph Lauren Center for Cancer Care and Prevention in Harlem, NY [40].

Navigation on the nursing front continued to develop as the Oncology Nursing Society in 2008 at their 33rd Annual Congress hosted a session on "Implementing the Nurse Navigator Role" [42]. In the same year, the National Coalition of Oncology Nurse Navigators (NCONN) incorporated but disbanded in 2014 [43]. They published "Core Competencies for the Oncology Nurse Navigator" in 2009, with the focus of this work to integrate the roles of healthcare promoter, educator, counselor, care coordinator, case manager, researcher, and patient advocate in the nurse navigator function [44].

Also in 2009, the Academy of Oncology Nurse Navigators (AONN) incorporated with the commitment to improve patient care and quality of life by defining, enhancing, and promoting the role of oncology nurse and patient navigators [45]. The 10th Annual Oncology Nursing Society Institutes of Learning had a presentation acknowledging nonclinical versus clinical navigators. An educational grant from Sanofi-Aventis, United States, enabled the Association of Community Cancer

Centers (ACCC) along with the Meniscus Educational Institute to introduce a comprehensive online resource to help cancer programs develop or enhance patient navigation services [46]. This was enhanced by their publication "Patient Navigation: A Call to Action," which was a resource for community cancer programs interested in implementing or expanding patient navigation services, and included some of the first published navigation tools such as pre-assessment forms, intake summaries, referral forms, navigation tracking forms, and patient satisfaction surveys [47].

In 2010, AONN established the *Journal of Oncology Navigation & Survivorship* (*JONS*) to promote the success and work of navigators [48]. The Oncology Nursing Society/Association of Social Work and the National Association of Social Workers published a joint position on the role of oncology nursing and oncology social work in patient navigation that recognized the teamwork of lay navigators, nurses, and social workers but called for navigation services delegated to lay navigators to be supervised by nurses or social workers [49].

Several national organizations in 2010 were addressing parallel issues to support nursing navigation in healthcare. The Patient-Centered Medical Home Model was being tried as a structured approach that strengthens the clinician-patient relationship by replacing episodic or reactive care with coordinated care where patients' needs are anticipated and decision-making is evidence-based and is coordinated and integrated [50]. Nurse navigators fit the focus of coordination across the complex healthcare system and the patient's community ensuring that the patients get the care they need in a culturally appropriate manner. The National Quality Forum released a portfolio of care coordination preferred practices and performance measures to evaluate access, continuity, communication, and tracking of patients across providers and settings in order to promote transitions in care settings [51]. Navigation oversight of patients who see multiple physicians and care providers can assist in reducing medication errors, hospital readmissions, and avoidable emergency department visits. The Health and Medicine Division of the National Academies of Sciences, Engineering, and Medicine (formerly the Institute of Medicine) released a report, "The Future of Nursing: Leading Change, Advancing Health," that supported nurses practicing to the full extent of their education and training and being partners with physicians and other healthcare professionals in redesigning healthcare in the United States [52].

In 2011, the first book on navigation was published by Jones and Bartlett— *Becoming a Breast Cancer Nurse Navigator* by Lillie Shockney—that was a primer for breast nurse navigators, but the tools and concepts could be applied to any cancer care navigation process [53].

AONN experienced a name change in 2013, to Academy of Oncology Nurse & Patient Navigators® (AONN+) to reflect support of the entire navigation community, whether nurses, social workers, lay professionals, administrators, or others [54]. *Seminars in Oncology Nursing* dedicated their May 2013 issue to "Patient Navigation in Cancer Care," and this was an overview of the navigation state of knowledge [55].

In 2014, ONS released the book, *Oncology Nurse Navigation: Delivering Patient-Centered Care Across the Continuum*, and in 2017 published, *Oncology Nurse Navigation Case Studies* as an education and navigation resource for nurse navigators [56].

In 2017, the American Cancer Society initiated work with leading organizations and individuals in the patient navigation field to form a National Navigation Roundtable (NNRT). The intent is to build a national coalition of public, private, and voluntary organizations, and invited experts dedicated to achieving access to quality equitable cancer care across the cancer continuum through various types of patient navigation. The ultimate goal of the NNRT is to increase access to evidence-based navigation services among the entire population for whom navigation is appropriate with the aim to do this through increased awareness, provider education, public education, systems changes, and health policy activities.

The leaders from the American Cancer Society are Katherine Sharpe, MTS, Senior Vice President with Patient and Caregiver Support, and Monica Dean, Director of the National Navigation Roundtable. Three task force groups are addressing training and certification, evidenced based promising practices and policy. Work is ongoing as this group meets monthly via web and in-person annually to focus on advancing navigation in a sustainable and unified manner (http://patientnavigator-training.org/colorado-leaders-help-launch-national-navigation-roundtable).

2.4   National Accreditation Programs Involving Navigation

In 2008, the National Accreditation Program for Breast Centers was created to establish evidence-based standards for the management of patients with breast cancer and benign breast disease, as well as to stipulate a process for elected cancer programs to monitor compliance [57]. It was the first organization to include a standard for navigation. Standard 2.2 states that a "patient navigation process is in place to guide the patient with a breast abnormality through provided and referred services" [58]. The standard recognizes that breast navigation will be unique based on community needs but requires the manner of practice to include "consistent care coordination throughout the continuum of care and an assessment of the physical, psychological and social needs of the patient with results for enhanced patient outcomes, increased satisfaction, and reduced costs of care" [58]. It does not specify a patient or nurse navigator to fulfill the role. Just as the breast care, cancer diagnosis, and treatment process differ from facility to facility, so do the definitions, activities, knowledge, and job descriptions of a breast patient navigator.

In 2012, the American College of Surgeons' Commission on Cancer (CoC) released a new standard that was reflective of their focus on enhancing patient-centered care [59]. The CoC clarified, "Patient navigation in cancer care refers to specialized assistance for the community, patients, families, and caregivers to assist in overcoming barriers to receiving care and facilitating timely access to clinical services and resources. Navigation processes encompass pre-diagnosis through all phases of the cancer experience. The navigation services implemented will depend upon the particular type, severity, and/or complexity of the identified barriers" [60]. The standard did not specify a patient or nurse navigator to fulfill the role. At the same time, the CoC included two other standards for accreditation that could impact the navigator role:

- Standard 3.2: Psychosocial Distress Screening
- Standard 3.3: Survivorship Care Plan

These standards would be required to be implemented by 2015 for all cancer facilities that wish to be accredited by the American College of Surgeons Commission on Cancer.

2.5   Delineation of Roles and Competencies for Navigators

At this point, the benefits of patient navigation had been recognized by different organizations, but the role of nurse or patient navigators, the terms used to describe them, and their functions within the oncology care team were not consistent. ONS published an Oncology Nurse Navigator Role Delineation Study in 2012 that assessed the job activities of the oncology nurse navigator from the feedback of 330 nurses and concluded there was overlap in knowledge with the general oncology nurse role that needed further exploration [61]. It was repeated again in 2016 since the role had expanded over the years, and concluded from 498 responses that the role required similar knowledge and skills of an oncology nurse but did recognize the difference in daily practice where the nurse navigator provides care coordination, guidance, education, and advocacy across care settings [62]. In 2013, Willis, Pratt-Chapman, and their team at The George Washington University Cancer Institute clarified roles between a nurse navigator, patient navigator, and community health worker in collaboration with national stakeholders in navigation and published the Patient Navigation Framework in *JONS* [63]. Willis and colleagues conveyed that patient navigators focused on barriers accessing the healthcare system and addressing general health disparities, while healthcare institution navigators such as nurses and social workers addressed clinical and service delivery barriers at the institutional or systemic level. The framework consists of 12 agreed-upon functional domains for navigation, and the role differences/similarities for each domain are explained in Table 2.2. This clarification of roles has potential to support competency development as well as future certification efforts.

In 2013, ONS published Oncology Nurse Navigator Core Competencies that were developed by using a literature review, a field review of 189 responses, and a team of 10 expert reviewers [64]. They defined a novice nurse navigator as having 2 years or less navigation experience and established four functional areas of professional role, education, coordination of care, and communication. They were updated again in 2017 using the same process and added a definition for an expert oncology nurse navigator as well as 12 expert core competencies [65].

During this same time, Willis and colleagues used the Patient Navigation Framework to create and publish competencies for patient navigators [66]. The process of literature review, national patient navigation focus groups, national experts, Accreditation Council for Graduate Medical Education competence domain structure, and a final survey response from 525 professional navigators resulted in 8 competency domains with 65 competency statements [66]. Table 2.3 shows the final competencies that have been used to develop a free online training funded by the

Table 2.2 Patient navigation framework: navigator function across domains

Domain	Community (Community Health Worker)	Community/ Healthcare Institution (Patient Navigator)	Healthcare Institution (Nurse Navigator/Social Work Navigator)
Professional Roles and Responsibilities: *The knowledge base and skills needed to perform job-related duties and tasks, including understanding scope of practice, supporting evaluation efforts, and identifying and exercising self-care strategies*	General knowledge base on health issues such as cancer, diabetes, obesity, heart disease, stroke, HIV/ AIDS, and other chronic diseases	Knowledge of cancer screening, diagnosis, treatment, and survivorship and related physical, psychological, and social issues	Knowledge and maintenance of knowledge (e.g., license, certification, continuing education) of cancer clinical impacts on patient, caregivers, and families and ability to intervene (e.g., symptom management, assessment of functional status and psychosocial health)
The following general skills are required:	Active documentation in client record	Active documentation of encounter with patient, barriers to care, and resources or referrals to resolve barriers, which may be noted in the client record and/or the medical record	Active documentation in medical record
Organizational skills *Office skills* *Interpersonal skills* *Time management* *Problem solving* *Multitasking* *Critical thinking*	Conduct evaluation focused on community needs assessment and health behaviors	Conduct evaluation focused on barriers to care, health disparities, and quality indicators	Conduct evaluation focused on clinical outcomes and quality indicators
Community Resources: *Ongoing identification, coordination, and referral to resources such as individuals, organizations, and services in the community*	Provide referral to evidence-based health promotion programs	Provide assistance with scheduling appointments and facilitate request and follow-up with specialist or supportive care based on clinical referral	Focus on clinically oriented resources, such as referrals for second opinions, treatment or testing that may not be offered at the patient's institution, as well as supportive or specialty referrals within or external to the institution (specific to nurse navigators)
	Provide assistance accessing health insurance	Provide assistance accessing health insurance, copay programs, patient assistance programs, and financial assistance	Provide assistance in identifying community resources to access psychosocial support throughout treatment (specific to social work navigators)

(continued)

Table 2.2 (continued)

Domain	Community (Community Health Worker)	Community/ Healthcare Institution (Patient Navigator)	Healthcare Institution (Nurse Navigator/Social Work Navigator)
Patient Empowerment: *Identifying problems and resources to help patients solve problems and be part of the decision-making process* [11]. *An important facilitator of patient empowerment is development of good patient rapport*	Motivate individual and community to make positive changes in health behaviors	Assist patient with identifying administrative, structural, social, and practical issues to participate in decision-making and solutions	Assist patients in decision-making regarding diagnostic testing and treatment options (specific to nurse navigators)
	Activate and empower individuals and communities to self-advocate and make healthy decisions	Empower patients by ensuring they know all their options; identify their preferences and priorities, and assist them to access healthcare services and self-manage their health	Provide patients with strategies to cope with disease, treatment, and stress (specific to social work navigators)
		Educate patients on their rights and preferences and ensure they are able to participate in the decision-making process throughout their care and into survivorship or end-of-life care	
Communication: *Ensuring appropriate communication with patient, healthcare and service providers, and community*	Facilitate communication with community about access and utilization of the healthcare system	Assist patient and provider with communicating expectations, needs, and perspectives	Provide translation and communication of clinical information
			Provide counseling through one-on-one communication and serve as a conduit between patient and providers to address emotional and psychosocial needs of patients (specific to social work navigators)

Table 2.2 (continued)

Domain	Community (Community Health Worker)	Community/ Healthcare Institution (Patient Navigator)	Healthcare Institution (Nurse Navigator/Social Work Navigator)
Barriers to Care/ Health Disparities: *Identifying and addressing barriers to care and reducing health disparities as defined by age, disability, education, ethnicity, gender, sexual identification, geographic location, income, or race in populations that often bear a greater burden of disease than the general population* [12]	Address barriers to accessing the healthcare system	Address structural, cultural, social, emotional, and administrative barriers to care	Address clinical and service delivery barriers to care
	Focus on reduction of general health disparities	Focus on reduction of cancer health disparities in medically underserved patients and timely access to care across the continuum	Provision of services to at-risk populations, which may be defined by individual need, high acuity, or high volume at institutional level
Education, Prevention, and Health Promotion: *Promoting healthy behaviors and lifestyle, including integrative and wellness approaches*	Provide general health promotion at the individual and community level, including physical activity, healthy eating habits, stress reduction, sunscreen use, tobacco cessation, and reduction of other risky behaviors to reduce risk of cancer and chronic disease	Educate patients on practical concerns and next steps in treatment with regard to what to expect	Assess educational needs of patient
		Identify the educational needs of patients to advocate on their behalf with the care team	Identify the educational needs of patients to advocate on their behalf with the care team
		Inform patients of the importance and benefit of clinical trials and connect them with additional resources	Inform patients of the importance and benefit of clinical trials and connect them with additional resources
			Provide clinical education about diagnosis, treatment, side effects, and posttreatment care (specific to nurse navigators)
			Educate patients and caregivers on their biopsychosocial concerns regarding their diagnosis and treatment (specific to social work navigators)

(continued)

Table 2.2 (continued)

Domain	Community (Community Health Worker)	Community/ Healthcare Institution (Patient Navigator)	Healthcare Institution (Nurse Navigator/Social Work Navigator)
Ethics and Professional Conduct: *Understanding scope of practice and professional boundaries, assuring confidentiality, and following legal requirements. Maintaining and adhering to the professional standards. Bringing accountability, responsibility, and trust to the individuals the profession services*	Abide by state-defined scope of practice	Understand difference in scope of practice between licensed professionals and nonlicensed professionals	Abide by the ethical principles in the profession's scope of practice and code of conduct according to licensure
Cultural Competency: *Healthcare services that recognize, respect, and respond to cultural and social differences within the context of beliefs, practices, behaviors, and needs of diverse community and/or population served* [13]	Act as community/ cultural liaison and mediator between community and healthcare system using culturally appropriate education materials	Provide navigation services in a culturally competent manner (e.g., National Culturally and Linguistically Appropriate Services [CLAS] Standards in Health and Health Care)	Provide clinical care and education materials in culturally competent manner
		Educate providers to increase their understanding of community's history, culture, and needs, as well as the cultural appropriateness of their approaches and educational materials	

Table 2.2   (continued)

Domain	Community (Community Health Worker)	Community/ Healthcare Institution (Patient Navigator)	Healthcare Institution (Nurse Navigator/Social Work Navigator)
Outreach: *Providing healthcare education to individuals and communities that address health disparities* [14, 15]	Work with the community to identify education needs and opportunities	Educate on cancer-related topics to reduce fears and barriers related to cancer screening Effectively link patients referred from the community to resources that can improve care coordination and timeliness to treatment	Consult and counsel patients on their unique risks
Care Coordination: *A method of organizing patient care activities to facilitate the appropriate delivery of healthcare services* [16]	Provide case management, service coordination, and system navigation	Identify the pathway in the continuum and document the next steps to ensure the patient's optimal outcomes Identify unmet needs and facilitate cancer care resources to eliminate barriers along the cancer continuum	Assess and facilitate coordination of psychosocial and medical/clinical care along the care continuum
Psychosocial Support Services/ Assessment: *Providing and/or connecting patients to resources for psychosocial support services*	Identify resources in the community for emotional and social support	Administer distress screening and provide assistance with administrative, practical, or social issues identified	Screen and assess for psychosocial distress Provide psychosocial support services such as counseling (specific to social work navigators)
Advocacy: *Advocating on behalf of patient within the community and healthcare system*	Speak up for individual and community needs	Educate providers on individual preferences of care and needs	Assure patients' needs and preferences are integrated into treatment and care delivery

Reprinted with permission from Willis A, Reed E, Pratt-Chapman M, et al. Development of a framework for patient navigation: delineating roles across navigator types. J Oncol Nav Surviv. 2013;4:20–26

Table 2.3 Core competencies for oncology patient navigator–certified generalists

Domain 1: Patient care

Facilitate patient-centered care that is compassionate, appropriate, and effective for the treatment of cancer and the promotion of health

- Assist patients in accessing cancer care and navigating healthcare systems. Assess barriers to care, and engage patients and families in creating potential solutions to financial, practical, and social challenges
- Identify appropriate and credible resources responsive to patient needs (practical, social, physical, emotional, spiritual) taking into consideration reading level, health literacy, culture, language, and amount of information desired. For physical concerns, emotional needs, or clinical information, refer to licensed clinicians
- Educate patients and caregivers on the multidisciplinary nature of cancer treatment, the roles of team members, and what to expect from the healthcare system. Provide patients and caregivers evidence-based information, and refer to clinical staff to answer questions about clinical information, treatment choices, and potential outcomes
- Empower patients to communicate their preferences and priorities for treatment to their healthcare team; facilitate shared decision-making in the patient's healthcare
- Empower patients to participate in their wellness by providing self-management and health promotion resources and referrals
- Follow up with patients to support adherence to agreed-upon treatment plan through continued nonclinical barrier assessment and referrals to supportive resources in collaboration with the clinical team

Domain 2: Knowledge for practice

Demonstrate basic understanding of cancer, healthcare systems, and how patients access care and services across the cancer continuum to support and assist patients. Note: This domain refers to foundational knowledge applied across other domains

- Demonstrate basic knowledge of medical and cancer terminology
- Demonstrate familiarity with and know how to access and reference evidence-based information regarding cancer screening, diagnosis, treatment, and survivorship
- Demonstrate basic knowledge of cancer, cancer treatment, and supportive care options, including risks and benefits of clinical trials and integrative therapies
- Demonstrate basic knowledge of health systems operations
- Identify potential physical, psychological, social, and spiritual impacts of cancer and its treatment
- Demonstrate general understanding of healthcare payment structure, financing, and where to refer patients for answers regarding insurance coverage and financial assistance

Domain 3: Practice-based learning and improvement

Improve patient navigation process through continual self-evaluation and quality improvement. Promote and advance the profession

- Contribute to patient navigation program development, implementation, and evaluation
- Use evaluation data (barriers to care, patient encounters, resource provision, population health disparities data, and quality indicators) to collaboratively improve navigation process and participate in quality improvement
- Incorporate feedback on performance to improve daily work
- Use information technology to maximize efficiency of patient navigator's time
- Continually identify, analyze, and use new knowledge to mitigate barriers to care

Table 2.3 (continued)

- Maintain comprehensive, timely, and legible records capturing ongoing patient barriers, patient interactions, barrier resolution, and other evaluation metrics, and report data to show value to administrators and funders
- Promote navigation role, responsibilities, and value to patients, providers, and the larger community

Domain 4: Interpersonal and communication skills

Demonstrate interpersonal and communication skills that result in the effective exchange of information and collaboration with patients, their families, and health professionals

- Assess patient capacity to self-advocate; help patients optimize time with their doctors and treatment team (e.g., prioritize questions, clarify information with treatment team)
- Communicate effectively with patients, families, and the public to build trusting relationships across a broad range of socioeconomic and cultural backgrounds
- Employ active listening and remain solution-oriented in interactions with patients, families, and members of the healthcare team
- Encourage active communication between patients/families and healthcare providers to optimize patient outcomes
- Communicate effectively with navigator colleagues, health professionals, and health-related agencies to promote patient navigation services, and leverage community resources to assist patients
- Demonstrate empathy, integrity, honesty, and compassion in difficult conversations
- Know and support National Standards for Culturally and Linguistically Appropriate Services (CLAS) in Health and Health Care to advance health equity, improve quality, and reduce health disparities
- Apply insight and understanding about emotions and human responses to emotions to create and maintain positive interpersonal interactions

Domain 5: Professionalism

Demonstrate a commitment to carrying out professional responsibilities and an adherence to ethical principles

- Apply knowledge of the difference in roles between clinically licensed and non-licensed professionals and act within professional boundaries
- Build trust by being accessible, accurate, supportive, and acting within scope of practice
- Use organization, time management, problem-solving, and critical thinking to assist patients efficiently and effectively
- Demonstrate responsiveness to patient needs within scope of practice and professional boundaries
- Know and support patient rights
- Demonstrate sensitivity and responsiveness to a diverse patient population, including but not limited to diversity in gender, age, culture, race, religion, abilities, and sexual orientation
- Demonstrate a commitment to ethical principles pertaining to confidentiality, informed consent, business practices, and compliance with relevant laws, policies, and regulations (e.g., HIPAA, agency abuse reporting rules, duty to warn, safety contracting)
- Perform administrative duties accurately and efficiently

Domain 6: Systems-based practice

Demonstrate an awareness of and responsiveness to the larger context and system of healthcare, as well as the ability to call effectively on other resources in the system to provide optimal healthcare

(continued)

Table 2.3 (continued)

• Support a smooth transition of patients across screening, diagnosis, active treatment, survivorship, and/or end-of-life care, working with the patient's clinical care team
• Advocate for quality patient care and optimal patient care systems
• Organize and prioritize resources to optimize access to care across the cancer continuum for the most vulnerable patients

Domain 7: Interprofessional collaboration

Demonstrate ability to engage in an interprofessional team in a manner that optimizes safe, effective patient- and population-centered care

• Work with other health professionals to establish and maintain a climate of mutual respect, dignity, diversity, ethical integrity, and trust
• Use knowledge of one's role and the roles of other health professionals to appropriately assess and address the needs of patients and populations served to optimize health and wellness
• Participate in interprofessional teams to provide patient- and population-centered care that is safe, timely, efficient, effective, and equitable

Domain 8: Personal and professional development

Demonstrate qualities required to sustain lifelong personal and professional growth

• Set learning and improvement goals. Identify and perform learning activities that address one's gaps in knowledge, skills, attitudes, and abilities
• Demonstrate healthy coping mechanisms to respond to stress; employ self-care strategies
• Manage possible and actual conflicts between personal and professional responsibilities
• Recognize that ambiguity is part of patient care and respond by utilizing appropriate resources in dealing with uncertainty

Reprinted with permission from Pratt-Chapman M, Willis M, Masselink L. Core Competencies for Oncology Patient Navigators. J Oncol Nav Surviv. 2015;6(2):16–21.

Centers for Disease Control and Prevention (http://gwcehp.learnercommunity.com/cancer-institute) [67]. For more information on navigation, please see the Navigation Training, Tools, and Resources chapter (Chapter 15).

From 2012 to 2015, the Patient Navigators, Community Health Workers (CHW), and Promotores de Salud Working Group in Colorado was also identifying and defining competencies in order to increase the opportunities for patient navigators, CHWs, and Promotores de Salud services to be eligible for reimbursement within the Affordable Care Act and other sources. The group included participation from the Native American Cancer Research Corporation, Sisters of Color, Community Research Education Awareness, Clinica Tepeyac, the Colorado Department of Public Health and Environment, the University of Colorado, the Colorado School of Public Health, and members of healthcare facilities, research institutions, service programs, medically underserved programs, as well as regional care collaborative organizations. The working group reviewed competencies from national programs and from states, as well as from peer-reviewed publications. Several generations of potential competencies and behavioral skills were drafted from 300 skills in 2012 and formatted into different models over the next 3 years. In August 2014, the document was finalized with the 11 performance-based competencies [68]. Table 2.4 is the list of the nine domains that relate to patient navigation, competencies, and examples of performance behaviors based on basic, intermediate, or advanced

Table 2.4   Patient navigation/community health workers/Promotores de Salud Working Group

Patient navigation domains, competencies, and performance behaviors living documentation
A. Domain: Health education and coaching
A1. Competency: Provide health education and coaching that enable patients to self-manage their health condition(s) using culturally tailored public health theory and strategies
Example of patient navigator basic-/entry-level behaviors
A.1 Gather data to assess patients' current management of their health conditions
Examples of patient navigator intermediate-level behaviors
A.2 Identify gaps in patients' knowledge regarding how to self-manage their health conditions
A.3 Help clients to identify their goals, barriers to change, and supports for change, including eliciting personal strengths and problem-solving abilities
A.4 Present pertinent information in a manner that is perceived as culturally and linguistically relevant to patients and their families
A.6 Provide and explain credible online and print materials that are culturally appropriate and at the patients' health literacy levels to facilitate learning
A.7 Refer patients back to providers when clinical expertise is needed
A.8 Establish accountability and negotiate responsibilities with the patient and/or healthcare team/family to complete plans of actions and fulfill healthcare needs (e.g., wellness care plans)
Examples of patient navigator advanced-level behaviors
A1.5 Effectively use coaching techniques (e.g., teach-back, demonstration, motivational interviewing, strength-based statements, role playing, discussing healthcare language) to maximize the patient's learning and skill transfer
A1.9 Document health education activities with patients appropriately and in a HIPAA compliant manner
B. Domain: Advocacy and community capacity building
B1. Competency: Communicate barriers and human rights violations that clients experience in the healthcare system to providers and staff in order to assure that these setbacks or discriminatory events are addressed and optimally resolved
Examples of patient navigator basic-/entry-level behaviors
B1.1 Elicit disclosure and feedback from patients regarding perceived barriers or human rights violations that impair or prevent using the healthcare system
B1.2 Assist patients in identifying what changes in services they believe are needed to diminish said barriers
B1.3 Present information and issues gathered from patients to members of the healthcare team, and advocate on the patients' behalf
B2. Competency: Seek and facilitate opportunities for community capacity building to address health inequities among populations
Examples of patient navigator intermediate-level behaviors
B2.1 Implement strategies that assist patients in identifying and prioritizing their personal, family, and community needs for new resources
B2.2 Develop relationships with relevant agencies and professionals in patients' communities to secure needed care and relevant resources to address health inequities
B2.4 Lead and/or undertake an active role in community and agency planning to bring needed resources into the community
B2.6 Provide information and support for patients to advocate for themselves over time and to participate in the provision of improved services
B2.7 Advocate on behalf of patients and communities, as appropriate, to assist them and relevant others to attain needed care or resources in a reasonable and timely fashion

Table 2.4 (continued)

Patient navigation domains, competencies, and performance behaviors living documentation

Examples of patient navigator advanced-level behaviors

B.1.4 Participate in healthcare team discussions about ways to proactively address patient barriers and improve overall patient care

B.1.5 Document changes in patient-service provisions in a HIPAA compliant manner

B2.3 Apply principles and skills needed for identifying and developing community leadership

B2.5 Share community assessment results with colleagues and community partners to inform planning and health improvement efforts for disadvantaged patients

C. Domain: Assessment and referral

C1. Competency: Assist clients in accessing additional services and programs as needed to self-manage their health condition(s)

Examples of patient navigator basic-/entry-level behaviors

C1 Identify patient needs for additional services and programs to self-manage their health condition(s)

C2 Assess quality and appropriateness of resources for patients (e.g., cultural appropriateness of staff behaviors, products, and services) and advocate for changes when needed

C3 Apply eligibility criteria in matching patients to available resources

C4 Determine patients' comprehension of needed and available resources and programs

C5 Ensure patients are enrolled in helpful or needed services for which they are eligible

C6 Identify patients' language needs and effectively use referral resources (interpreters, English as second or third language)

Examples of patient navigator intermediate-level behaviors

C7 Periodically reassess patient strengths and needs for referrals, taking into account changes in their personal or family circumstances

D. Domain: Communication

D1. Competency: Demonstrate the ability to effectively communicate with clients, families, and members of the healthcare team

Examples of patient navigator basic-/entry-level behaviors

D1 Explain role and function of PN to clinical/research staff, patients, and families

D3 Explain to the healthcare team what specific traditional/cultural care patients may use or prefer in order to improve the effectiveness of services provided

D4 Provide support for patients' healthcare decisions when interacting with healthcare professionals

D6 Effectively adjust (i.e., accommodate) communication style to the needs of the audience, such as patients, their families, or similar small groups (e.g., explaining basic disease-specific content)

D7 Use text and visual materials to convey information clearly and accurately

D8 Use nonjudgmental language that conveys respect and empathy

D9 Identify discrepancies between patients' verbal and nonverbal behaviors and explore meaning with patients

D12 Clarify mutual rights and obligations, as necessary, such as patient confidentiality or reporting responsibilities

D14 Maintain appropriate boundaries that balance professional and personal relationships while recognizing dual roles as both PN and community member

Examples of patient navigator intermediate-level behaviors

(continued)

Table 2.4   (continued)

Patient navigation domains, competencies, and performance behaviors living documentation
D2 Demonstrate skill in navigating emotionally charged or high-stakes issues with other healthcare professionals, staff, patients, and families
D5 Translate patients' culturally specific issues into scientific and healthcare terminology to effectively communicate with providers
D11 Demonstrate writing skills appropriate to each task at hand (easy-to-understand information for patients and technical language for patient updates to other members of healthcare team)
D13 Facilitate discussion with the family or small group to address new patient and/or family needs
E. Domain: Care coordination and case management
E1. Competency: Facilitate the appropriate and efficient delivery of services to bridge gaps, both within and across systems, to promote person-centered, optimal outcomes
Examples of patient navigator basic-/entry-level behaviors
E1 Assist patients to ensure completion of specialty appointments through barrier reduction, monitoring, and follow-up
E2 Monitor, follow up, and respond to change of care plan(s)
E3 Maintain patient confidentiality and privacy when working with clinical and professional staff both within and outside of systems of care and community-based programs
E4 Document the attainment or receipt of appropriate healthcare
E5 Collaboratively and accurately complete required forms with patients, attaching required documentation, and submit to appropriate programs, staff, or organizations
E7 Obtain and share up-to-date information about health insurance programs and eligibility, public health and social service programs, and additional resources to protect and promote health
E9 Provide information and support for people in using agency and institutional services
E10 Provide support for patients to follow professional caregiver instructions or advice
E12 Coordinate one's roles with other local programs to prevent duplication of services
Examples of patient navigator intermediate-level behaviors
E6 Advocate for care for patients
E8 Provide care coordination, including basic care planning (prepare questions to ask provider, treatment options clarifications) with individuals and families based on engagement and needs assessments, and facilitate care transitions
E11 Use assessment information to develop a plan to address health and related patient needs in cooperation with the patient and based on patient priorities
F. Domain: Reporting, evaluation, and tracking
F1. Competency: Demonstrate effective "documentation" techniques including reporting, evaluating, monitoring, revising, and tracking data related to client care
Examples of patient navigator basic-/entry-level behaviors
F.6 Obtain and document patient data within the scope and boundaries of the PN role in the context of the agency team and agency policy
F.7 Ensure documentation complies with applicable privacy laws and policies (e.g., Health Insurance Portability and Accountability Act [HIPAA])
Examples of patient navigator intermediate-level behaviors
F.1 Collect interview or survey data in a culturally competent manner that complies with the given methodological design of the protocol

(continued)

Table 2.4 (continued)

Patient navigation domains, competencies, and performance behaviors living documentation
F.2 Develop, maintain, and utilize an organizational system to record and update healthcare, cultural relevance, health literacy, and linguistically appropriate resources for patients and their communities
F.3 Track, document, and report both externally and internally relevant PN activities for internal administration and funders
F.4 Use appropriate technology, such as computers and database systems, for work-based communication in accordance with employer requirements
F.5 Document program evaluation and sustainability data to help patients achieve their goals
F.8 Document and follow up on issues related to abuse, neglect, and criminal activity that may be reportable by law and under regulation according to agency policy and report activities when required
Examples of patient navigator advanced-level behaviors
F.9 Use both quantitative and qualitative data in developing and evaluating program priorities
G. Domain: Cultural responsiveness
G1. Competency: Demonstrate skills, establish and follow protocols, and exemplify behaviors that exhibit the value of diversity and intentionally promote effective and productive exchanges among clients and all employees or contractors of myriad cultural backgrounds within the healthcare system and its various settings
Examples of patient navigator basic-/entry-level behaviors
G.3 Assess and refer patients to appropriate, culturally relevant experts to assist with ceremonies or special services (e.g., gifting, tobacco ties for American Indian traditional healer) beyond one's personal level of expertise
G.6 Demonstrate culturally respectful behaviors when assisting patients with ceremonies or special services (e.g., gifting, tobacco ties for AI traditional healer) that are pertinent to the patients' cultural healthcare values, beliefs, and practices
G.8 Demonstrate cultural knowledge and sensitivity in all aspects of work, including (1) seeking to understand and acting in accordance with specific cultural norms when appropriate, (2) awareness of potential bias in one's own culture and life experience, and (3) awareness of the influence of diverse beliefs and practices on thinking and behavior across cultures, communities, and organizations
G.10 Explain reasons for health behavior change and patient options in a culturally sensitive manner
G.13 Make accommodations to address communication needs accurately and sensitively with people whose language(s) one cannot understand
G.17 Demonstrate the ability to identify and suggest alternatives that respect patients' privacy and modesty (e.g., during a Pap smear, some patients may prefer to maintain wearing a blouse or shirt)
Examples of patient navigator intermediate-level behaviors
G.4 Assist patients with ceremonies or special services in a culturally respectful manner (e.g., conducting a cultural ceremony in compliance with a given protocol)
G.5 Effectively communicate cultural assets (e.g., barriers that interfere with participation alongside priorities of caring for family) with providers and funders
G.11 Employ techniques for interacting sensitively and effectively with people from cultures or communities that differ from one's own (e.g., demonstration of cultural humility in instances when cultural competence is not possible)
G.12 Employ practices that assist service organizations and the patients and communities they serve to better understand one another's perspectives

(continued)

Table 2.4   (continued)

Patient navigation domains, competencies, and performance behaviors living documentation

G.14 Advocate for and promote the use of culturally and linguistically appropriate services and resources within organizations and with diverse colleagues and community partners

G.15 Advocate for patients' self-determination, personal motivations, and dignity

G.16 Gather and integrate information from different sources to better understand patients, their families, and their communities (sources may include—but are not limited to— performing interviews and researching community resources and conditions and participating in peer-reviewed publications describing the specific population)

H. Domain: Outreach methods and strategies

H1. Competency: Comprehend and demonstrate the ability to implement multipronged approaches to engage un- and underserved communities through a variety of innovative strategies, as well as using established best practices (i.e., effective health promotion/behavior practices)

Examples of patient navigator basic-/entry-level behaviors

H.2 Use standard knowledge of basic health and social indicators

H.3 Effectively engage patients and families in ongoing assessment efforts

H.7 Identify and share appropriate information, referrals, and other resources to help individuals, families, groups, and organizations meet their respective needs

H.11 Identify factors that affect health and resources that will benefit community members

H.12 Bring information and services to communities where patients reside, including where they work and spend their time (e.g., grocery stores, parks)

Examples of patient navigator intermediate-level behaviors

H.4 Gather and combine information from different sources to better understand patients, their families, and their communities (sources may include—but are not limited to—performing interviews and researching community resources and conditions)

H.9 Use outreach methods to engage individuals and groups in diverse settings

Examples of patient navigator advanced-level behaviors

H.5 Share community assessment results with colleagues and community partners to inform planning and health improvement efforts

H.6 Implement outreach plans based on individual and community strengths, needs, and resources, all of which are developed in collaboration with other stakeholders

H.10 Conduct baseline and ongoing needs assessments of communities and their members with clearly defined goals and objectives

I. Domain: Use of public health concepts and approaches

I1. Competency: Demonstrate an understanding of the larger, more complex issues of public health and their relation to the healthcare system in order to promote prevention, problem-solving, and policy change to achieve better health outcomes

Example of patient navigator basic-/entry-level behaviors

I.13 Describe ways PN roles in prevention strategies and implementation promote health equity

Examples of patient navigator intermediate-level behaviors

I.5 Communicate with health systems staff and social service organizations to help them understand and accept community and individual conditions, culture, and behavior with the goal of developing policies and plans that support individual and community health efforts

I.7 Explain the principles of public health and its relevance for helping patients, their families, and the community

(continued)

Table 2.4 (continued)

Patient navigation domains, competencies, and performance behaviors living documentation
I.8 Educate patients on the role of prevention, education, and advocacy and community participation in their healthcare
I.9 Identify how the social determinants of health (e.g., poverty, transportation, safety, housing) impact a client's ability to access healthcare
Examples of patient navigator advanced-level behaviors
I.1 Apply information from patient and community assessments to develop and/or validate existing health education strategies
I.10 Describe ways social determinants of health (e.g., food deserts, violence, poor infrastructure) impact the individual, family, and community
I.11 Explain the relationship between public health and social justice
I.12 Describe ways of prevention in public health and the role of policy change in preventing injury and disease to promote health equality. Adapted from: http://natamcancer.org/PDFs/2015-03-02_TOC_Def_PN_Behaviors_Ranked_w-i_competency-rs.pdf.

skills. This is a "living document" that is refined quarterly to integrate innovative evidence-based methods as they develop in rural and underserved communities. The document is for patient navigation programs in oncology as well as others to use evidence-based practice to promote efficiency as well as cost-effectiveness and integrate training efforts [68].

The clarification of roles and competencies has a dual effect of allowing clinically licensed navigators to function at the top of their license and protect patient navigators and institutions from liability issues [66]. This evolution of patient and nurse navigation has allowed AONN+ to develop general navigation certification for the patient and nurse navigators.

2.6 Navigation Certification

Certification is a way competency is measured against a set of standards in a specialized field. In 2008, the NCBC recognized the need for a standardization of the breast navigator's role and formed a peer committee to define the function of breast navigators that provide care throughout the continuum and develop a certification program to validate the skill sets of breast patient navigators [69]. In 2010, they became the first national organization to offer a certification for navigation, and more than 900 breast healthcare professionals received their designations as certified breast patient navigators [69]. There are six different levels of navigator certification that cover from advocacy in the community through diagnostic and clinically licensed professionals in the breast care continuum [70].

In 2016, AONN+ launched an oncology nurse navigator–certified generalist certification examination as well as an oncology patient navigator-certified generalist certification examination [71]. AONN+ created the certifications in recognition of the development of role delineation and competencies in the navigation field as well as the desires of their membership. The educational criteria and curriculum were developed by the AONN+ Certification Task Force that was made up of experienced leaders within both patient and nurse navigator fields [72]. These certification examinations are for anyone involved in navigation as outlined in the framework for navigation role delineation and core competencies for oncology patient navigators. The individual designations are Oncology Nurse Navigator–Certified Generalist™ (ONN-CG) and Oncology Patient Navigator–Certified Generalist™ (OPN-CG) [73].

2.7   Metrics

In 2010, the National Quality Forum issued practice and performance measures for care coordination that fits in with the navigation concept to blend patient-centered care processes, teamwork, and coordinated action [74]. To promote the value of navigation, The Advisory Board Company has consistently shared best practices of navigation and the importance navigation brings to an organization in finances, healthcare utilization, and patient satisfaction [74]. Also in 2010 the ACS hosted the National Patient Navigation Leadership Summit and brought together leaders in the field to establish common measures for navigation across the cancer continuum [75]. The 115 participants represented over 65 organizations and included clinicians, researchers, public health experts, funders, and patient navigators. Results published in the fall 2011 issue of *Cancer Epidemiology, Biomarkers & Prevention* laid out a framework for the principles of navigation; defined measures for navigation across the cancer continuum including prevention and early detection, diagnosis and treatment, posttreatment survivorship, and palliative care; as well as discussed partnership approaches, patient-centered outcomes, and cost measures [76]. In 2016, Strusowski and Stapp further stratified navigation value by identifying three main categories of navigation—business performance, clinical outcomes, and patient experience based on a literature review [77].

In 2013, the Institute of Medicine report, "Delivering High-Quality Cancer Care: Charting a New Course for a System in Crisis," concluded that cancer treatment in the United States lacks in consistent quality and is neither patient-centric nor well-coordinated [78]. The old fee-for-service oncology payment model never emphasized value or quality of care. It was a volume-driven model. But the Affordable Care Act (2010) established the Center for Medicare and Medicaid Innovation to incorporate value in the delivery of healthcare with innovative payment models [79]. The Oncology Care Model which launched on July 1, 2016, is a program that hopes to shift reimbursement and payment to value-based quality care, and one of the six fundamental transformation processes is patient navigation [80]. Some immediate solutions to value are improving access to care and avoiding unnecessary emergency department visits and hospitalizations. These improvements fit in with the metrics that navigation has shown to effect with their patient-centered care approach.

In 2016, AONN+ announced that their Evidence into Practice Metrics Subcommittee had created 35 evidenced-based national navigation metrics that all programs would be able to utilize in their navigation model [81]. The evidence-based metrics were identified as an extensive literature search that took several months to complete and the team utilized the eight AONN+ certification domains as well as the categories of patient experience (PE), clinical outcomes (CO), and return on investment (ROI). The AONN+ navigation certification domains were applied; AONN+ has been recognized by the CoC to be the content experts for oncology navigation. For detailed information, please refer to Chapter 14, "Measuring the Impact Navigation Has on Patient Care by Supporting the Multidisciplinary Team."

2.8   Oncology Nurse Navigators and Patient Navigators Working as a Collaborative Team

According to Domingo et al, "although all navigators want to help patients through the cancer care continuum (from screening, suspicious finding, diagnosis, treatment, post-treatment, and survivorship), generally hospital based navigators accrue clients at the point of suspicious finding or cancer diagnosis and discharge them after treatment, unless they have specific screening or survivorship navigation programs. Community-based navigators, on the other hand, may work with clients to get them to screening, working in concert with hospital-based navigators through diagnosis and treatment, and then follow through with the clients and their family's post-treatment" [82]. Patient and nurse navigators can work effectively together providing a higher-quality and less stressful experience for underserved cancer patients and their families.

One example is from the NCI Community Cancer Centers Program (NCCCP) that was piloted from 2007 to 2010 with a goal of expanding cancer research capacity to more community settings and delivering the latest cancer care to Americans in the communities in which they live [83]. A network of community hospitals and hospital systems were committed to six goals in which three were to reduce disparities in cancer care, increase patient participation in clinical trials, and improve the quality of cancer care [84]. Navigation as a part of multidisciplinary care was strategic in promoting the concept of research as the patient moved through the cancer continuum in the culturally diverse communities [85]. An overall example is that the patient navigator who is knowledgeable in clinical trials can facilitate and promote the patient experience from the initial diagnosis by assisting with specific trial referrals for underserved populations, and the nurse navigator can then proactively encourage patient education and referrals to clinical trial team members. After the NCCCP pilot, the program ran until 2014 when aspects were integrated into the newer NCI Community Oncology Research Program [84]. More examples around clinical trial navigation can be found in Chapter 12.

In Connecticut's highest known area for breast cancer mortality, patient and nurse navigators work collaboratively to increase breast cancer screening in an underserved area [86]. Bilingual trained patient navigators make contact with this population at community events such as job training programs, parent groups, programs for the homeless, and a church food pantry with culturally appropriate educational material. The nurse navigator works with them to encourage women into breast screening. Patients were scheduled for care at the point of community contact and assessed to see if they completed the scheduled appointment. Additional information such as financial counseling to access other benefits and assistance in connecting with a primary care physician was provided.

At the Johns Hopkins Hospital in Baltimore, Maryland, where the local population is comprised of low-income African Americans, trained patient navigators work alongside the nurse navigators to optimize breast care services [34]. Patient navigators can assist patients to access resources for care within and outside the institution and then a nurse navigator can initiate care at the point of diagnosis to provide comprehensive patient and family education and psychosocial support through the continuum to survivorship. The navigation network has reduced length of stay, improved quality of life, and increased patient satisfaction.

Northside Hospital in Atlanta, Georgia, uses cancer care liaisons (CCLs) as patient navigators to enhance care and support the nonclinical needs of patients and allows the oncology nurse navigators to direct their time and efforts to clinical aspects of care [87]. The complementary role of the CCL has provided patients with increased means to financial assistance, expanded resources to embellish their activities of daily living, as well as resolved numerous barriers to care. The coordination with the nurses on symptoms or clinical issues has decreased emergency room visits. The consistent contact of the CCLs through the care continuum has allowed patients to share concerns that might not otherwise be discussed with the nurse navigator.

Conclusion As a healthcare delivery support strategy, navigation has evolved over the decades with better role definitions for navigator types, a framework that outlines functional domains of care and development of core competencies. As oncology care has transitioned to the outpatient setting with increasing personalized clinical care decisions, each navigation model has held fast to the concept of patient-centered care. This has been promoted by decreasing barriers, increasing patient resources to care access, as well as continuing resource support throughout the continuum. Care pathways involving patient and nurse navigation to promote improved patient outcomes, better patient adherence to treatment, and care coordination at transition points have allowed individualized healthcare systems to become less fragmented. Navigation will continue to evolve as patient engagement and care coordination patterns change in the future. The focus of navigation fits in with the quality value of future oncology care.

References

1. American Cancer Society. The history of cancer. 2014. www.cancer.org/acs/groups/cid/documents/webcontent/002048-pdf.pdf.
2. Gibbons MC. Common ground: exploring policy approaches to addressing racial disparities from the left and the right. J Health Care Law Policy. 2006;9:48–76.
3. Freeman HP. The Harold P. Freeman Patient Navigation Institute. 2009. www.hpfreemanpni.org.
4. www.patientnavigation.com/why-is-it-important.
5. Freeman H, Rodriguez R. History and principles of patient navigation. Cancer. 2011; 117(15):3539–42. https://doi.org/10.1002/cncr.26262.
6. Freeman HP. Cancer in the socioeconomically disadvantaged. CA Cancer J Clin. 1989;39:266–88.

7. American Cancer Society. A summary of the American Cancer Society Report to the Nation: cancer in the poor. CA Cancer J Clin. 1989;39(5):263–5. https://doi.org/10.3322/canjclin.39.5.263.
8. Freeman H. Patient navigation: a community centered approach to reducing cancer mortality. J Cancer Educ. 2006;21(1 Suppl):S11–4. https://doi.org/10.1207/s15430154jce2101s_4.
9. Freeman HP. A model patient navigation program. Oncol Issues. 2004;19:44–6.
10. Hede K. Agencies look to patient navigators to reduce cancer care disparities. J Natl Cancer Inst. 2006;98:157–9.
11. American Cancer Society. Cancer patients can more easily navigate health care system thanks to the American Cancer Society and AstraZeneca. Atlanta, GA: American Cancer Society; 2008. www.cancer.org/docroot/MED/content/MED_2_lx_Cancer_Patients_Can_More_Easily_Navigate_Health_Care_System_Thanks_to_the_American_Cancer_Society_and_AstraZeneca.
12. http://pressroom.cancer.org/MerckFoundationgrant.
13. Long Island College Hospital. Breast health navigator program. In: HANYS Breast Cancer Demonstration Project®, editor. Best practices strategy guide. Rensselaer, NY: Healthcare Association of New York State; 2002. www.hanys.org/bcdp/upload/Long-Island-College-Hospital-Breast-Health-Navigator-Program.pdf.
14. US Department of Health and Human Services, Voices of a broken system: real people, real problems, DHHS, National Cancer Institute, September 2001. https://deainfo.nci.nih.gov/advisory/pcp/archive/pcp00.
15. https://prescancerpanel.cancer.gov/.
16. US Department of Health and Human Services, President's Cancer Panel 2002 Annual report, facing cancer in Indian Country: The Yakama Nation and Pacific Northwest Tribe: US DHHS: NIH: NCI: December 2003.
17. Freeman HP. Voices of a broken system: real people, real problems. President's Cancer Panel Report of the Chairman 2000–2001. Bethesda, MD: National Institutes of Health; 2001.
18. Trans-HHS Cancer Health Disparities Progress Review Group. Making Cancer Health Disparities History. Submitted to the Secretary, HHS, March 2004. Washington, DC: HHS.
19. www.cancer.gov/about-nci/organization/crchd/about-health-disparities/definitions.
20. Trans-HHS Cancer Health Disparities Progress Review Group. Making cancer health disparities history. Submitted to the Secretary, HHS, March 2004. Washington, DC: HHS. Appendix B
21. H.R. 1812—109th congress: patient navigator outreach and chronic disease prevention act of 2005. www.GovTrack.us. 2005. June 12, 2017. www.govtrack.us/congress/bills/109/hr1812. www.congress.gov/bill/109th-congress/house-bill/1812.
22. Hopkins J, Mumber MP. Patient navigation through the cancer care continuum: an overview. J Oncol Pract. 2009;5(4):150–2. https://doi.org/10.1200/JOP.0943501.
23. Patient Navigator Outreach and Chronic Disease Prevention Act of 2005, HR 1812, 109th Cong, 2005.
24. National Cancer Institute. The patient navigator research program (PNRP). 2006. http://crchd.cancer.gov/attachments/pnrp_brochure.pdf.
25. https://grants.nih.gov/grants/guide/rfa-files/RFA-CA-05-019.html.
26. Freund KM, Battaglia TA, Calhoun E, et al. National Cancer Institute patient navigation research program: methods, protocol and measures. Cancer. 2008;113(12):3391–9. https://doi.org/10.1002/cncr.23960.
27. www.cancer.gov/about-nci/organization/crchd/disparities-research/pnrp#PNRP.
28. Burhansstipanov L, Dresser CM. Native American Monograph #1: Documentation of the Cancer Research Needs of American Indians and Alaska Natives. National Cancer Institute. Bethesda, MD. NIH Pub. No. 94-3603. 1994.
29. Matsunaga DS, Enos R, Gotay CC, Banner RO, DeCambra H, Hammond OW, Hedlund N, Ilaban EK, Issell BF, Tsark JU. Participatory research in a Native Hawaiian Community: The Wai'anae cancer research project. Cancer. 1996;78(7 Suppl):1582–6.
30. www.cancer.gov/about-nci/organization/crchd/about-health-disparities/resources/CNPC.
31. www.cancer.gov/about-nci/organization/crchd/disparities-research/cnp.
32. www.cms.gov/CCIIO/Programs-and-Initiatives/Health-Insurance-Marketplaces/Downloads/navigator-list-10-18-2013_2.pdf.

33. Shockney L. Evolution of patient navigation. Clin J Oncol Nurs. 2010;14(4):405–7. https://doi.org/10.1188/10.CJON.405-407.
34. Shockney LD, Haylock PJ, Cantril C. Development of a breast navigation program. Semin Oncol Nurs. 2013;29(2):97–104. https://doi.org/10.1016/j.soncn.2013.02.006.
35. Shockney LD. Becoming a breast cancer nurse navigator. 1st ed. Sudbury, MA: Jones and Bartlett Publishers; 2011.
36. Shockney LD. Evolution of patient navigation. Clin J Oncol Nurs. 2010;14(4):405–7. https://doi.org/10.1188/10.CJON.405-407.
37. Perry Nell. A recycled mom. South Carolina Nursing Matters, 1992 April, 5–8.
38. Kneece J. Fulfilling a mission. Cope. 1994 March/April, 6–7.
39. Kneece J. Breast health navigator: a paradigm shift in breast care. Semin Breast Dis. 2008;11:13–9.
40. www.hanys.org/quality/clinical_operational_initiatives/bcdp/patient_navigation/.
41. www.patientnavigation.com/home?LMenuId=100.
42. Oncology Nursing Society. Implementing the nurse navigator role session at 33rd Annual Congress. 2008. https://onf.ons.org/file/4295/download.
43. National Coalition of Oncology Nurse Navigators. www.nconn.org.
44. www.oncnursingnews.com/publications/oncology-nurse/2011/october-2011/core-competencies-for-the-oncology-nurse-navigator.
45. https://aononline.org/about.
46. www.accc-cancer.org/mediaroom/press_releases/2009/ACCC-Launches-Patient-Navigation-Website-6.1.09.asp.
47. Association of Community Cancer Centers. New cancer program guidelines released by association of community cancer centers. 2009. www.accc-cancer.org/mediaroom/press_releases/2009/New-Cancer-Program-Guidelines-3.6.09.asp.
48. Academy of Oncology Nurse & Patient Navigators® http://www.jons-online.com/.
49. Oncology Nursing Society. Oncology Nursing Society, the Association of Oncology Social Work, and the National Association of Social Workers Joint Position on the Role of Oncology Nursing and Oncology Social Work in Patient Navigation. 2010. www.ons.org/advocacy-policy/positions/education/patient-navigation.
50. Carver M, Jessie A. Patient-centered care in a medical home. Online J Issues Nurs. 2011;16(2):4. https://doi.org/10.3912/OJIN.Vol16No02Man04.
51. www.qualityforum.org/Publications/2010/10/Preferred_Practices_and_Performance_Measures_for_Measuring_and_Reporting_Care_Coordination.aspx.
52. www.nationalacademies.org/hmd/Reports/2010/The-Future-of-Nursing-Leading-Change-Advancing-Health.aspx.
53. Shockney L. Becoming a breast cancer nurse navigator. Burlington: Jones & Bartlett Learning; 2010.
54. Academy of Oncology Nurse & Patient Navigators®. www.aononline.org/about/faq/.
55. Seminars in Oncology Nursing Volume 29, Issue 2, Pages 71–156 (May 2013) Patient Navigation in Cancer Care. Edited by Pamela J. Haylock and Cynthia Cantril.
56. www.ons.org/store/books?combine=navigation&tid=All&=Search.
57. Bensenhaver J, Winchester D. Surgical leadership and standardization of multidisciplinary breast center care: the evolution of the National Accreditation Program for Breast Centers. Surg Oncol Clin N Am. 2014;23(3):609–16. https://doi.org/10.1016/j.soc.2014.03.005.
58. National Accreditation Program for Breast Centers. Breast center standards manual. 2014. p.35. www.facs.org/~/media/files/quality%20programs/napbc/2014%20napbc%20standards%20manual.ashx.
59. American College of Surgeons: Commission on Cancer. Cancer program standards 2012: ensuring patient-centered care. www.facs.org/~/media/files/quality%20programs/cancer/coc/programstandards2012.ashx%20ACS%20CoC;%202012.
60. www.facs.org/~/media/files/quality%20programs/cancer/coc/programstandards2012.ashx.
61. Brown C, Cantril C, McMullen L, Barkley D, et al. Oncology nurse navigator role delineation study: an oncology nursing society report. Clin J Oncol Nurs. 2012;16(6):581–5.

62. Lubejko B, Bellfield S, Kahn E, Lee C, Peterson N, Rose T, Murphy CM, McCorkle M. Oncology nurse navigation: results of the 2016 role delineation study. Clin J Oncol Nurs. 2017;21(1):43–50. https://cjon.ons.org/oncology-nurse-navigation-results-2016-role-delineation-study.
63. Willis A, Reed E, Pratt-Chapman M, Kapp H, Hatcher E, Vaitones V, Collins S, Bires J, Washington E. Development of a framework for patient navigation: Delineating roles across navigator types. J Oncol Navig Surviv. 2013;4(6):20–6.
64. Oncology Nursing Society. ONS Oncology Nurse Navigator Core Competencies. 2013. www.ons.org/practice-resources/competencies.
65. www.ons.org/sites/default/files/2017ONNcompetencies.pdf.
66. Pratt-Chapman M, Willis M, Masselink L. Core competencies for oncology patient navigators. J Oncol Navig Surviv. 2015;6(2):16–21.
67. GW Cancer Center's Online Academy. oncology patient navigator training: the fundamentals. Accessed tinyurl.com/GWOnlineAcademy.
68. http://natamcancer.org/PDFs/2015-03-02_TOC_Def_PN_Behaviors_Ranked_w-i_compe-tency-rs.pdf.
69. www2.bpnc.org/about-bpnc/.
70. www2.bpnc.org/certification/.
71. www.jons-online.com/issue-archive/2016-issue/april-2016-vol-7-no-3/making-progress-with-patient-navigation-certification/.
72. www.aonnonline.org/certification/certification-task-force.
73. www.jons-online.com/issue-archive/2016-issue/june-2016-vol-7-no-5/certification-a-winwin-for-navigators-employers-and-patients/.
74. National Quality Forum (NQF). Preferred practices and performance measures for measuring and reporting care coordination: a Consensus Report. Washington, DC: NQF; 2010.
75. Esparza A, Calhoun E. Measuring the impact and potential of patient navigation. Cancer. 2011;117(S15):3536–8. https://doi.org/10.1002/cncr.26265.
76. Martinez M, Thompson B, editors. Patient navigation in cancer care. Cancer Epidemiol Biomark Prev. 2012;21(10):1613–700. https://doi.org/10.1158/1538–7755.DISP14-IA38.
77. Strusowski P, Stapp J. Patient navigation metrics: measuring the impact of your patient navigation services. Oncol Issues. 2016;31(1):56–63.
78. Institute of Medicine. In: Levit L, Balogh E, Nass S, et al., editors. Committee on improving the quality of cancer care: addressing the challenges of an aging population. Delivering high-quality cancer care: charting a new course for a system in crisis. Washington, DC: National Academies Press; 2013. www.ncbi.nlm.nih.gov/books/NBK202150.
79. https://innovation.cms.gov/About.
80. Maharshi P, Kashyap P. The oncology care model: aligning financial incentives to improve outcomes. Oncol Pract Manag. 2016;6(12). http://oncpracticemanagement.com/issue-archive/2016/december-2016-vol-6-no-12/the-oncology-care-model-aligning-financial-incentives-to-improve-outcomes/.
81. www.aonnonline.org/education/articles/10-aonn-announces-standardized-navigation-metrics.
82. Domingo JB, Davis EL, Allison AL, Braun KL. Cancer patient navigation case studies in Hawai'i: the complimentary role of clinical and community navigators. Hawaii Med J. 2011;70(12):257–61.
83. Clauser S, Johnson M, O'Brien D, Beveridge J, Fennell N, Kaluzny A. Improving clinical research and cancer care delivery in community settings: evaluating the NCI community cancer centers program. Implement Sci. 2009;4:63. https://doi.org/10.1186/1748-5908-4-63.
84. Hirsch B, Locke S, Abernethy A. Experience of the National Cancer Institute Community Cancer Centers Program on community-based cancer clinical trials activity. J Oncol Pract. 2016;12(4):e350–8. https://doi.org/10.1200/JOP.2015.005090.
85. Swanson J, Strusowski P, Mack N, et al. Growing a navigation program: using the NCCCP navigation assessment tool. Oncol Issues. 2012;27(4):36–45.
86. Cascella S, Keren J. Mujer a Mujer/woman to woman. J Oncol Navig Surviv. 2012;3(2):20–6.
87. Bickes D. Integrating lay navigators within an existing nurse navigation program. In: Daugherty P, Gamblin K, Rummel M, editors. Oncology nurse navigation case studies. Pittsburgh, PA: Oncology Nursing Society; 2017. p. 11–40.

Quality Cancer Care

3

Mandi Pratt-Chapman

3.1   Cancer Care in Crisis

In 2015, there were a reported 17.5 million cancer cases worldwide, an increase of 33% within a decade [1]. Nearly 9 million people died from cancer that year, the second leading cause of death globally [1]. Personalized medicine and the establishment of longitudinal cancer survivorship as a distinct part of the cancer care continuum have improved cancer outcomes for many. However, great disparities persist, with minority populations within industrialized nations and residents of low and middle income countries (LMICs) suffering disproportionately. Racial and ethnic minorities, sexual and gender minorities, those of lower socioeconomic status, and residents living far from cancer centers both in the USA and abroad face a multitude of barriers that impact access to early detection of cancer, evidence-informed treatment, survival, and quality of life [2].

In 1999, the Institute of Medicine (IOM) defined quality cancer care as "providing patients with appropriate services in a technically competent manner, with good communication, shared decision making and cultural sensitivity" [3]. Two years later in its *Crossing the Quality Chasm*, the IOM defined quality care as safe, effective, patient-centered, timely, efficient, and equitable [4]. This report challenged American healthcare stakeholders to align payment and regulatory incentives, organize patient-centered teams, effectively leverage information technologies, and coordinate care. However, more than a decade later, the IOM reported that the cancer care system was in "crisis." Reminiscent of the 2001 report, in 2013 the IOM recommended six critical components to transform the US healthcare system for cancer patients. These components included engaged

M. Pratt-Chapman, M.A.
Institute for Patient-Centered Initiatives & Health Equity, The George Washington University Cancer Center, Washington, DC, USA
e-mail: mandi@gwu.edu

© Springer International Publishing AG, part of Springer Nature 2018   43
L. D. Shockney (ed.), *Team-Based Oncology Care: The Pivotal Role of Oncology Navigation*, https://doi.org/10.1007/978-3-319-69038-4_3

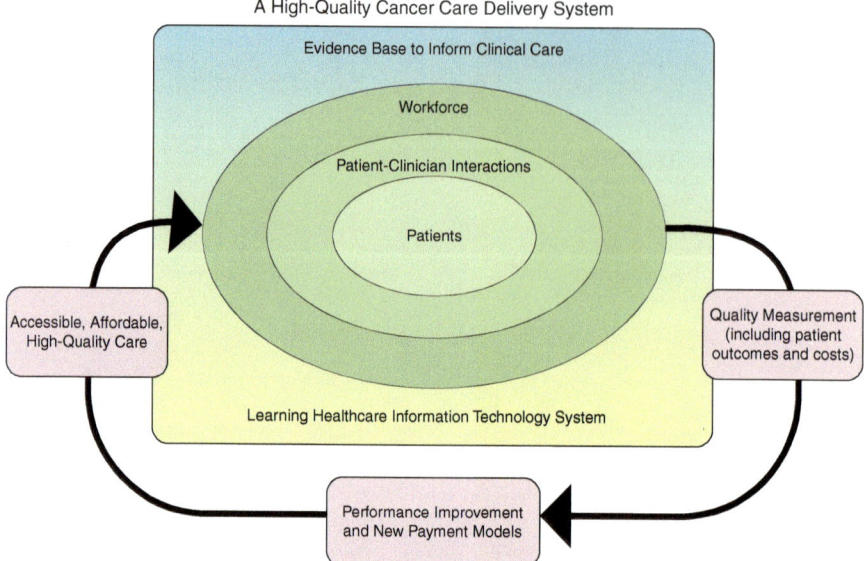

Fig. 3.1 Conceptual framework for a high-quality cancer care delivery system [45] (Reprinted with permission from the National Academies Press. 2013)

patients, an adequate workforce, evidence-based care, a learning healthcare information technology system, translation of evidence to practice, and accessible, affordable care (see Fig. 3.1) [5].

Navigators have a key role to play in achieving high-quality care. In this chapter, quality cancer care is defined as equitable, patient-centered, effective and safe, and timely—with equity serving as the primary and central value. Further, quality must keep pace with new scientific findings, technological innovations, and patient expectations. As such quality improvement must be continuous.

3.2 Quality Cancer Care Is Equitable

Most definitions of quality give a nod to health equity. The IOM lists equity as one of its six criteria for quality care in 1999 [4] and less explicitly acknowledges equity as a quality pillar by asserting the importance of affordable, accessible care in 2013 (see Table 3.1) [5]. This chapter proposes that consideration of population needs, resource stewardship, and ethics demand equity to be a central pillar of a quality cancer care system. It would be difficult to imagine quality cancer care as compatible with bigotry. Discrimination based on race, ethnicity, sex, gender identity, religion, socioeconomic status, nationality, or geographic residence has no place in a quality healthcare system. To achieve health equity, however, nondiscrimination is only the first step. Without turning the current healthcare system on its head by making equity the central component of quality care, the system will continue to be in a state of crisis: a system that relegates a significant portion of those in need to charitable care fails to account for its context as well as its purpose.

Table 3.1 Goals of the IOM recommendations [47]

1.	Provide patients and their families with understandable information about cancer prognosis, treatment benefits and harms, palliative care, psychosocial support, and costs
2.	Provide patients with end-of-life care that meets their needs, values, and preferences
3.	Ensure coordinated and comprehensive patient-centered care
4.	Ensure that all individuals caring for cancer patients have appropriate core competencies
5.	Expand the breadth of data collected in cancer research for older adults and patients with multiple comorbid conditions
6.	Expand the depth of data collected in cancer research through a common set of data elements that capture patient-reported outcomes, relevant patient characteristics, and health behaviors
7.	Develop a learning healthcare information technology system for cancer that enables real-time analysis of data from cancer patients in a variety of care settings
8.	Develop a national quality reporting program for cancer care as part of a learning healthcare system
9.	Implement a national strategy to reduce disparities in access to cancer care for underserved populations by leveraging community interventions
10.	Improve the affordability of cancer care by leveraging existing efforts to reform payment and eliminate waste

Reprinted with permission from the National Academies Press, 2013.

At the population level, quality cannot exist without equitable access to care for all. Consider the evidence-based medicine (EBM) movement. EBM is typically heralded as the first component of quality care—and understandably so. Healthcare should be based on tested science to ensure that treatments will be therapeutic and as safe as possible. Yet clinical care guidelines—critical for guiding clinician decisions about the benefits and risks of a particular intervention—are based on meta-analyses of research studies that are not representative of the diverse populations clinicians serve [6]. In the USA, less than 10% of clinical trial participants are racial minorities [7]. Guidelines are most helpful to the population represented in the research informing the creation of the guideline. They are less helpful to patients not represented in clinical trials. The Federal Drug Administration named 2016 the "Year of Diversity in Clinical Trials" to begin to address this challenge [8].

Minorities in the USA experience disparities in cancer staging, aggressiveness, and health outcomes. There are striking and sustained disparities between white and black Americans. Black women in the USA present with later stages of breast cancer and have lower 5-year survival (78%) compared to their white counterparts (90%) [9]. Black prostate and lung cancer patients also present with more advanced disease than white Americans [9]. American Indians have more emergencies after a cancer diagnosis than other Americans, a clear indicator of suboptimal quality of care [10]. It is difficult to make any conclusive statements about sexual and gender minority cancer disparities, since data are not routinely collected on these populations. To bridge this data gap, in 2011, the Institute of Medicine called for the expansion of research to address sexual and gender minority needs [11], and in 2016, the director of the National Institute on Minority Health and Health Disparities announced the new Sexual and Gender Minority Research Office [12]. Sexual and gender minority patients face unique cancer care risks and challenges due to a history of social stigma, heavy tobacco marketing, healthcare system discrimination, and near-invisibility in medical curricula [2].

In addition to recruiting diverse populations into clinical research, it is critical that researchers publish data stratified by the subpopulations included. The promise of EBM is not realized if biological and sociodemographic differences among studied individuals are ignored for the sake of bolstering the chances that the overall results are statistically significant. Stating that an intervention works because differences are not examined and analyzed does not make that intervention work better— it simply makes it more likely that reports of overall efficacy elide important differences that might alter therapeutic benefit and safety. Recruitment of diverse subpopulations in clinical trials with transparent data reporting of results within and between subgroups is important, even if those analyses prove less significant from a statistical standpoint. As Bluhm notes, "when the putative differences between subgroups have a potential effect on patient safety (as when a particular subgroup appears more likely to suffer adverse effects from the treatment regimen), it may well be better to err on the side of caution and take the effect seriously" [13].

Conducting research without collecting inclusive sociodemographic information is inefficient at best. A recent editorial in *JAMA* argued that exclusion of sexual orientation and gender identity data in research is an inefficient and unethical use of federal research dollars [14]. Since data specific to sexual and gender minorities could be collected, published, and pooled to more quickly assess the unique needs of these populations, continued reluctance to include sexual orientation and gender identity measures wastes research dollars. By not including and reporting these data, studies will need to be replicated when dollars could be better spent addressing already identified needs.

In addition to stewardship of research dollars, examination of the broader set of healthcare resources and their distribution is important to achieving a quality cancer care system. A quality cancer care system would disseminate and implement what research has identified as effective prevention, screening, treatment, and supportive care strategies to all populations who could benefit. On a global scale, as a result of grossly inequitable resource distributions, LMICs suffer from inadequate training opportunities for healthcare professionals as well as insufficient and poorly distributed healthcare resources and infrastructure that result in severely restricted access to healthcare services for much of their populations. Cancer patients in LMICs have less access to radiotherapy and basic palliative care while enduring more invasive surgeries with more complications [15]. The infrastructure for quality cancer screening, early detection, treatment, and posttreatment survivorship care simply does not exist for most of the world [2]. Additionally, inadequate surveillance infrastructure makes it impossible to accurately document global cancer incidence, prevalence, and mortality. Patients who do not have access to early detection programs are typically symptomatic before going to see a doctor, resulting in significantly worse survival and quality of life.

Patient navigation was initially established for the purpose of addressing cancer disparities in staging and survival outcomes among black breast cancer patients in Harlem, New York—with remarkable success [16]. Navigators continue to play a vital role in outreach to underserved communities by bridging access to cancer screening, early detection, treatment, and care coordination for those who are most vulnerable to falling through the cracks of a confusing, inefficient healthcare labyrinth. A challenge for navigators is meeting all of the needs patients have, because the needs are so great. Two ways to address this challenge are (1) prioritizing equity as a value to guide resource stewardship and (2) making resources go further by sharing hard-earned lessons with peers across the world through innovations like telehealth consultations.

3.3   Quality Cancer Care Is Patient-Centered

Quality cancer care is defined differently depending on the perspective of the stakeholder. Cancer center executives may define quality care, in part, by patient adherence and reductions in no-show rates. Accreditation bodies set standards based on stated metrics that are meant to ensure a quality care experience (e.g., Commission on Cancer, National Accreditation Program for Breast Centers). Payers in a fee-for-service environment and hospitals in a value-based purchasing environment may include reduction in emergency department visits and unplanned hospital readmissions as proxy measures for quality.

In 1999, the IOM acknowledged these diverse perspectives on quality, including the potential gap between patient and provider views:

> Patients tend to evaluate care in terms of its responsiveness to their individual needs and may expect and value access to, and choice of services, doctors, and treatments that maximize their ability to work and enjoy life. Physicians may view quality in terms of their ability to exercise their medical judgment to optimize outcomes for patients. [3]

In contrast to the patient perspective, researchers often define cancer care as successful if there is no evidence of disease or if the patient has progression-free survival. This is not to say that patients do not value curative therapy or progression-free survival. However, patients may not value progression-free survival at the expense of functional living or relief from chronic pain.

While oncologists are experts on what cancer therapies and supportive care can do for a patient, the patient is the expert of their own body, mind, and priorities. Many leading health authorities, including the American College of Physicians [17], the American Medical Association [18], the American Association of Colleges of Nursing, the American Association of Colleges of Osteopathic Medicine, the American Association of Colleges of Pharmacy, the American Dental Education Association, the Association of American Medical Colleges [19], and the National Academy of Sciences [4] advocate for shared decision-making or a model where physicians and patients decide together on the best course of treatment. Patient concerns may include functional and financial priorities not always at the top of medical provider considerations for care. Ethically, patients should be asked how they want treatment decisions to be made, how much information they wish to know, what would help clarify questions about their health and treatment options, and who they want to be included in medical appointments and care decisions. For patients to be able to share their values and preferences for care, their healthcare team must ask them these important questions. A recent ethical commentary suggested that the axiom "do no harm" best be considered in the context of patient autonomy, since assessments of the benefits and risks of therapy vary widely [20]. While autonomy is valued differently across cultures and prioritized more in Western cultures, asking the patient how they want care decisions to be made and who they want involved can bridge potential differences between patient wishes and provider assumptions.

Patients are best equipped to engage in care decisions when they are encouraged to do so through clear communication and time for thoughtful consideration of options. Peek et al. developed a useful conceptual framework for shared decision-making in order to improve patient engagement in care, treatment adherence, and health outcomes (see Fig. 3.2) [21]. In the model, shared decision-making requires

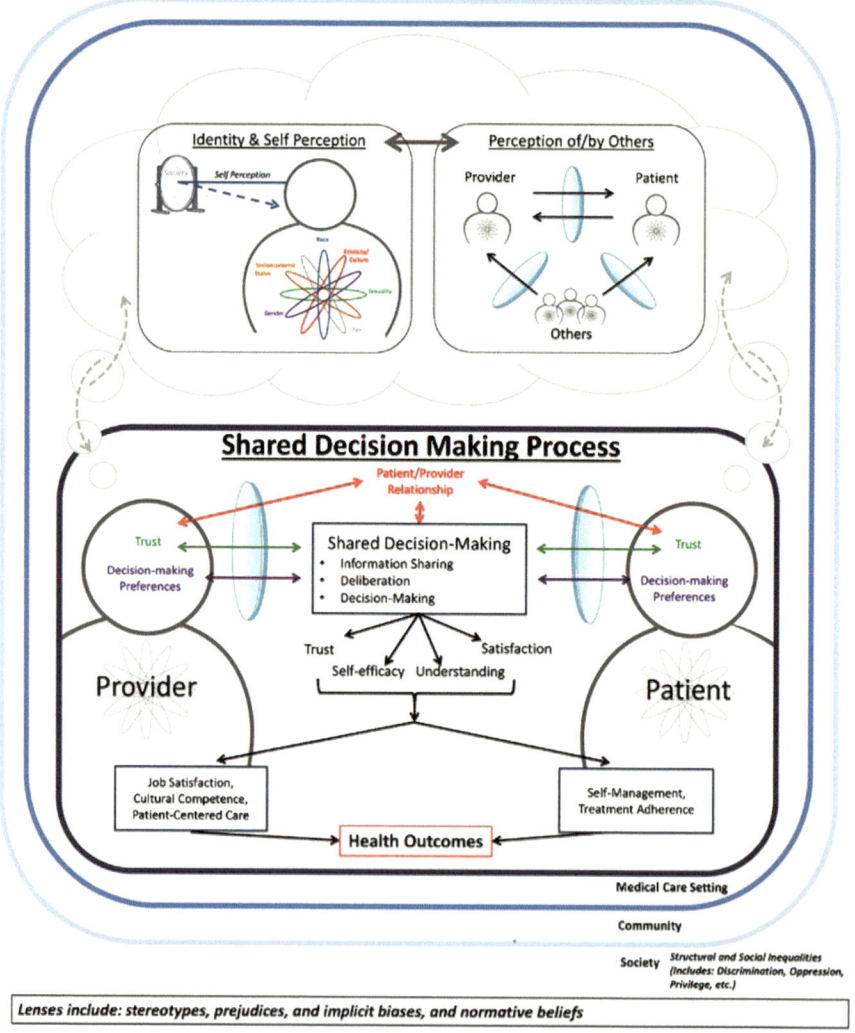

Fig. 3.2 Conceptual model of shared decision-making [21] (Reprinted with permission from the *Journal of General Internal Medicine*)

trust between patients and providers with time for information sharing, deliberation, and decision-making. Patient capacity to self-manage aspects of their care and treatment adherence are intended outcomes of shared decision-making and mediators of eventual patient health outcomes. Provider job satisfaction, cultural competence, and delivery of patient-centered care are provider outcomes of shared decision-making and mediators of patient health outcomes. Identity and self-perception are factors outside of the patient–provider encounter that also influence the shared decision-making process. Self-perception is influenced by treatment from others, since this is internalized to varying degrees. Implicit bias and normative beliefs influence patient and provider perceptions of self and others. Reinforcing the importance of embedding equity in every aspect of quality, Peek et al. identify sexual orientation and gender identity as mediating factors that negatively impact patient-provider relationships and shared decision-making. Further, qualitative research suggests that patients who are of minority race and a sexual or gender minority may perceive greater discrimination in the healthcare system, which has a negative impact on shared decision-making [21].

In order to make informed decisions, patients must understand their disease, treatment options, goals of therapy, and the potential consequences of treatment. The Committee on Improving the Quality of Cancer Care reported that 65%–80% of patients with advanced disease mistakenly believe their disease can be cured [5], indicating a breakdown in patient–provider communication. Providers can increase patient understanding by reducing use of medical jargon when providing information about the clinical evidence of risks and benefits of treatment options. In a recent focus group of cancer survivors, one participant indicated that the best way providers could ensure patient understanding was by frequently creating space for patient questions throughout the care process [22]. Multidisciplinary care can also support shared decision-making as nurses, social workers, case managers, and patient navigators often have more time to provide information about practical, psychosocial, and financial services available as well as to listen to patient concerns. Navigators can also help patients prioritize their questions for their doctor. Finally, navigators can be mindful of patients' pain levels, advocate for appropriate palliation, and encourage patients to complete and share an advanced directive with their healthcare team to ensure clarity about their care preferences across the cancer care continuum.

Finally, technology is a barely tapped opportunity for longitudinal patient engagement. With wearable devices and accelerometers programmed into smartphones, individuals have the ability to collect physical activity, heart rate, weight, blood pressure, and other data that can be helpful to that individual's healthcare team as well as researchers pooling large data sets [23]. Given that 78% of Americans are willing to contribute health data through wearable technology, there is a lost opportunity in not leveraging these data for clinical care improvements [24]. The willingness of patients to engage with their healthcare teams through data sharing provides unprecedented opportunities for primary and tertiary cancer prevention. Tapping these data is a key opportunity for a quality cancer care system.

3.4   Quality Cancer Care Is Safe and Effective

One of the greatest challenges for oncology healthcare professionals today is assessing, managing, translating, and applying research findings in an age where information is more readily available than can be digested. In this environment of information overload, EBM arose as a potential solution. EBM prioritizes highly controlled, randomized controlled trials (RCTs) of quantitative design as the gold standard for clinical decision-making.

An outgrowth of the EBM movement has been the development of clinical care guidelines for cancer prevention and risk reduction, early detection, biomarker testing, cancer treatment by tumor site, symptom management and supportive care, and cancer survivorship. See Table 3.2 for the major oncology organizations issuing clinical care guidelines, including the National Comprehensive Cancer Network (NCCN), the American Society of Clinical Oncology (ASCO), and the American Cancer Society (ACS).

Guidelines are critical to help oncology clinicians wade through existing evidence quickly as they juggle busy clinical practice with greater time constraints than ever before.

The ASCO Quality Oncology Practice Initiative has also issued quality metrics that can be used when considering clinical and safety measures in a value-based purchasing environment. These metrics include standards for pathology, recommendations for genetic testing, therapeutic standards for adjuvant chemotherapy, attention to emotional well-being of patients, patient relief from pain, and considerations for end-of-life (see Table 3.3).

Despite these critical contributions, the EBM movement continues to be controversial. Within scientific debates, RCTs provide important information about cause and effect in a simplified, controlled environment; however, they produce only one aspect of knowledge critical for clinical excellence [25]. As a counterpoint, Miles and Loughlin advocate for evidence-informed medicine [26]. Sturmberg and Martin acknowledge the complexity of real-world patient contexts and advocate for an approach that bridges EBM and patient-centered care [25]. Evidence-informed medicine provides a model for this bridging by considering scientific research knowledge in conjunction with patient values, preferences, and priorities for care.

Table 3.2 Clinical care guidelines overview

	NCCN [48]	ASCO [49]	ACS [50, 51]
Assays and predictive markers		✓	
Prevention and risk reduction	✓		✓
Detection of cancer	✓		✓
Treatment by tumor site	✓	✓	
Symptom management	✓	✓	
Age-related concerns	✓		
Cancer survivorship	✓	✓	✓
Palliative care	✓	✓	

Table 3.3 ASCO patient-centered oncology payment quality measures [52]

Quality oncology practice initiative measures in PCOP

Measures of quality of treatment planning for a new patient

- Pathology report confirming malignancy and staging documented within 1 month of first visit (1, 2)
- Documented plan for chemotherapy and intent (curative or non-curative) before or within 2 weeks of treatment (9, 10)
- Patient emotional well-being assessed by the second office visit (24)
- Test for HER2/neu overexpression or gene amplification for female patients with breast cancer who are candidates for HER2/neu-directed therapy (54)
- KRAS testing for patients with metastatic colorectal cancer who receive anti-EGFR MoAb therapy (74)
- Infertility risks discussed prior to chemotherapy with patients of reproductive age (33)
- Fertility preservation options discussed or referral to specialist (34)
- Patient ratings of their experience of care

Measures of quality of care during treatment

All patients

- Pain addressed (6)
- Oral chemotherapy education provided prior to the start of therapy (13oral12)
- Oral anticancer therapy monitored on visit/contact following start of therapy (13oral13)
- Antiemetic therapy prescribed appropriately with moderate/high emetogenic risk chemotherapy (29)
- Patient ratings of their experience of care

Breast cancer patients

- Chemotherapy recommended within 4 months of diagnosis to women under 70 with AJCC stage I (Tlc) to III ER-/PR-negative breast cancer (52)
- Trastuzumab recommended to patients with AJCC stage I (Tlc) to III HER2/neu-positive breast cancer (55)
- Tamoxifen or AI recommended within 1 year of diagnosis to patients with AJCC stage I (Tlc) to III ER- or PR-positive breast cancer (58)

Colon and rectal cancer patients

- Adjuvant chemotherapy recommended within 4 months of diagnosis for AJCC stage III colon cancer (67)
- Adjuvant chemotherapy recommended within 9 months of diagnosis for AJCC stage II or III rectal cancer (71)
- Colonoscopy before or within 6 months of curative colorectal resection or completion of primary adjuvant chemotherapy (73)

Lung cancer patients

- Adjuvant chemotherapy recommended for patients with AJCC stage II or IIIA non-small cell lung cancer (79)
- Platinum doublet first-line chemotherapy or EGFR-TKI (or other targeted therapy with documented DNA mutation) recommended to patients with initial AJCC stage IV or distant metastatic non-small cell lung cancer with performance status of 0–1 without prior history of chemotherapy (85)

(continued)

Table 3.3 (continued)

Quality oncology practice initiative measures in PCOP
Measures of quality of care following completion of treatment
• Avoiding chemotherapy within 14 days prior to death (48)
• Enrolling patients in hospice more than 7 days before death (45a)
• Ensuring patients' pain is addressed appropriately (38)
• Patient/family ratings of their experience of care

Note: Numbers in parentheses indicate ASCO QOPI measures
Reprinted with permission of ASCO.

Clinical pathway programs exemplify the complexity of developing an evidence-informed approach. Clinical pathways programs are controversial, since they are perceived by some as limiting physician flexibility and autonomy as well as patient choice. Also, some pathway programs are connected to payment incentives that are not always transparent. Nevertheless, clinical pathways have shown remarkable improvements in quality indicators in a variety of settings. Incorporating clinical pathways in a Chinese study yielded improvements in preoperative core biopsy or fine needle aspiration for breast cancer patients and more complete pathology reports to inform treatment planning [27]. A Belgian study implementing a breast cancer treatment clinical pathway program resulted in an increase in guideline-adherent sentinel node biopsy, preoperative staging tests, breast-conserving surgery, adjuvant chemotherapy, and anti-hormonal treatment. Patient satisfaction and progression-free survival also rose significantly [28]. A rectal cancer pathway developed by a multidisciplinary team in Spain also had dramatic results in just the pilot phase: time to diagnostic resolution and time to treatment were shortened significantly, use of neoadjuvant chemotherapy rose from 2% to 71%, short-course radiotherapy was eliminated, preoperative MRI rose tenfold, and anal sphincter preservation—an important patient quality of life indicator—rose, as well (though not significantly) [29].

Acknowledging the complexity and potential of clinical pathway programs, ASCO issued a policy statement on clinical pathways in oncology. Recognizing that reducing variability results in more consistent quality and efficiency, ASCO generally supported pathways in their statement but called for a collaborative, national approach to avoid proliferation of numerous institution-specific pathway efforts. ASCO also called for a consistent, transparent, and inclusive process of clinical pathway development, use of the best-available evidence for the full spectrum of cancer continuum of care services, robust pathway certification criteria, and use of data to improve care and outcomes for patients. ASCO's statement acknowledged that patients have autonomy and suggested that clinical pathway programs allow for a range of options that are reflective of standard of care based on patient-specific goals of therapy, comorbidities, and other patient-centered considerations [30]. In brief, evidence-informed protocols—if created through transparent, inclusive processes and updated regularly—offer a solid base from which physicians can consciously depart based on patient-specific considerations of care [31]. See Table 3.4 for ASCO's guiding principles on clinical pathway development.

Table 3.4 ASCO guiding principles for the development of clinical pathways in oncology [30]

Practicing oncologists should play a central role in developing and revising oncology pathways
The quality of the evidence used in developing an oncology pathway, and the process for continuously updating and enhancing the recommendations in the oncology pathway, should be robust and transparent. This process should be set up in such a way as to ensure that oncology pathway updates are implemented as soon as practice-changing scientific information becomes available
Full disclosure of methodologies, with associated conflicts of interest, should be provided for oncology pathways committee members, vendors, insurers, and any other individuals or entities that contribute to the development of pathway content
Clinical pathway programs in oncology should identify the following key parameters
The proportion of patients the oncology pathway is intended to cover, within the type of cancer on which the oncology pathway focuses
The expected adherence rate and the actual adherence rate with the most recent version of the oncology pathway
The measured outcomes associated with adherence to the oncology pathway (in absolute terms and/or relative to other oncology pathways)
The costs of care associated with adherence to the oncology pathway (in absolute terms using the Medicare payment standards, including the normal 20% patient copay) relative to other oncology pathways
The following mechanisms should be put into place to guide communication between the provider and payer when offpathway (sic) or on-pathway modification decisions are being considered
An appeal process and mechanism for arbitration should be in place for use when there are disagreements between the physician's desired care plan and the oncology pathway care plan
A treatment approval process should be in place to guide decision-making for uncommon cancers where they (sic) may be no guidelines in place
Mechanisms should be available to address dose modifications of regimens/agents while receiving therapy
Mechanisms should be in place to monitor and improve prior authorization processes

Reprinted with permission of ASCO.

In summary, EBM has been critical in moving important quality indicators forward into practice. Newer comparative effectiveness research (CER) and pragmatic trials provide more of an evidence-informed rather than strict EBM approach. The Patient-Centered Outcomes Research Institute (PCORI), a primary funder of CER and pragmatic trials, requires stakeholder engagement in research prioritization, design, planning, implementation, and interpretation with the goal of aligning clinical and research expertise with outcomes valuable to the patients they serve [32]. PCORI also prioritizes research that compares evidence head-to-head to more quickly advance science outside of the RCT model, including analyses on the heterogeneity of treatment effects across subgroups. Finally, PCORI requires dissemination planning, which is essential for expedited translation of scientific knowledge to clinical practice.

3.5   Quality Cancer Care Is Timely

Patients who have cancer detected early and are able to quickly access cancer therapies have the best chance for survival. Quality cancer care should be both accessible and affordable to facilitate timely care regardless of individual background. To be accessible and affordable, a number of components need to be in place: critically, these components include universal access to healthcare and an adequate oncology workforce.

Of all industrialized nations, the USA is the only one that fails to provide universal health insurance, yet its healthcare spending ranks higher than any other industrialized country with no better health outcomes [33]. Health insurance is not the only mechanism for universal healthcare access, but it is critical to expand access to health insurance as long as it remains the primary means of obtaining healthcare. In the USA, the Patient Protection and Affordable Care Act (ACA) issued a variety of consumer protections important for quality cancer care, making it illegal for health insurance plans to refuse coverage to those previously diagnosed with cancer or issue lifetime caps on coverage. The ACA also expanded coverage for services by guaranteeing certain essential health benefits and providing 100% coverage for preventive services rated an A or B by the US Preventive Services Task Force. Finally, the ACA assumed universal expansion of Medicaid with federal cost-sharing; however, this was subsequently rendered optional by a Supreme Court decision in June 2012 [34]. The ACA also provided new insurance options through marketplaces for those previously unable to obtain health insurance [35]. Debate is ongoing regarding health reform refinements; however, retaining these protections is critical to ensuring a quality cancer care system in the USA.

Another critical component for timely care is an adequate oncology workforce. With an aging population and more cancer survivors than ever, the oncology system simply cannot run business as usual. A major reason for the "crisis" in cancer care in the twenty-first century is a strained workforce with misaligned payment incentives [5]. In its 2013 report, the IOM recommended four major strategies to build an adequate oncology workforce. These included:

- *Recruiting and retaining oncology professionals.* The IOM notes that job stress and dissatisfaction deter professionals from staying in oncology careers. System pressures, expectations for high patient volume, short patient visits, and onerous documentation lead to burnout and dissatisfaction. Factors that influence retention of oncology staff include salary and benefits, work culture, promotion potential, and flexibility in work schedules.
- *Providing team-based care.* Patients benefit from a coordinated, multidisciplinary approach to care. Team-based care can also improve clinician and staff satisfaction by spreading responsibility for care across skilled professionals. Interprofessional education is key to this strategy.

- *Providing adequate training opportunities.* The IOM recommends that all oncology professionals be trained based on clear competencies that fit their scope of practice and assigned responsibilities in patient care.
- *Leveraging telemedicine.* To reach those in areas more remote from cancer care settings, telemedicine has shown great promise. However, reimbursement for telehealth collaborations remains a challenge [5].

Team-based care can extend beyond multidisciplinary teams in one setting. Shared care models are emerging in cancer survivorship to spread responsibility for follow-up care across oncology and primary care providers with nurse practitioners playing a major role in filling longitudinal cancer survivorship care needs. Another major success that has begun to expand global capacity to deliver healthcare services to those in need is Project ECHO (Extension for Community Healthcare Outcomes). Project ECHO is "a clinician-to-clinician remote mentoring program in which community primary care clinicians in low-resource areas connect with specialists from academic hubs in order to discuss patient cases, learn new information and receive feedback and guidance in delivering specialty care" [36]. Originally designed to expand capacity for hepatitis treatment in New Mexico, the project has expanded to offer new co-learning opportunities globally [37].

3.6   Quality Cancer Care Requires Transparent Information Sharing for Ongoing Quality Improvement

A major obstacle to quality cancer care is lack of transparency of information, ranging from lack of public reporting of drug development costs, drug acquisition costs, and practice-specific reimbursement rates; hospital, practice, pharmaceutical, and insurance company revenue margins; physician and C-suite salaries for all stakeholder organizations; and insurance company algorithms for premiums and cost-sharing. Additionally, restrictions on the interoperability of electronic health records (EHRs) and proprietary EHR codes create obstacles and waste resources better spent on the provision of patient-centered care.

Recent value-based purchasing pilots in US oncology settings are attempting to shift traditional fee-for-service arrangements to episodic payments for a full course of a patient's care (with some exclusions, such as for drug regimens that vary widely). These pilots also seek to reward clinical practices that choose less expensive therapeutically equivalent options for chemotherapy [38]. Medicare's oncology medical home (OMH) provides $160 per patient per month for 6 months to help practices invest in infrastructure and staff for better care coordination. OMH experiments show great promise, yielding savings from reduced emergency department visits [38]. The Anthem Cancer Quality Care Program provides $350 per patient per month for pilot practices that follow approved clinical pathways and enter supplemental data not typically available from claims into the Anthem oncology database. Supplemental data include demographics, tumor type, stage of cancer, and biomarker information. In exchange, Anthem provides reports on quality metrics to show practices their hospitalization and emergency department use rates compared to benchmark rates [38]. The UnitedHealthcare pilot also requires practices to submit data on genetic tests and goals of therapy (curative or palliative). The UnitedHealthcare pilot has yielded substantial savings for both the insurance company and providers [38]. The Accountable Care Organization (ACO) is another innovative model. ACOs put the onus on providers to manage all care for a pool of patients rather than paying for patient-specific episodes or bundles. ACOs have showed significant quality improvements and some small cost savings [39].

Key to these experimental models is information sharing. Currently physicians operate with little information from billing departments, and quality departments are separate from oncology and finance. With new value-based purchasing pilots, practices commit to sharing supplemental information to payers, and in return, payers provide timely and meaningful feedback that can be used for ongoing performance improvement. This information sharing is crucial. In the fee-for-service world, quality reports from payers are not the norm. Without data transparency about costs of therapies, physicians cannot know the cost of treatment plans nor the potential financial toxicity for patients choosing expensive regimens. Without clinical data, practices cannot evaluate their performance compared to peers or strive for improvements. Without data transparency about costs and revenues, Medicaid and Medicare cannot create payment algorithms that keep clinical practices afloat and protect patient therapeutic needs. Without transparency of insurance algorithms for payment, consumers cannot be guaranteed that increased premiums and cost-sharing are the result of spreading risk rather than higher margins for health plans with strong bargaining power. If we could muster political consensus to do so, establishing an independent, nongovernmental body to assess new therapies based on clinical advantage compared to existing options and to negotiate pricing accordingly could provide relief from ever-escalating, irrational drug price escalation [40].

Finally, a shift in the approach of EHR vendors from selling proprietary licenses to meeting consumer needs is critical to ensure a quality cancer care system. Information technology has extraordinary capacity to help patients better manage their health and healthcare and to help healthcare teams better coordinate care for patients. Lack of transparent and accessible health information causes healthcare waste, including inefficient use of staff time obtaining records from multiple locations and duplicate healthcare tests and services for patients. Lack of information across providers also increases the chances for uninformed treatment planning and uncoordinated care. Open-source software development and licensing provide an alternative to proprietary EHR options. While some have argued that open-source software is vulnerable to hackers, a counterpoint is the active engagement of open-source coders for rapid and easier bug fixes [41]. The promise of open-source EHRs is tremendous cost-savings to the healthcare system and potential access to EHRs for the many institutions still without them. Investing in open-source programming rather than proprietary software will allow systems to invest limited resources to improve patient health rather than into annual software licenses. Further, each health system would not need to reinvent templates for quality protocols—centers could collaborate on what works, more rapidly improving data capture and reporting so that the focus is returned where it should be, on patient care.

3.7   Implications for Navigators

Patient navigators, nurse navigators, social workers, and other patient-centered support caregivers are critical to achieving quality cancer care. Navigation, initially envisioned as a strategy for health equity among breast cancer patients in Harlem, now spans the cancer care continuum from outreach through treatment to survivorship and palliative care. Navigators—in their varied professional roles—can play a critical role in the achievement of a quality cancer care system.

Navigators are a primary point of contact for patients, serving as an advocate for timely, patient-centered care and a coordinating force for patients who often need to access multiple modalities of treatment from multiple clinicians in a variety of treatment settings. Navigators are often gatekeepers of resources. They can support equity in cancer care by prioritizing patients in greatest need—those with multiple comorbidities, with little social support, and/or with meager financial means. Navigators proactively troubleshoot challenges to getting to appointments and adhering to medication regimens. Navigators can also advocate for resources for patients in financial need. Navigators can coordinate multidisciplinary team meetings to ensure provider-to-provider communication and team-based cancer care planning.

Clinically licensed navigators, like nurses and social workers, can fill care coordination needs. Nurse navigators can be a key to clinical pathway improvements, monitoring safety indicators and elevating awareness of variations in clinical practice. Through pathway monitoring, nurse navigators can provide information to multidisciplinary cancer care teams on potential quality care gaps to allow teams to identify and collaboratively implement quality improvements. Social workers can address important psychosocial concerns of cancer patients. Social workers are often best positioned to identify quality improvement efforts that could alleviate patient, staff, and clinician stress. Social workers are often tasked with supporting the mental health of colleagues who serve, as they do, in a profession that is challenging, exhausting, and grief-laden when patients succumb to disease. Additionally, both social workers and nurses often lead the multidisciplinary team through inclusive patient intake processes and communication strategies to ensure respect of all patients regardless of background. Finally, nurse practitioners (NPs), though not technically a navigating profession, play a crucial role in leading longitudinal quality care for posttreatment cancer survivors. NP leadership in cancer survivorship care is both clinically efficient and optimal for ensuring holistic care for survivors posttreatment (see Fig. 3.3).

Through innovative collaborations and a commitment to mentoring, nurses have the potential to radically change the global landscape of palliative care by sharing knowledge with peers in rural areas of the USA and in less resourced LMICs to support palliation for those who suffer with advanced disease.

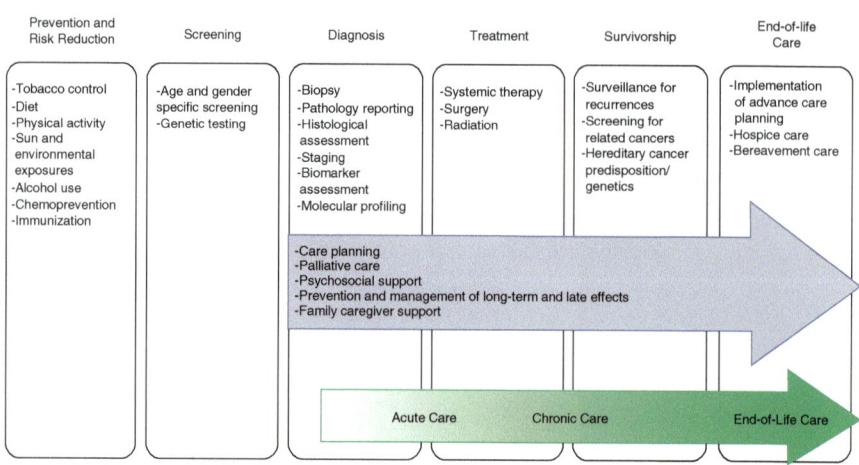

Fig. 3.3 Domains of the cancer care continuum with examples of activities in each domain [46] (Reprinted with permission from the National Academies Press, 2013)

3.8   A Road Map to Quality Cancer Care

In the USA, a suspension of self-interest is critical for the vision of quality cancer care to be achieved. Nearly a decade ago, Berwick, Nolan, and Whittington asserted that "the remaining barriers to integrated care are not technical; they are political" [33]. It is important to point out that self-interest and equity are not intrinsically at odds. The drive to protect the interests of more privileged persons at the expense of those with less economic means perpetuates an inefficient system with high administrative costs that are passed on to patients. The result is higher than necessary premiums and out-of-pocket costs for the insured. While argued to be untenable in the USA, a single-payer healthcare system would obviate the need for such extreme administrative juggling to shore up business interests [42]. It would also logically shift focus to preventive services, as improved preventive care in Medicaid expansion states has started to demonstrate. According to the Kaiser Family Foundation, 26% of newly insured beneficiaries under Medicaid expansion went from not having a primary care checkup in 2013 to having one in 2014 [43]. Medicaid expansion has been "particularly effective at increasing prescription drug utilization for common and potentially costly chronic medical conditions" [43]. Opponents of expanded coverage complain about increased costs to the consumer—but this argument falls flat both logically and ethically. Logically, insurance is intended to cover healthcare services when they are needed, not to ensure that the consumer breaks even financially on an annual basis. Ethically, this argument ignores millions of newly insured people that go missing in the calculation of cheaper healthcare before the ACA. Put otherwise, increased costs are a result of increased coverage for more people. Longtime subsidies of health insurance coverage for white-collar workers belie actual healthcare costs. Spreading these costs across consumers to put healthcare in reach of those formerly without access makes ethical and financial sense.

Globally, a recent vision statement by the Union for International Cancer Control Young World Cancer Leaders representing 12 countries and 6 healthcare sectors provides a blueprint for quality going forward [44]. The authors point out that while impressive, advances in cancer prevention, screening, and treatment cannot be declared successful without access to quality care for all. Currently, scientific progress benefits those of higher socioeconomic status in economically advanced nations, while those of less privilege in industrialized nations and the majority of individuals in LMICs disproportionately suffer from cancer. The authors issue a call to action to:

- Reframe cancer care to attain universal health coverage with a foundation in primary care and holistic patient care.
- Expand cancer outcome measures beyond survival and progression-free survival to include patient-reported outcomes (PROs).
- Expand access to quality care for all populations regardless of race, ethnicity, sexual orientation, gender identity, religion, nationality, or socioeconomic status.
- Steward resources and incorporate social values into decisions about what to fund for whom.
- Provide ethical, supportive care to include financial counseling, palliative care, and transparency of options [44].

With aligned incentives, transparency, collaboration, and an ethical commitment to extend what is known to work to all who can benefit, this vision can be accomplished.

Conclusion
Quality cancer care is care that is equitable, patient-centered, safe, effective, and timely. A commitment to team-based care, transparency, and information sharing can yield improved access to quality cancer care for all. Navigation, launched as a strategy to increase health equity among cancer patients, will play a critical role in achieving this vision.

Acknowledgments Special thanks to Donna Vigue and Sara Rosenbaum for providing feedback on an earlier draft.

References

1. Global Burden of Disease Cancer Collaboration. Global, regional and national cancer incidence, mortality, years of life lost, years lived with disability, and disability-adjusted life years for 32 cancer groups, 1990 to 2015: a systematic analysis for the global burden of disease study. JAMA Oncol. 2016;3(4):524–48. https://doi.org/10.1001/jamaoncol.2016.5688.

2. Pratt-Chapman M. Approaches to cancer survivorship in unique populations: solutions and creative problem-solving. In: Cancer survivorship: transdisciplinary, patient-centered approaches to the seasons of survival. Pittsburg, PA: Oncology Nursing Society; in press.

3. National Cancer Policy Board. In: Hewitt M, Simone JV, editors. Ensuring quality cancer care. Washington, DC: National Academy Press; 1999. p. 79.

4. Committee on Quality of Health Care in America, Institute of Medicine. Crossing the quality chasm: a new health system for the 21st century. Washington, DC: National Academies Press; 2001.

5. Committee on Improving the Quality of Cancer Care, Institute of Medicine. In: Levit LA, Nass SJ, Ganz PA, editors. Delivering high-quality cancer care: charting a new course for a system in crisis. Washington, DC: National Academies Press; 2013.

6. Sackett DL, Straus SE, Richardson WS, Rosenberg WMC, Haynes RB. Evidence-based medicine: how to practice and teach EBM. 2nd ed. Edinburgh, Scotland: Churchill Livingstone; 2000.

7. Levine D, Greenberg R. More minorities needed in clinical trials to make research relevant to all. AAMC News. 2016. https://news.aamc.org/diversity/article/more-minorities-needed-clinical-trials-research.

8. Califf RM. 2016: The year of diversity in clinical trials. U.S. Food & Drug Administration. 2016. https://blogs.fda.gov/fdavoice/index.php/2016/01/2016-the-year-of-diversity-in-clinical-trials.

9. O'Keefe EB, Melzer JP, Bethea TN. Heath disparities and cancer: racial disparities in cancer mortality in the United States: 2000–2010. Front Public Health. 2015;3:1–15. https://doi.org/10.3399/fpubh.2015.00051.

10. Guadagnolo BA, Petereit DG, Coleman CN. Cancer care access and outcomes for American Indian populations in the United States: challenges and models for progress. Semin Radiat Oncol. 2017;27:143–9. https://doi.org/10.1016/j.semradonc.2016.11.006.

11. Institute of Medicine. The health of lesbian, gay, bisexual and transgender people: building a foundation for better understanding. Washington, DC: National Academies Press; 2011.

12. Director's message: sexual and gender minorities formally designated as a health disparity population for research purposes. National Institute on Minority Health and Health Disparities. 2016. https://www.nimhd.nih.gov/about/directors-corner/message.html.

13. Bluhm R. From hierarchy to network: a richer view of evidence for evidence-based medicine. Perspect Biol Med. 2005;48(4):535–47. https://doi.org/10.1353/pbm.2005.0082.

14. Clayton JA, Tannenbaum C. Reporting sex, gender, or both in clinical research. JAMA. 2016;316(18):1863–4.

15. Ganz PA, Cheng HY, Gralow JR, Distelhorst SR, Albain KS, Anderson B, Bevilacqua JL, de Azambuja E, El Saghir NS, Kaur R, McTiernan A, Partridge AH, Rowland JH, Singh-Carlson S, Vargo MM, Thompson B, Anderson BO. Supportive care after curative treatment for breast cancer (survivorship care): resource allocations in low- and middle-income countries. A breast health global initiative 2013 consensus statement. Breast. 2013;22:606–15.

16. Freeman H, Rodriguez RL. The history and principles of patient navigation. Cancer. 2011;117(5):3539–42. https://doi.org/10.1002/cncr.26262.

17. American College of Physicians. American College of Physicians endorses shared decision making approach for prostate cancer screening. 2013. www.informedmedicaldecisions.org/2013/04/09/american-college-of-physicians-endorses-shared-decision making-approach-for-prostate-cancer-screening.

18. American Medical Association. Getting the most for our health care dollars: shared decision making. 2010. www.allhealth.org/briefingmaterials/AMASharedDecisionMaking-1936.pdf.

19. Interprofessional Education Collaborative. Core competencies for interprofessional collaborative practice. 2011. www.aamc.org/download/186750/data/core_competencies.pdf.

20. Sokol DK. "First do no harm" revisited. BMJ. 2013;347:f6426. https://doi.org/10.1136/bmj.f6426.

21. Peek ME, Lopez FY, Williams HS, Xu LJ, McNulty MC, Acree ME, Schneider JA. Development of a conceptual framework for understanding shared decision making among African-American LGBT patients and their clinicians. J Gen Intern Med. 2016;31(6):677–87.

22. Pratt-Chapman M. TEAM study. Unpublished focus group. August 23, 2017.

23. Lai AM, Hsueh P-YS, Choi YK, Austin RR. Present and future trends in consumer health informatics and patient-generated health data. IMA Yearb Med Inform. 2017;26(1):152–9. https://doi.org/10.15265/IY-2017-016.
24. Safavi K, Ratli R, Webb K, MacCracken L. Patients want a heavy dose of digital [presentation]. 2016. www.accenture.com/_acnmedia/PDF-8/Accenture-Patients-Want-A-Heavy-Dose-of-Digital-Infographic-v2.pdf
25. Sturmberg JP, Martin CM. The complex nature of knowledge. In: Sturmberg JP, Martin C, editors. Handbook of systems and complexity in health. New York, NY: Springer; 2014. p. 39–62.
26. Miles A, Loughlin M. Models in the balance: evidence-based medicine versus evidence-informed individualized care. J Eval Clin Pract. 2011;17(4):531–6.
27. Bao H, Yang F, Su S, Wang X, Zhang M, Xiao Y, Jiang H, Wang J, Liu M. Evaluating the effect of clinical care pathways on quality of cancer care: analysis of breast, colon and rectal cancer pathways. J Cancer Res Clin Oncol. 2016;142:1079–89. https://doi.org/10.1007/s00432-015-2106-z.
28. Van Dam PA, Verheyden G, Sugihara A, Trinh XB, Van Der Mussele H, Wyuts H, Verkinderen L, Hauspy J, Vermeulen P, Dirix L. A dynamic clinical pathway for the treatment of patients with early breast cancer is a tool for better care: implementation and prospective analysis between 2002–2010. World J Surg Oncol. 2013;11:70.
29. Uña E, López-Lara F. Pilot study of a clinical pathway implementation in rectal cancer. Clin Med Insights Oncol. 2010;4:111–5.
30. Zon RT, Frame JN, Neuss MN, Page RD, Wollins DS, Stranne S, Bosserman LD. American Society of Clinical Oncology policy statement on clinical pathways in oncology. J Oncol Pract. 2016;12(3):261–7.
31. Cohen R. Guideline-adherent care vs quality care in cancer patients: twins or distant cousins? JAMA Intern Med. 2013;173(7):596–70.
32. Roundtable on the Promotion of Health Equity and the Elements of health Disparities; Board on Population Health and Public Health Practice; Institute of Medicine; National Academies of Sciences: Engineering and Medicine. Achieving health equity via the affordable care act: promises, provisions, and making reform a reality for diverse patients [workshop summary]. Washington, DC: National Academies Press; 2015.
33. Berwick DM, Nolan TW, Whittington J. The triple aim: care, health, and cost. Health Aff. 2008;27(3):759–69.
34. National Federation of Independent Business v. Sebelius, 567 US 519. 2012; 183 L. Ed.
35. Patient Protection and Affordable Care Act, 42 U.S.C. § 18001. 2010.
36. National Cancer Policy Forum. In: Balogh RE, Patlak M, Nass S, editors. Cancer care in low-resource areas: cancer treatment, palliative care and survivorship care [workshop summary]. Washington, DC: National Academies Press; 2017. p. 36.
37. University of New Mexico School of Medicine. (n.d.). Project ECHO: a revolution in medical education and care delivery. https://echo.unm.edu.
38. Robinson J. Value-based physician payment in oncology: public and private insurer initiatives. Milbank Q. 2017;95(1):184–203.
39. Song Z, Fisher ES. The ACO experiment in infancy—looking back and looking forward. JAMA. 2016;316(7):705–6.
40. Chalkidou K, Tunis S, Lopert R, Rochaix L, Sawicki P, Nasser M, Xerri B. Comparative effectiveness research and evidence-based health policy: experience from four countries. Milbank Q. 2009;87(2):339–67.
41. Webster PC. The rise of open-source electronic health records. Lancet. 2011;377:1641–2.
42. Lopez A. The economic case for single payer health care in the US. Institute for Economic Thinking. 2017. www.ineteconomics.org/perspectives/blog/the-economic-case-for-single-payer-health-care-in-the-us.
43. Antonisse L, Garfield R, Rudowitz R, Artiga S. The effects of Medicaid expansion under the ACA: updated findings from a literature review. Kaiser Family Foundation. 2017. www.kff.org/report-section/the-effects-of-medicaid-expansion-under-the-aca-updated-findings-from-a-literature-review-table-2.

44. Ilbawi AM, Ayoo E, Bhadelia A, Chidebe RC, Fadelu T, Herrera C, Htun HW, Jadoon NA, James OW, May L, Maza M, Murgor M, Nency YM, Oraegbunam C, Pratt-Chapman M, Qin X, Rodin D, Tripathi N, Wainer Z, Yap M. Advancing access and equity: the vision of a new generation in cancer control. Lancet Oncol. 2017;18(2):172–5. https://doi.org/10.1016/S1470-2045(17)30041-4.
45. Committee on Improving the Quality of Cancer Care, Institute of Medicine. In: Levit LA, Nass SJ, Ganz, PA, editors. Delivering high-quality cancer care: charting a new course for a system in crisis. Washington, DC: National Academies Press; 2013. p. 5.
46. Committee on Improving the Quality of Cancer Care, Institute of Medicine. In: Levit LA, Nass SJ, Ganz, PA, editors. Delivering high-quality cancer care: charting a new course for a system in crisis. Washington, DC: National Academies Press; 2013. p. 4.
47. Committee on Improving the Quality of Cancer Care, Institute of Medicine. In: Levit LA, Nass SJ, Ganz, PA, editors. Delivering high-quality cancer care: charting a new course for a system in crisis. Washington, DC: National Academies Press; 2013. p. 7.
48. National Comprehensive Cancer Network. (n.d.) NCCN guidelines. www.nccn.org/professionals/physician_gls/f_guidelines.asp.
49. American Society of Clinical Oncology. (n.d.). Guidelines, tools, & resources. www.asco.org/practice-guidelines/quality-guidelines/guidelines.
50. American Cancer Society. (n.d.) American Cancer Society prevention and early detection guidelines. www.cancer.org/healthy/find-cancer-early/cancer-screening-guidelines/american-cancer-society-guidelines-for-the-early-detection-of-cancer.html.
51. American Cancer Society. (n.d.) American Cancer Society survivorship care guidelines. www.cancer.org/health-care-professionals/american-cancer-society-survivorship-guidelines.html.
52. American Society of Clinical Oncology. Patient-centered oncology payment: payment reform to support higher quality, more affordable cancer care. Alexandria, VA: American Society of Clinical Oncology; 2015. www.asco.org/paymentreform.

Building a Navigation Program

4

Mandi Pratt-Chapman, Linda Burhansstipanov, and Lillie D. Shockney

4.1 Introduction

The US healthcare system is complex and fragmented. Efforts to shift from volume- to value-based payment models are on the rise subsequent to the passage of the Patient Protection and Affordable Care Act [1]. Patient navigation has emerged as a critical component of accreditation as well as a requirement for some experimental payment models, including the Oncology Care Model (OCM) [2–4]. The Centers for Medicare & Medicaid Services (CMS) initiated the OCM to improve the effectiveness and efficiency of specialist care with a focus on better care, smarter spending, and healthier people. Patient navigation is integrated into the OCM to help patients coordinate appointments, maintain communication with providers, ensure medical records are available at appointments, arrange transportation, coordinate follow-up services, and facilitate access to clinical trials [5].

Navigators—a term used throughout this chapter inclusive of community patient navigators, patient navigators situated in clinics, and nurse navigators—can do a great deal for patients to improve satisfaction and outcomes and also make clinician time more efficient. However, navigators need a system of support in order to do their job well. This requires thoughtful program planning when building a

M. Pratt-Chapman, MA (✉)
Institute for Patient-Centered Initiatives & Health Equity, The George Washington University Cancer Center, Washington, DC, USA
e-mail: mandi@gwu.edu

L. Burhansstipanov, MSPH, DrPH
Native American Cancer Research Corporation, Pine, CO, USA
e-mail: lindab@natamcancer.net

L. D. Shockney, RN, BS, MAS, ONN-CG
Johns Hopkins University School of Medicine, Baltimore, MD, USA
e-mail: shockli@jhmi.edu

© Springer International Publishing AG, part of Springer Nature 2018
L. D. Shockney (ed.), *Team-Based Oncology Care: The Pivotal Role of Oncology Navigation*, https://doi.org/10.1007/978-3-319-69038-4_4

navigation program, ensuring champions are in place for navigators, and monitoring the program to improve protocols and systems with an eye to patient-centered and culturally tailored care. This chapter provides highlights of program planning considerations. For detailed guidance on program planning, see the GW Cancer Center's Executive Training on Navigation and Survivorship online training and its corresponding program development guide and workbook [6, 7].

4.2   Building a Program

4.2.1   Needs Assessment

Establishing a solid navigation program requires an ongoing process of assessment, planning, implementation, and evaluation (see Fig. 4.1.).

Whether in a community or a clinical setting, it is important to begin with a needs assessment. This helps clarify priorities, resources available within and outside the clinical setting, staffing, and coordination factors. A rigorous needs assessment identifies both the patient and organizational needs. Needs assessments identify major gaps or problem areas to focus the program and clarify the role of the navigator, which should directly correspond to evaluation metrics in order to document success.

Needs assessment involves identifying the needs and interests of the many stakeholders who stand to benefit from the navigation program, including patients, family members, physicians, nurses, front desk staff, and other healthcare team members. Needs assessment includes community assessment, patient and caregiver assessments, provider and staff assessments, an institutional analysis (if the patient navigator is operating within an organization or clinical setting), and resource mapping.

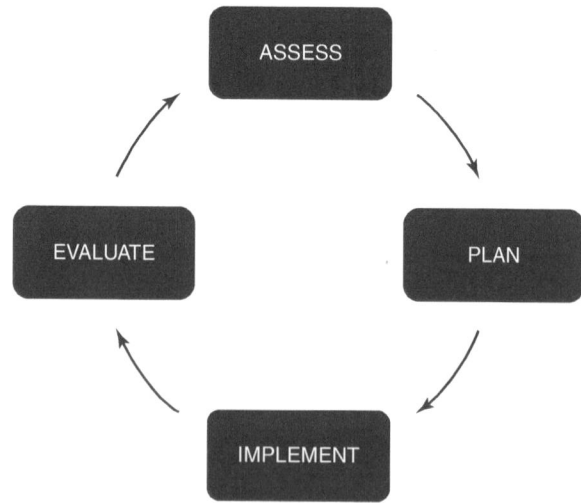

Fig. 4.1 Program planning cycle (Reprinted with permission of the GW Cancer Center [12])

Community assessment refers to the needs of the local service area. What are the demographics of the local service area (e.g., age, race, ethnicity, sexual orientation, gender identity, languages, socioeconomic status)? What data already exist that program staff can use for the community assessment? Tax-exempt hospitals are required to conduct a community health needs assessment every 3 years. The Centers for Disease Control and Prevention (CDC) funded a forum to help institutions create community health needs assessments. The report of forum proceedings emphasizes the importance of "shared ownership of community health among diverse stakeholders." Creating shared ownership means creating consensus around a common agenda and how progress will be measured [8, 9].

The needs of patients and their families also must be evaluated to ensure that the navigation program is serving the specific needs of the patient population. First, consider who are the patients needing navigation? Or, if the patient navigator is in a community organization, who are the clients, and what are the needs of the family members? What barriers do the clients or patients experience in accessing screening, diagnosis, treatment, or supportive care services? For the patient and caregiver assessment, data may already exist if the local organization captures patient satisfaction data. Other ways to obtain information about what patients and their families want and need are by talking to them. Assessments can be formal or informal. Formal methods of obtaining patient and caregiver feedback include interviews, focus groups, and surveys.

Program staff should also consider what impact the patient navigation program will have on clinicians and staff. How will the program impact clinical workflow, provider efficiency, and staff? How will patients be introduced to the navigator? Where will the navigator sit? What will navigators be responsible for? Where does the navigator role stop and other roles begin? Consideration of the needs of the local community, the patient population, and providers and staff can help in tailoring the patient navigation program to address these needs.

A SWOT analysis provides a helpful structure to guide the institutional analysis. SWOT stands for strengths, weaknesses, opportunities, and threats. When considering strengths and weaknesses, consider human resources—are the program staffing levels sufficient? What talent does the program have on the team? What talent is missing? Does the program have physical space for a navigator? Where will navigators interact with patients and family members? Is the institution in good financial standing? How are services financed? Is there internal support for the program? Threats and opportunities are external to the organization, such as accreditation standards and payer policies. In what ways can the program staff leverage navigation requirements from the American College of Surgeons Commission on Cancer and the National Accreditation Program for Breast Centers to increase support for the local patient navigation program? Consider referencing the OCM and the shift to value-based payments when advocating for the patient navigation program. Are there other national, state, or regional forces that could strengthen or threaten the local program?

The SWOT analysis gives the program a start on resource mapping. The program's strengths may include a variety of internal resources to support the patient navigation program. Consider external resources available to both the program and to patients, as well. For example, what relationships does the institution or organization have with other clinics and community-based service organizations?

There are literally hundreds of needs assessment tools: some are very short and simple and help the administration acknowledge issues, such as patients migrating from their clinic to other facilities. Others include patient navigation specific questions, such as, "For which cancer type(s) are the staff considering implementing a patient navigation program? (Check all that apply)." (See Fig. 4.2. for a sample needs assessment tool) [7, 10].

4.2.2 Designing the Navigation Program

Recent research conducted as part of the NCI-funded Patient Navigation Research Program found that patient navigation focused on the highest-risk populations to address known challenges to healthcare were most successful [11]. High-risk populations included those with comorbidities, low income, and low educational attainment [11]. A 2017 scoping review identified 11 elements that influenced the successful implementation of navigation programs, including meeting an assessed need, effective training of navigators, role clarity, adequate resources, strong relationships, clear communication, and program evaluation (see Fig. 4.3 for all 11 components) [12].

Models of patient navigation vary by location and focus. For example, some models are linked with specific tumor types, such as breast or thoracic cancers. Other models focus on the point of client or patient entry, such as outreach to drive community members to risk-appropriate screenings, at the time of diagnosis, at the time treatment begins, or posttreatment survivorship. Models may be described based on volume, or the number of patients per navigator, or based on risk stratification (e.g., stage I colorectal cancer versus undefined stage of pancreatic cancer).

The model the program staff select should be based on the needs identified in the needs assessment—or put another way, the problem the program is trying to solve. A program could focus on logistical barriers to care, symptom management, or transitions of care within and between institutions based on the gaps in services and needs elevated throughout the needs assessment process. There is no single perfect way but rather several strategies to get a patient navigation program started, supported, and sustained. Here are some things to consider when designing the patient navigation program model:

- What problem is the patient navigation program trying to solve for patients?
- What services does the program want to offer?
- What are the program goals?
- How will administrative staff know if the program is successful?
- How will patients be introduced to the navigator?

Do you have difficuilty obtaining your medicines due to finances? ☐ Yes ☐ No

Do you feel there is a language barrier between you and your provider? ☐ Yes ☐ No

What services and information would be most helpful to you?

☐ A treatment plan

☐ Asking for help

☐ Communicating with my employer

☐ Communicating with my family and friends about my diagnosis and treatment

☐ Communication with my healthcare team

☐ Coping with a cancer diagnosis

☐ Coping with physical changes

☐ Coping with work issues

☐ Counseling for psychological or practical issues

☐ Dealing with emotional effects of cancer

☐ Dealing with employment issues

☐ Dealing with financial issues

☐ Dealing with insurance issues

☐ Dealing with school issues

☐ Education about community resources

☐ Education about my cancer

☐ Employment/career/job counseling

☐ Exercise information

☐ Fitness and exercise

☐ Genetic counseling

☐ Healthy behaviors

☐ Help dealing with insurance company

☐ Help getting insurance

☐ Help with coordination of appoinments and communication with providers

☐ Help with financial issues

☐ Help with scheduling appoinments

☐ Identifying treatment options

☐ Identifying treatment preferences

☐ Information about clinical trials and other treatment options

☐ Information about completion of treatment

☐ Information at diagnosis

☐ Information during the treatment decision making process

☐ Information during treatment

☐ Information for family/caregivers

☐ Language assistance

☐ Managing distress

☐ Managing side effects

☐ Managing stress

☐ Managing treatment side effects

☐ Meeting others with cancer

☐ Nutrition and healthy living

☐ Nutrition information

☐ Someone to go with me to my appointment

☐ Spirituality finding meaning

☐ Talking to family and children about cancer

☐ Tips for caregivers

☐ Transportation assistance

☐ Understanding the timeframe for making decisions

☐ Other _____

I understand my treatment plan and how side effects from my treatment will be managed.
☐ Strongly agree ☐ Agree ☐ Not sure ☐ Disagree ☐ Strongly disagree
I understand my plan for follow up care and health related screenings.
☐ Strongly agree ☐ Agree ☐ Not sure ☐ Disagree ☐ Strongly disagree

Fig. 4.2 Sample needs assessment tool (Adapted with permission from the GW Cancer Center [7])

Factors	Elements describing each factor
1. Patient characteristics	• Complexity of clients/patients • Need to address clients/patients basic needs (eg, shelter) first • Caregivers of clients/patients are patients themselves • Geographic restrictions (eg, access to services in rural communities) • Language barriers • Respect for cultural values
2. Effective Recruitment and Training of Navigators	• Recruitment of lay navigators supported by word of mouth • Maintenance of ongoing training to support: Growth and development of navigators • Role transitions • Problem solving for complex cases • Collaboration and mutual support among navigators • Orientation to the needs of the population being served by navigators
3. Role Clarity	• Clear boundaries set for navigators (particularly lay navigators) in their role • Clarifying role boundaries with patients/clients as well as physicians • Valuing role clarification • Management of anxiety when taking on new navigation role to build confidence
4. Effective and Clear Operational Processes	• Careful development of planning processes • Development of policies and procedures to support program activities • Establishment of documentation mechanisms such as clinical intake forms • Use of consensus decision-making approaches • Provision of clinical supervision and steering committee oversight • Regular communication between agencies for planning purposes • Mechanisms to address scheduling and referral challenges

Fig. 4.3 Factors and their elements influencing implementation and maintenance of navigation programs (Reprinted with permission from BioMedical Central (2017) [12])

5. Adequate Human, Financial, and Tangible Resources including Technological Resources	Provision for: • Human resources • Dedicated, committed, engaged and adequately trained clinical staff • External availability of experts such as attorneys • Financial resources • Secured external funding • Technological resources • Internet resources to locate resources and support complex cases • Electronic health records (EHR) to support documentation of evidence based care plans, patient assessments • EHR to support access to community resources, coordinate transitions, and promote self-management • Email or phones to support communication with physicians • Adequate time to support transitional care and provide comprehensive care to a large caseload.
6. Strong Inter and In tra Organizational Relationships/Partnerships	• Encouraging commitment from all professionals involved • Establishment of self-governing team environment in the practice (supports role development) • Development of strong relationships with community agencies by: • Development of a community center development of navigators • Establishment of a community-based steering committee • Development of communication strategies with partner agencies • Mechanisms to address inter-organizational issues with power differentials and other tensions between agencies
7. Lack of Available Services in a Community	• Addressing the problem of "navigation to nowhere" (inadequate or non-existent local services)
8. Effective Communication between Providers	• Encouragement of consistent attendance at regular meetings by staff (monthly) • Sharing of updates related to patient/client progress (through EHR) regularly • Involvement of physicians in meetings regularly • Communication between all care providers
9. Program Uptake and Buy In by End Users of the Program	• Selling/getting buy in to the navigation program with consumers • Use of diverse strategies for recruitment to programs • Recruitment strategies are not successful with all population groups (i.e., outreach) need to be tailored • Addressing potential stigma in getting participation in mental health navigation programs

Fig. 4.3 (continued)

10. Valuing of Navigators	• Valuing navigators by providing them with opportunities to be recognized and heard
11. Evaluation of Navigation Programs	• Team for ongoing evaluation • Developing evaluation plan with • Considering community-based participatory research approaches • Focusing on program related processes (degree to which mission/goals are met) • Considering using pre-identified indicators • Addressing potential problems with lack of access to data, monitoring health status changes over time attribution of outcomes to navigation interventions

Fig. 4.3 (continued)

- How will the program staff communicate and market the program?
- What human and financial resources will support the program?
- How will the program be evaluated?
- How will the program staff use the evaluation findings?

See below for potential services to consider offering through the navigation program (reprinted with permission from the GW Cancer Center) [13].

- Accompany patients to appointments.
- Address health literacy challenges.
- Assist in appointment scheduling.
- Assess family/caregiver needs.
- Coordinate care (internal).
- Coordinate care with referring physicians.
- Help to recruit patients for clinical trials.
- Conduct informational classes.
- Coordinate clinic or multidisciplinary conference.
- Conduct distress screenings.
- Assist with employment needs and referrals.
- Assist with external/community resource referrals.
- Assist with financial assessment and referrals.
- Assist with genetic counseling referrals.
- Improve timeliness of care.
- Assist with insurance coverage issues.
- Coordinate language assistance.
- Address logistical barriers (e.g., housing utilities, dependent care).
- Assist with nutrition referrals.

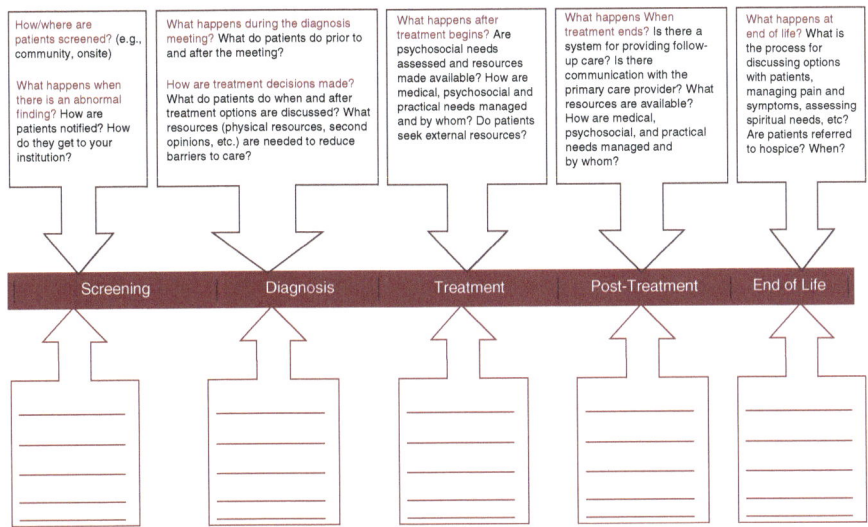

Fig. 4.4 Determining patient flow (Reprinted with permission from the GW Cancer Center [7])

- Provide patient education.
- Provide or refer for psychosocial support.
- Coordinate transportation assistance.
- Coordinate treatment planning.
- Coordinate vocational/career counseling.

For additional examples of needs assessment and program planning tools, see Chapter 15 of this book, "Patient Navigation Training, Tools, and Resources."

Leadership will want to consider patient flow and how the navigation team will interact with patients at each stage of the cancer care continuum. The National Cancer Institute (NCI)-funded Patient Navigation Research Program found that direct in-person contact with navigators yielded the best outcomes for patients and healthcare providers (See Fig. 4.4 for a simple visual to help map what happens at each stage of the continuum for patients) [14].

4.2.3 The Role of Champions

For navigation programs to succeed, administrators need to champion the program, and supervisors must provide clinical and administrative support [15]. The NCI Community Cancer Centers Program (2011) created a Navigation Assessment Tool that associates the strength of the program directly with the level and breadth of physician and administrator support for the program [16].

One of the most successful large-scale patient navigation programs to date, the Patient Care Connect Program of the University of Alabama, established site-specific teams that included "trained lay navigators, a registered nurse site manager, a physician medical director, and an administrative champion" [17]. This structure ensured clinical supervision of patient navigators by a nurse and physician-level and administrator-level champions for each site. This multidisciplinary, multilevel approach helped with navigator integration on the care team and problem-solving as challenges arose. The physician champion's role was to encourage other physicians to integrate the navigators into the multidisciplinary team and to participate in quality improvement efforts as quality-of-care challenges were identified [17].

4.3   Monitoring for Quality Improvement

Quality improvement is critical for high-quality healthcare [18]. The NCI National Community Cancer Centers Program (2011) Navigation Assessment Tool rates the strongest navigation programs as having multiple quality improvement (QI) initiatives that can also be leveraged for demonstrating the impact of the program and securing sustained financial support.

Quality improvement is connected to ongoing evaluation of the program. There are several widely used quality improvement frameworks, including Plan-Do-Study-Act (PDSA), the Lean Process, and Six Sigma. PDSA is a framework used to test a change in a healthcare system by planning, implementing (doing), observing (studying), and then deciding what needs to be changed (acting). The Institute for Healthcare Improvement provides a Plan-Do-Study-Act worksheet to help institutions plan quality improvement initiatives [19]. A 2017 report of a pragmatic clinical trial testing colorectal cancer screening improvements used the PDSA process to structure the trial [20]. The clinics that participated in the trial were able to select their own quality improvement initiatives such as changing workflow or tailoring outreach materials [20]. The University Hospital of North Norway used the Lean Process to reduce median time to diagnosis for lung cancer patients from 64 days to 16 days and median time from chest X-ray to CT scan from 10 days to 5.5 days by eliminating steps that were unnecessary from clinical workflow [21]. The Lean Process uses the following steps: sort, set in order, shine, standardize, and sustain—also known as the 5S approach. A recent nurse-led initiative used Six Sigma to streamline clinical workflow and reduce variations in practice [22]. Six Sigma steps include define, measure, analyze, improve, and control (DMAIC). The focus of the Six Sigma study was improvement of patient scheduling and accuracy of orders and lab data [22]. In all three quality improvement initiatives listed here, a variety of stakeholders were used to inform workflow improvements.

Evaluation metrics for navigation quality improvement could include targeted improvements to patient health behaviors or adherence to treatment, efficiency of healthcare services, shortened time to diagnostic resolution or treatment commencement, improved patient adherence to treatment appointments or oral medication, efficiency of healthcare services provided, or patient-reported outcome (PRO) measures ranging from satisfaction to distress level, quality of life, or symptom relief. See Chapter 14 of this book, "Measuring the Impact Navigation Has on Patient Care by Supporting the Multidisciplinary Team," for a comprehensive review of value metrics to consider for the patient navigation program.

4.4 Extended Case Study: A Community-Based, American Indian Patient Navigation Program

The Native American Cancer Research Corporation's "Native Sister" program evolved over many years through the support of local, national, and government funding. The program relied on community advisory committees, local and state needs assessments, and research findings from multiple grants. New partnerships and resources were necessary to cultivate throughout the years of evolution. This case study maps the evolution of the program from initiation through training, evaluation, and sustainability.

4.4.1 Development

The Native Sister program was initiated after hearing Dr. Harold Freeman's talk at the National Cancer Institute (NCI) in 1989 and 1990, followed by one-on-one telephone conversations between Dr. Freeman and an American Indian who was at that time staff within the NCI. American Indian leaders and elders in Denver and Los Angeles were engaged and agreed that navigation sounded appropriate for addressing needs of their greatly underserved communities. A patient navigation collaborative project among the AMC Cancer Research Center in Denver, the Denver Indian Center, Denver Indian Health and Family Services, and the American Indian Clinic in Compton, CA, was funded by the Robert Wood Johnson Foundation in 1994. The "navigators" of the "Native American Women's Wellness through Awareness" (NAWWA) program were called "Native Sisters," and the program focused on breast cancer screening and education [23, 24]. Two community advisory committees and focus groups ensured broader engagement to refine the navigation intervention. Per the request of the funder, NAWWA initially recruited unpaid volunteers as navigators.

4.4.2   Training for NAWWA (1994–1996)

American Indian women were trained to provide logistical and emotional support to others throughout the cancer care continuum. Training topics included breast cancer education, protection of human subjects, navigation strategies, communication strategies, resource acquisition, and desktop computer skills. Upon completion of the initial training, three of the four trained Native Sisters at the Denver setting were offered higher paying jobs with HIV/AIDS and diabetes programs due to their newly acquired skills. Keeping the trained navigators was difficult, because the program could not pay the navigators. To support navigator salaries, funding proposals were submitted to nine additional community organizations and foundations. These proposals also sought funding for breast cancer screening for women without insurance and treatment costs for those diagnosed. Native Sisters often had to negotiate between Medicaid, Medicare, indigent care options, and the Indian Health Service since more than one of these funders claimed to be the payer of last resort, leading to substantial delays in treatment.

4.4.3   Research

Later, through NCI funding, phone-based versus in-person navigation was compared with the goal of improving American Indian women's adherence to mammography screening in Denver and Los Angeles. Native Sisters tailored breast health information and accompanied patients to screening appointments. The study showed major improvements in screening for both groups [25, 26]. Subsequently, the American Cancer Society sponsored the "Partnerships In Cancer Control Among Underserved Populations" (PICCUP) national initiative in 1997. Among the major issues of concern to this group were breast health screening, accessing culturally acceptable services, and providing appropriate cultural and medical follow-up care for women who receive abnormal screening results. Of primary focus were gaps in the continuum of care for medically underserved women living in the greater Denver area. Three of the community organizations involved in the MUP Committee within PICCUP (Native American Cancer Research Corporation, Clínica Tepeyac, and Exempla/Saint Joseph Hospital) initiated a collaborative, community-based participatory research (CBPR) study that focused on medically underserved populations residing in the greater Denver metropolitan area. The Native Sister model was expanded through a new study designed to work with African-Americans, Latinas, Native Americans, and impoverished white women who had not been rescreened in more than 18 months and were living in the Denver metropolitan area. Education materials were tailored to the individual participants but were culturally modified for each underserved community with great success increasing adherence to recommendations for rescreening mammograms.

4.4.4   Expansion

In 1996, the NAWWA program expanded its focus to survivorship through six new studies supported by the Susan G. Komen for the Cure® Foundation, Mayo Clinic, and NCI. Through this support, the Native Sisters conducted culturally specific outreach and education. Notably, of the 579 Native survivors in the NCI-funded project, more than one-third ($n = 213/579$; 36.8%) had difficulty getting treatments. For almost one-third ($n = 176/579$; 30.4%), there were no local clinics that would provide care for them, and almost one-third ($n = 176/579$; 30.4%) had difficulty completing paperwork to access cancer care [27]. However, quality of life indicators were equivalent to controls due to the Native Sister intervention. Other changes to the program included expansion of the curriculum to palliative care and clinical trials recruitment. In 2002, palliative care was incorporated into training for Native Sisters given the dearth of in-home hospice services, lack of hospital hospice care, and lack of awareness of palliative care options within American Indian communities. This new program addressed the needs of those who lived on reservations and/ or could not pay for expensive in-hospital care. Through the intervention, trained family members increased their capacity to support dying relatives. Clinical trial recruitment efforts offered new access to novel therapies for American Indian patients [28].

4.4.5   Evaluation

Process and outcome evaluation was essential throughout every step of the Native Sisters Community Patient Navigation Program. During the initial years in particular, the project team conducted biweekly debriefings to try to figure out if the program was working. The Native Sisters identified gaps in services, and everyone tried to come up with better strategies and solutions. For example, resources were insufficient to support navigator time and the gasoline needed to transport patients from home to healthcare facilities and back. Written qualitative and quantitative assessments were conducted with the Native Sisters to evaluate their cancer knowledge and knowledge, attitudes, and behaviors for each task they conducted. The Native Sisters started taking part in peer evaluation using observational assessment forms to help one another improve in 2002. Project administrators also shadowed Native Sisters on the job to identify new topics for quarterly in-service trainings and individual performance improvement. Evaluation findings helped to support new financing arrangements to sustain the program: clinics now outsource navigation services for indigenous patients through subcontracts to Native Sisters (see Table 4.1).

Table 4.1 Barriers

Logistics/financial
• Trouble getting transportation
• Unable to pay for the trip/motel/food
• Clinic too far away (time to travel)
• Housing (homeless, unsafe, need rent/mortgage assistance)
• Gasoline
• Food
• Utilities
• Clothing assistance
• Logistics—others
Clinic staff
• No healthcare provider
• Clinic staff was unable to communicate in my primary language
• Clinic staff were disrespectful
• Clinic staff treated me poorly (racism)
• Lack of confidence/trust in healthcare providers
• No clinic staff who are from my cultural group
• Only male providers available at the clinic
• Only female providers available at the clinic
• Healthcare provider did/has not referred for care
• Doctor not at clinic most days
• Clinic staff—others
Clinic
• No cancer services available at local clinic
• Clinic hours inconvenient
• Had to wait too long in office or clinic for scheduled appointment
• No childcare available for while I am in with doctor
• No eldercare available for while I am in with doctor
• Too much paperwork
• Medical records were lost/misplaced at the clinic
• IHS Purchased/Referred Care (formerly known as "Contracted Health Service") issues
• Insufficient insurance (medical, dental, prescription)
• Clinic—others
Cultural
• Age
• Gender identity
• Sexual orientation
• Race/ethnicity
• Socioeconomic status
• Geographic isolation (rural setting with no resources or support)

Table 4.1 (continued)

• Beliefs (spiritual, health practice beliefs)
• Traditional cultural practices
• Emotional issues (fear, guilt related to cancer diagnosis)
• Cultural perceptions of cancer screening, diagnosis, etc.
• Communication styles and issues and cultural connotations of words/phrases
• Language
• Job (e.g., blue collar; cannot get off work to take part in cancer screening or care)
Others
Language/literacy
• Language preference
• Reading literacy
• Health literacy
• Math literacy
• Visual literacy
• Others
Functional
• Daily living assistance (bathing, dressing)
• Mobility needs (walker, wheelchair)
• Disabled (physical, vision, hearing, mental functioning)
• In-home caregiving services
• Fragility
• Competing life demands
Others   Write-in space

Conclusion

Patient navigation programs, whether in the community or housed within cancer centers, require thoughtful planning prior to implementation. A stakeholder analysis and comprehensive needs assessment can drive program focus and evaluation metrics for success. Programs will evolve over time but need program champions and data for ongoing quality improvement to optimize impact and success.

National Community Cancer Program Assessment Tool

	Level 1	Level 2	Level 3	Level 4	Level 5
Key stakeholders	Administrative support	At least one physician champion referring to navigation program	Two physicians involved and referring to navigation program; one is not an oncologist	Most specialty physicians support the navigation program	The navigation program receives referrals from employed and non-employed MDs PCPs or community partners
Community partnerships	Navigator works with departments outside of cancer but within own facility	Plus, works with at least one national group such as NCI, ACS, LLS, wellness community, Susan G. Komen for the Cure, or LIVESTRONG	Plus supports state cancer control goals and objectives	Plus connects with other local community partners such as churches, community centers, other community organizations	Includes a formal connection to national/state/local organizations as an active committee or board member
Acuity system/patient risk factor	No risk factor or acuity system available	Some patients assessed but no formal tool is used. Acuity based on dependence of patient vs actual patient risk factors	Use of a formal tool which may be disease specific	Utilizing formal assessment tool has a well-defined referral process for identified issues	Provides periodic reevaluation as a proactive approach to intervene or prevent issues and ensure quality of care during specific treatment points
Quality improvement measures	None in place	Brainstorming and discussion regarding metrics and reporting within the multidisciplinary team or cancer committee	One quality improvement (QI) initiative in place measured and reported to all stakeholders on hardcopy file annually	QI initiatives developed in collaboration with patient feedback and/or patient satisfaction surveys reported to administration	Multiple QI initiatives in place monitored to demonstrate program improvement and financial contribution and cost savings services of navigation (i.e., compliance to POC)

	Level 1	Level 2	Level 3	Level 4	Level 5
Marketing of the navigation program	Occurs by word of mouth	Includes level 1 as well as some basic written material, i.e., pamphlet	Plus, navigator participation at health fairs, cancer screening events as a means of marketing cancer program	Plus, effort made to promote navigation in some media form	Plus, multiple sources of media used to support navigation (video, print, audio, web, etc.)
Percentage of patients offered navigation	0–20% of defined tumor site	21–40%	41–60%	61–80%	>80%
Continuum of navigation	One functional area within the cancer navigation continuum	Two functional areas navigated within the continuum	Three functional areas navigated within the continuum	Four functional areas navigated within the continuum	Navigation across all functional levels of the continuum
Support services available and used by the navigation team	No resources available	Hospital resources (SW and/or case manager) are available to assist with cases	Outpatient social services available within cancer program	Level 3 plus a minimum of two additional outpatient oncology-specific services available	All services available or can be accessed within the community or organization dietitian, social work, psychologist, clinical trials, speech therapy physical/ occupational/pastoral care, oncology rehab, financial counselor's, palliative care, volunteer dept., genetic counselor, survivorship
Tools for reporting navigator statistics	No reports or tools. Paper record (patient chart) narrative of services provided for patients and their family	Basic Homegrown Access file/Word, Excel basic info tracked, i.e., number of patients, disease site, supportive services provided	High-level Homegrown Access database created by hospital IT dept. Collects stats and support services provided for patient/family	Formal hospital system EMR database utilized to collect support services and stats. Not a database specific for navigation	Reporting of all support services provided to the patient via EMR specific for navigation including outcome information. Document all support services

(continued)

	Level 1	Level 2	Level 3	Level 4	Level 5
Financial assessment	No financial assessment performed	Financial assessment and assistance only available in the in-patient setting	Plus, financial assessment and assistance available for outpatients within cancer program	Plus, proactive financial assessment completed for all oncology patients	Plus, data collection completed on types of services provided and number of patients assisted on a regular basis
Focus on disparities	None defined	Underserved Population Defined	At least one culturally sensitive activity devoted to reaching underserved population provided annually	Patient service mechanism defined to integrate underserved patients into the program	Cultural sensitivity assessment completed on cancer center staff with cultural objectives created on at least an annual basis
Navigator responsibilities	Navigator is unaligned with any physician and responsible only for support of the patient	Plus, navigator coordinates care between multiple disciplines within the cancer program	Plus, navigator participation in support groups, family/patient center programs	Plus, navigator maintains an active role in disease-specific MDC/tumor conferences	Plus, navigator is an integral part of quality improvement, audits, and strategic planning
Patient identification process	No formal patient identification. Pathology reports, daily schedule, radiology reports used to identify patients	N/A	Patients self-refer or are referred by oncology provider	N/A	Primary care provider and/or specialist (GI, pulmonary, interventional radiology) refers at the time of abnormal finding
Navigator training	No formal training in place	Core competencies of navigation defined	Local/in-house training curriculum developed specific to navigator core competency and development of navigator role	Local/in-house training program completed by all navigators—or are certified in oncology in their respective disciplines	Navigators formally trained by nationally recognized training program and certified

	Level 1	Level 2	Level 3	Level 4	Level 5
Engagement with clinical trials	Navigator shares basic understanding of clinical trials in cancer	Navigator has greater depth understanding of clinical trials, has completed specific training (NCI, ONS, etc.)	Navigator shares information regarding the availability of clinical trials in their community cancer center with patients	Navigator engages with research team in providing general referrals	Navigator engages with research team and assists with specific trial referrals for underserved populations
Multidisciplinary care/conference involvement	Basic Commission on Cancer requirements met. Including discussion of NCCN guidelines or other National Oncology Standards	Navigator attends tumor conference but doesn't participate, documents physician discussion of plan of care in narrative note but not formal part of patient record	Navigator assists with case finding for MDC presentations. No treatment plan documented, dictation completed by MD re plan of care	Navigator provides formal review of discussion of MDC with patient after case presentation	Patient informed of presentation at MDC with full formal report on treatment planned discussion shared with patient referring MD and primary care, formal audits completed

Reprinted with permission of the National Cancer Institute

References

1. Patient Protection and Affordable Care Act, 42 U.S.C. § 18001. 2010.
2. American College of Surgeons. Accreditation Committee Clarifications for Standard 3.3 Survivorship Care Plan. 2014. www.facs.org/publications/newsletters/coc-source/special-source/standard33.
3. National Accreditation Program of Breast Centers. Clarifications/Changes to NAPBC Standards. 2016. www.facs.org/quality-programs/napbc/standards/changes.
4. Centers for Medicare and Medicaid Services. Oncology Care Model. 2017. https://innovation.cms.gov/initiatives/oncology-care/.
5. Centers for Medicare and Medicaid Services. Oncology Care Model Request for Applications. 2015. https://innovation.cms.gov/Files/x/ocmrfa.pdf.
6. GW Cancer Institute. Executive training on navigation and survivorship: finding your patient focus: guide for program development. Washington, DC: The George Washington University; 2014.
7. GW Cancer Institute. Executive training on navigation and survivorship: finding your patient focus: program development workbook. Washington, DC: The George Washington University; 2014.
8. Barnett K. Best practices for community health needs assessment and implementation strategy development: a review of scientific methods, current practices and interviews of experts. Report of proceedings from a public forum and interviews of experts. The Public Health Institute, Oakland; 2012 p. iv. www.phi.org/uploads/application/files/dz9vh55o3bb2x56lcrzy-el83fwfu3mvu24oqqvn5z6qaeiw2u4.pdf.
9. Barnett K. Best practices for community health needs assessment and implementation strategy development: a review of scientific methods, current practices and interviews of experts. Report of proceedings from a public forum and interviews of experts. The Public Health Institute, Oakland; 2012. www.phi.org/uploads/application/files/dz9vh55o3bb2x56lcrzyel83f-wfu3mvu24oqqvn5z6qaeiw2u4.pdf.
10. Catholic Health Initiatives. (n.d.) Navigation program resource guide: best practices for patient navigation programs. p. 15. https://mdpnn.files.wordpress.com/2013/04/chi-navigation-pro-gram-resource-guide-_final-012013_.pdf.
11. Freund KM. Implementation of evidence-based patient navigation programs. Acta Oncol. 2017;56:123–7.
12. Willis A, Hoffler E, Villalobos A, Pratt-Chapman M. Advancing the field of cancer patient navigation: a toolkit for comprehensive cancer control professionals. Washington, DC: The George Washington University Cancer Institute; 2016.
13. Gunn C, Battaglia TA, Parker VA, Clark JA, Paskett E, Calhoun E, Snyder FR, Bergling E, Freund KM. What makes navigation most effective: defining useful tasks and networks. J Health Care Poor Underserved. 2017;28:663–76.
14. McCoy M, Caron SE, Battaglia TA. Prevention and early detection case study: patient navigation in the breast health program at Boston Medical Center. In: Calhoun E, Esparza A, editors. Patient navigation: overcoming barriers to care. New York, NY: Springer; 2017. https://doi.org/10.1007/1978-1-4939-6979-1.
15. National Cancer Institute. National community cancer program assessment tool. 2011. http://www.accc-cancer.org/oncology_issues/supplements/NCCCP-Navigation-Matrix-Tool.pdf.
16. Rocque GB, Partridge E, Pisu M, Martin MY, Demark-Wahnfriend W, Acemgil A, Kenzik K, Kvale EA, Meneses K, Li X, Li Y, Halilova KI, Jackson BE, Chambless C, Lisovicz N, Fouad M, Taylor R. The patient care connect program: transforming health care through lay navigation. J Oncol Pract. 2016;12:e633–42. https://doi.org/10.1200/JOP.2015.008896.
17. Marley KA, Collier DA, Goldstein SM. The role of clinical and process quality in achieving patient satisfaction in hospitals. Decis Sci. 2004;35:349–69. https://doi.org/10.1111/j.00117315.2004.02570.x.
18. Institute for Healthcare Improvement. (n.d.). Plan-Do-Study-Act (PDSA) Worksheet. http://www.ihi.org/resources/Pages/Tools/PlanDoStudyActWorksheet.aspx.

19. Coury J, Schneider JL, Rivellie JS, Petrik AF, Seibel E, D'Agostin B, Taplin SH, Green BB, Coronado GD. Applying the Plan-Do-Study-Act (PDSA) approach to a large pragmatic study involving safety net clinics. BMC Health Serv Res. 2017;17:411–21. https://doi.org/10.1186/s12913-017-2364-3.

20. Aasebø U, Strøm HH, Postmyr M. The Lean method as a clinical pathway facilitator in patients with lung cancer. Clin Respir J. 2012;6(3):169–74. https://doi.org/10.1111/j.1752-699X.2011.00271.x.

21. Dydyk D, Franco T, Lebsack J. The cancer service line's use of Six Sigma in the health care setting: creating standardized processes and helping nurses become more efficient with less work while improving staff and patient satisfaction. Oncol Nurs Forum. 2007;34:516–7.

22. Burhansstipanov L, Bad Wound D, Capelouto N, Goldfarb F, Harjo L, Hatathlie L, Vigil G, White M. Culturally relevant "Navigator" patient support: the Native Sisters. Cancer Pract. 1998;6:191–4.

23. Burhansstipanov L, Dignan MB, Bad Wound D, Tenney M, Vigil G. Native American recruitment into breast cancer screening: the NAWWA project. J Cancer Educ. 2000;15:29–33.

24. Burhansstipanov L, Christopher S, Schumacher A. Lessons learned from community-based participatory research in Indian country. Cancer Control. 2005;12:70–6.

25. Dignan MB, Burhansstipanov L, Hariton J, Harjo L, Rattler T, Lee R, Mason M. A comparison of two Native American Navigator formats: face-to-face and telephone. Cancer Control. 2005;12:28–33.

26. Kaur JS, Coe K, Rowland J, Braun KL, Conde FA, Burhansstipanov L, Heiney S, Kagawa-Singer M, Lu Q. Enhancing life after cancer in diverse communities. Cancer. 2012;118:5366–73. https://doi.org/10.1002/cncr.27491.

27. Burhansstipanov L, Krebs LU, Bradley A, Gamito E, Osborne K, Kaur JS. Lessons learned while developing "Clinical Trials Education for Native Americans" Curriculum. Cancer Control. 2003;10:29–36.

28. Valaitus RK, Carter N, Lam A, Nicholl J, Feather J, Cleghorn L. Implementation and maintenance of patient navigation programs linking primary care with community-based health and social services: a scoping review. BMC Health Serv Res. 2017;17:116. https://doi.org/10.1186/s12913-017-2046-1.

Navigation Across the Continuum of Care

5

Danelle Johnston, Tricia Strusowski, Cheryl Bellomo, and Linda Burhansstipanov

5.1 Health Disparities in Cancer Care

The elimination of healthcare disparities is essential in the care and management of cancer patients. A critical element in navigation competencies is to understand the reasons for cancer disparities in order to implement appropriate interventions to overcome disparities and eliminate barriers to care. The *Theoretical Model of Cancer Health Disparities* identifies how the barriers can impact processes and outcomes of cancer care [1]. This theoretical model identifies factors that can be impacted by patient navigation. In summary, the areas that navigation can impact care are adherence to treatment, timely access to care, quality of cancer treatments, quality of life, patient satisfaction, referrals to community resources, patient engagement and empowerment, and removal of barriers to care [1] (Fig. 5.1).

5.2 Care Transitions

It is imperative that navigators facilitate seamless care transitions across the cancer care continuum to ensure patients receive timely access to care. Coleman defines care transitions as "the movement patients make between healthcare practitioners

D. Johnston, MSN, RN, OCN, ONN-CG (✉)
Academy of Oncology Nurse and Patient Navigators, The Lynx Group, Cranbury, NJ, USA
e-mail: djohnston@the-lynx-group.com

T. Strusowski, MS, RN
Oncology Solutions LLC, Decatur, GA, USA

C. Bellomo, MSN, RN, OCN, ONN-CG
Oncology Nurse Navigator, Intermountain Cancer Centers, Cedar City Hospital, Cedar City, UT, USA

L. Burhansstipanov, MSPH, DrPH
Native American Cancer Research Corporation, Pine, CO, USA
e-mail: lindab@natamcancer.net

© Springer International Publishing AG, part of Springer Nature 2018
L. D. Shockney (ed.), *Team-Based Oncology Care: The Pivotal Role of Oncology Navigation*, https://doi.org/10.1007/978-3-319-69038-4_5

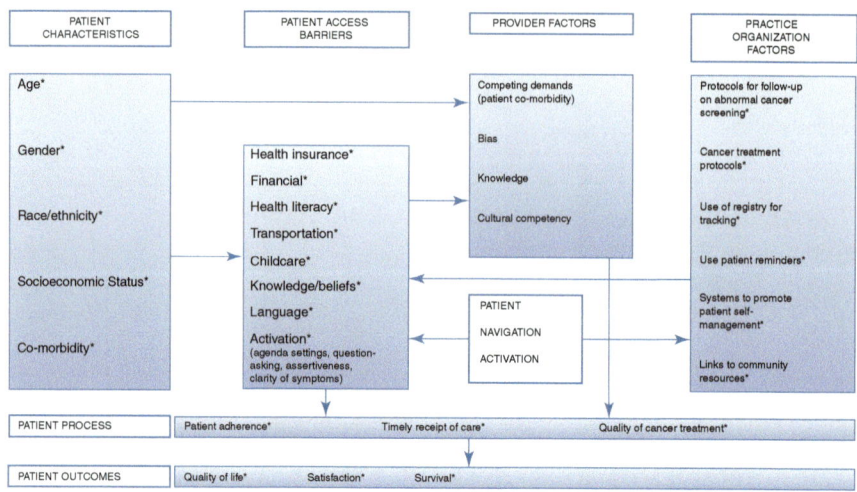

Fig. 5.1 Theoretical model of cancer health disparities. Reprinted with permission from [1]

and settings as their condition and care needs change during the course of a chronic or acute illness" [2]. Inadequate communication between healthcare providers can lead to poor patient outcomes [3]. Information exchanged with each transition between the patient and the healthcare providers is necessary to ensure execution of the plan of care and appropriate coordination of care.

Transitions theory is a process of how one experiences and moves through the changes [4]. The transitions framework has three expected stages that occur: endings, the neutral zone, and beginnings. Endings are the letting go of relationships, roles, and connections before creating new ones. The ending is leaving the known and may be accompanied by a sense of loss or grief [4]. The neutral zone is a time of reflection and insight that is met with confusion, anxiety, and feeling lost [5]. The final stage of transition is the beginning, which offers the opportunity to create new commencement [5]. The navigator needs to recognize the stages of transition as the cancer survivor moves from diagnosis, to acute treatment, into long-term survivorship/end of life in order to provide assistance and guidance.

Poorly coordinated care transitions can lead to increased utilization of the emergency room and hospital readmission rates, which leads to increased healthcare costs [6]. Patients with chronic conditions can follow up to 16 different providers in 1 year [3]. Patients who have complex healthcare conditions experience more care transitions, especially with the elderly, who are subject to being the most vulnerable population. Navigators greatly help facilitate care transitions, which translate to improved quality care [6].

The National Transitions of Care Coalition (NTOCC) has identified the following ways to facilitate transitions: improve communication between providers and patients, electronic medical record, pharmacist involved in medication reconciliation, professional care coordination, and the development of performance measures, which improve patient outcomes [7]. Fragmented systems and poor communication across the care continuum heighten the risk for failure to meet the patient needs during transitions. The Agency for Healthcare Research and Quality (AHRQ) conducted a survey with hospitals and discovered that 42% reported fragmented care [8]. This occurred due to a poor communication process. Inadequate care transitions caused confusion on the patient's condition and care, duplicated tests, medication errors, inconsistent patient monitoring, delay in diagnosis, and lack of appropriate follow-up care, which lead to concerns with patient safety, quality of care, and health outcomes [8]. The Centers for Medicare and Medicaid (CMS) has an initiative to improve quality care across settings by improving transitions between settings [9]. The navigator is instrumental in facilitation of care transitions to safeguard patients from experiencing gaps in care delivery, which can lead to poor patient outcomes.

5.3   The Cancer Care Continuum

Navigators bring a unique and powerful perspective to the patient's care as there is oversight of the patient's comprehensive care needs across the care continuum and across care settings interfacing with the multidisciplinary care team. In 2010, the Oncology Nursing Society (ONS) and the National Association of Social Workers (NASW) published a joint position statement on patient navigation that stated survivors should be offered individualized assistance to help with eliminating barriers to care throughout the cancer care continuum [10]. The IOM identified that oncology nurses are underutilized as a communication resource and that patients who receive care from these nurses can influence quality of life [11]. Case defines navigation as "…a process by which nurses assess individual needs, plan for education, coordination, communication and support, implement effective transitions through the illness trajectory; and evaluate the effect on patient, family and organizational outcomes" [12]. Navigation by definition is to provide individualized assistance to the patients, families, and caregivers to overcome barriers ensuring timely access to quality care throughout the cancer care continuum [13].

The navigator moves with the patient and family/caregiver through the cancer control continuum to facilitate seamless care transitions in all phases of care. In Section 5.7 each phase of the cancer control continuum will be addressed in detail (Fig. 5.2).

5.4   Chronic Care Model

The Chronic Care Model is designed to drive quality and improve outcomes [15]. The model defines six elements—community resources, healthcare system, patient self-management, decision support, delivery system redesign, and clinical information

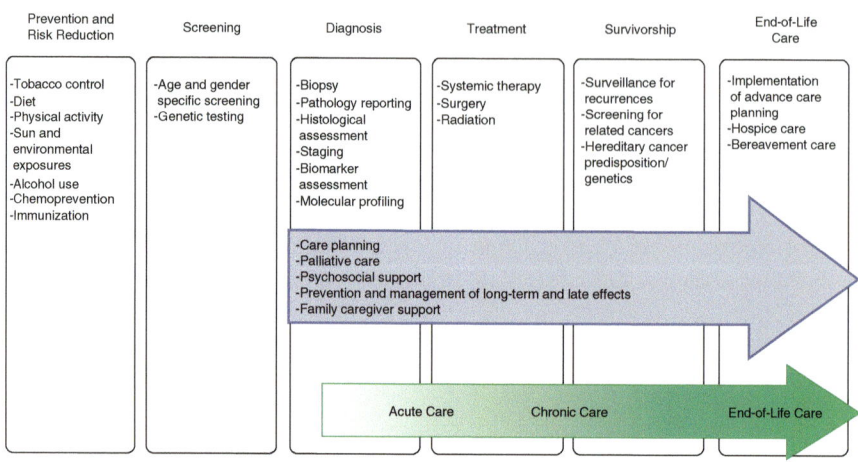

Prevention and Risk Reduction	Screening	Diagnosis	Treatment	Survivorship	End-of-Life Care
-Tobacco control -Diet -Physical activity -Sun and environmental exposures -Alcohol use -Chemoprevention -Immunization	-Age and gender specific screening -Genetic testing	-Biopsy -Pathology reporting -Histological assessment -Staging -Biomarker assessment -Molecular profiling	-Systemic therapy -Surgery -Radiation	-Surveillance for recurrences -Screening for related cancers -Hereditary cancer predisposition/genetics	-Implementation of advance care planning -Hospice care -Bereavement care

-Care planning
-Palliative care
-Psychosocial support
-Prevention and management of long-term and late effects
-Family caregiver support

Acute Care   Chronic Care   End-of-Life Care

Fig. 5.2 Cancer control continuum. Reprinted with permission from [14]

systems. This model highlights the importance of care coordination within and across care settings with three overlapping domains: entire community, healthcare systems, and provider organizations. In order to achieve improved outcomes, this necessitates productive interactions between the patient and the care team.

The navigator works fluidly across all three domains to ensure the patient is informed, empowered, and engaged in care. The role of the navigator is a bidimensional care concept: patient-centered and health system–oriented. Fundamental to the navigator role is to facilitate effective interprofessional collaboration, ensure quality care delivery, promote patient satisfaction, and effectively utilize resources to drive down cost across care settings and improve patient outcomes [16].

The six domains can lead to system reform. The navigator facilitates **community partnerships** to support and develop interventions for the patient and family/caregiver that address barriers to care. The organization of a healthcare goal is to provide safe and high-quality care delivery and patient outcomes. The navigator works across **health organizations** to facilitate seamless care coordination across the cancer care continuum. **Self-management** support is facilitated by the navigator to ensure that the patient is empowered and prepared to be engaged and active in decision-making and health outcomes. **Decision support** is driven by the navigator's professional practice that is built on evidenced-based clinical practice guidelines. The navigator works **across delivery systems** to provide care coordination and services. The final element is **clinical information systems** to augment data collection, outcome metrics, benchmarks, and performance improvement initiatives, and facilitate patient tracking and documentation. The six elements within this model are activated and work synergistically within the three domains, which translate to productive interactions with improved outcomes (Fig. 5.3).

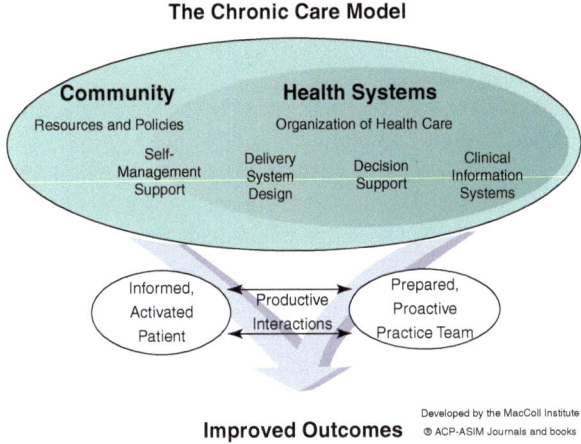

Fig. 5.3 Chronic Care Model. Reprinted with permission from [15]

5.5 Goals of Navigation

The goals of navigation are to educate, remove barriers, facilitate timely access to care and resources, assess needs, and provide emotional support. Education is provided throughout the continuum to the patient, family, and caregiver to address cancer diagnosis, treatment, side effects, and clinical trials. A comprehensive patient, family, and caregiver assessment is crucial to identify barriers to care and patient life goals to direct care decisions. Health system partnerships and multidisciplinary team relationships are imperative to coordinate timely access to support services, appointments, tests, and procedures. The navigator is the "friend on the inside" who becomes the trusted advocate and provides emotional support. It is vital the cancer survivor receives seamless care throughout the cancer trajectory. Early identification and intervention are essential to positively impact quality of life and patient outcomes. The roles and responsibilities of the navigator are outlined in Section 5.6, which drive the navigation goals. Navigation has increased patient satisfaction, decreased barriers to care, improved continuity of care, improved timely access to care, increased emotional support, improved symptom management, and improved patient empowerment [17]. The navigator is the consistent healthcare provider who can coordinate care along the continuum.

5.6 Roles and Responsibilities

It is the position of the Oncology Nursing Society (ONS), Association of Oncology Social Work (AOSW), and National Association of Social Workers (NASW) that [10]:

- Patient navigation processes, whether provided on-site or in coordination with local agencies or facilities, are essential components of cancer care services.

- Patient outcomes are optimal when a social worker, nurse, and lay navigator (defined as a trained nonprofessional or volunteer) function as a multidisciplinary team.
- Patient navigation programs in cancer care must address underserved populations in the community.
- Patient navigation programs must lay the groundwork for their sustainability.
- Nurses and social workers in oncology who function in patient navigator roles do so based on the scope of practice for each discipline. Educational preparation and professional certification play roles in regulating the practice of both disciplines.
- Nationally recognized standards of practice specific to the discipline and specialty also define safe and effective practice.
- Nurses and social workers in oncology who perform navigator services should have education and knowledge in community assessment, cancer program assessment, resolution of system barriers, the cancer continuum, cancer health disparities, cultural competence, and the individualized provision of assistance to patients with cancer, their families, caregivers, and survivors at risk.
- Additional research to explore, confirm, and advance patient navigation processes, roles, and identification of appropriate evidence-based outcome measures must be supported.
- Ongoing collaboration to identify and/or derive metrics that can be used to clarify the role, function, and desired outcomes of navigators must be supported and promoted.
- Navigation services can be delegated to trained nonprofessionals and/or volunteers and should be supervised by nurses or social workers.

5.6.1   Generalized Roles and Responsibilities: Overview Role Delineation

The definition of delineation is to describe, portray, or set forth with accuracy or in detail [18]. Role delineation includes a comprehensive, clearly defined list of critical tasks that are to be included in the roles and responsibilities for a specific job.

As outlined by the Commission on Cancer, Chapter 3, Continuum of Care, Standard 3.1, the navigation process first starts with the community needs assessment [19]. It is essential that the navigation program addresses the needs of the patients served. Essentially, a community assessment seeks to identify a group's strengths and needs to guide in establishing priorities that impact its health status [20].

Cancer programs needed direction in regard to the essential job responsibilities or competencies required by a navigator. In 2013, the Oncology Nursing Society (ONS) created Oncology Nurse Navigator Competencies, which included the categories of professional role, education, coordination or care, and communication.

The oncology nurse navigator (ONN) demonstrates professionalism within both the workplace and community through respectful interactions and effective teamwork. He or she works to promote and advance the role of the ONN and takes responsibility to pursue personal professional growth and development. The ONN provides appropriate and timely education to patients, families, and caregivers to facilitate understanding and support informed decision-making. The ONN facilitates the appropriate and efficient delivery of healthcare services, both within and across systems, to promote optimal outcomes while delivering patient-centered care. The ONN demonstrates interpersonal communication skills that enable exchange of ideas and information effectively with patients, families, and colleagues at all levels. This includes writing, speaking, and listening skills [21].

Cancer centers often hire either oncology nurse navigators or lay patient navigators, each functioning within his or her own scope of training, skills, credentialing, and practice requirements [22]. Essential job functions and scope of practice are vital to the understanding of the navigator role and must be conveyed to multidisciplinary team; refer to Tables 5.1, 5.2, and 5.3.

5.6.2   Nurse, Social Worker, and Lay Navigator Essential Job Functions/Scope of Practice

Table 5.1 Nurse navigator summary of essential job functions/scope of practice

- To provide education related to oncology diagnosis, treatment, cancer center support services, and community resources
- To facilitate timely coordination of appointments, tests, and procedures communicating any concerns to the appropriate physician(s)
- To provide a comprehensive assessment of the oncology patient, family, and/or caregiver needs at pivotal medical visits across the continuum, including assessing barriers to care and distress screening, refer to appropriate disciplines (Commission on Cancer, Chapter 3, Standard 3.2)
- To develop assessment tools, guidelines, pathways, and algorithms across the continuum of care
- To educate the patient, family, and/or caregiver to clinical trials and coordinate with Cancer Research Department (Commission on Cancer E9, Clinical Trial Information)
- To coordinate patient multidisciplinary clinic (MDC) visit, document treatment plan summary, and disseminate to patient, appropriate departments, and physicians. Coordinate all appointments and referrals after the MDC visit
- To participate in the multidisciplinary tumor conference and document recommendations as outlined by Commission on Cancer standards. To monitor recommendations for appropriateness with NCCN or other national guidelines (Commission on Cancer, Standard 1.7)
- To participate in navigation tool development for assessing patient, family, and/or caregiver needs
- To review national NCCN or other national oncology standards with the multidisciplinary team on a yearly basis

(continued)

Table 5.1 (continued)

- To utilize tumor registry for any specific data requests for program development or performance improvement initiatives
- To participate in the completion of the cancer-focused community needs assessment, present to cancer committee per Commission on Cancer standards, and review on an annual basis. Navigation program needs to be modified based on the changes to the community needs assessment (Commission on Cancer Standard 3.1)
- To participate in performance improvement activities to enhance the patient, family, and/or caregiver experience across the continuum (Commission on Cancer Standards 4.5, 4.7, and 4.8)
- To develop in conjunction with support staff support groups and education programs for the patient, their families, and/or caregivers
- To participate in the Patient Advisory Committee and/or Patient and Family Centered Care Committee

Table 5.2 Social work navigator summary of essential job functions/scope of practice

- To provide psychosocial screening for the patient, family, and/or caregiver at pivotal medical visits across the continuum: prevention, diagnosis, treatment, survivorship, palliative care, end-of-life care, and bereavement (Commission on Cancer Standard 3.2)
- To provide counseling and education regarding cancer diagnosis and treatment with the patient, family, and/or caregiver, facilitating referrals to appropriate disciplines and community resources
- To assess and remove barriers to care across the continuum and coordinate with appropriate resources (Commission on Cancer Standard 3.1)
- To participate on the working group for the cancer-focused community needs assessment (Commission on Cancer Standard 3.1)
- To evaluate patient, family, and/or caregiver coping styles and support system, and provide counseling/education to decrease emotional barriers
- To develop support groups and educational programs to meet the needs of the patients, their families, and/or caregivers. To coordinate with community agencies/programs to meet these needs
- To assess gaps in services within the cancer program and community agencies
- To create screening tools to address psychosocial, social, cultural, and spiritual factors
- To participate in the multidisciplinary center (MDC) visits with the patients and MDC team to provide education and support regarding psychosocial issues
- To participate in cancer center tumor boards and provided education and support regarding psychosocial issues
- To participate in the cancer center cancer committee on a quarterly basis (Commission on Cancer Standard 1.7)
- To understand and be aware of clinical trials and educate patient, family, and/or caregiver about clinical trials
- To participate on the survivorship program or coordinate referral to survivorship services/program
- To collaborate with other professional staff on Patient and Family Centered Care Committee or Patient Advisory Committee
- To participate in performance improvement activities and research
- To assess and educate the patient, family, and/or caregiver on the following
  - Social Security Disability
  - Medicaid and Medicare Guidelines

Table 5.2   (continued)

– Medicare Part D
– COBRA Insurance
– Family Medical Leave Act (FMLA)
– Financial resources
– Transportation resources
– Advance directives, power of attorney for healthcare and wills
– Home care, hospice, and end-of-life resources
– Medications and pharmaceutical indigent programs
– Hospital charitable applications

5.7   Phases of the Continuum

5.7.1   Introduction: Phases of the Continuum

The navigation pathway/workflow is bidimensional in nature, being patient centered as well as healthcare system–oriented [23]. Considering the needs of patients, along with system characteristics, promotes continuity of care. Navigators may work in the outreach/screening entry of the care continuum and oversee nonclinical staff to increase cancer screening rates [24–26]. Or they may interact with patients at diagnosis, navigating them throughout the treatment phase and the transition into survivorship or end-of-life care [27–29]. The cancer care continuum consists of the phases of community outreach and education/prevention, screening and early detection, diagnosis, treatment, survivorship, and end of life. Navigators may work with patients throughout any or all phases of the cancer continuum depending upon their work setting and role. No matter their role along the care continuum, navigators must possess oversight of the comprehensive care needs, provide education and advocacy for patients, provide or refer patients to networks of professional and community resources, and act as a distinct contact to enhance psychosocial care [30].

5.7.2   Community Outreach and Education/Prevention

The role of navigation was originally developed to help eliminate barriers to care and to promote timely diagnosis and treatment for cancer in underserved populations. Since its inception in the 1990s with the Freeman model of community outreach and prevention, the role has grown across the disease trajectory and has helped to identify and eliminate communication, logistical, emotional/social, financial, and treatment-related barriers. Along the continuum of cancer care for many patient populations, navigators play an essential role in community outreach and education/prevention. Outreach is the process of contacting, engaging with, and helping people to learn about and to use resources to improve their health and well-being. Outreach may be conducted with individuals, groups, organizations, and at the community level. Outreach efforts can be conducted through cultural and educational

Table 5.3 Phases 4–7 of the cancer continuum

	4. Diagnosis and staging	5. Treatment	6. Survivorship (quality of life [QOL])	7. End of life
Description (components of what is included)	Palliation			
	Diagnosis through	• Surgery	Assessment of QOL (tools)	Advance directives
	• History and physical exam	• Radiation therapy	• Physical QOL	Final will and testament (legal document)
	• Radiologic studies	• Chemotherapy	– Self-rating	Legal power of attorney
	• Magnetic resonance imaging (MRI)	• Immunotherapy	– Side effects	Final wishes (burial/cremation, ceremony logistics)
	• Ultrasound	• Targeted therapy	– Late effects	Do not resuscitate (DNR) orders
	• Nuclear Medicine scans	• Precision medicine	– Long-term effects	Hospice services (hospital, hospice facility, in-home hospice care)
	• Positron emission tomography (PET) scans	• Hormone therapy	– Comorbidities	Spirituality services for patient, family, and loved ones
	• Computed tomography (CT or CAT) scans	• Stem-cell transplant	– Fertility/reproduction	
	• Visualization (endoscopy)	• Unproven/alternative therapies	– Daily functionality	
	• Laboratory studies		– Health behaviors	
	• Tumor markers		Tobacco	
	Types of staging		Marijuana	
	• Clinical staging		Other substances (cocaine, meth)	
	• Pathological staging		Exercise	
	• TNM staging		Diet	
	• Staging for recurrence		• Mental-emotional QOL	
			– Self-rating	

- Body image
- Distress/Stress
- Satisfaction
- Hope
- Isolated
- Depressed
- Useful
- Purpose for living
- Ability to concentrate
- Practical problems (child/elder care, housing)
- Family problems
- Emotional problems
- Social QOL
- Self-rating
- Social support
- Cancer creates issue with job
- Cancer creates issue with relationships
- Intimacy with loved one

• Spiritual QOL
- Self-rating
- Activities
- Abilities
- Religious issues

(continued)

Table 5.3 (continued)

Examples of patient navigator (PN) roles or functions	*The PN is likely to perform each of the following tasks within Phases 4–7*
	• Identify barriers (transportation, insurance, financial, cultural, gender, poverty-related, etc.) and solutions to address each
	• Educate patient and/or family members on cancer care relevant to this phase
	• Evaluate outcomes and explain pros and cons with oncology team to patient and/or family members
	• Conduct motivational interviewing or comparable strategies to help patient take leadership role on cancer care decisions
	• Help schedule and complete appointments (schedule appointments, provide transportation services, provide lodging, child/elder care services)
	• Help patient address cultural issues that may interfere with compliance to Western medical protocols
	• Track/document intervals between recommended appointments to completion of appointments
	• Clarify factors that interfered with timely completion of recommended appointments (system understaffed and appointments' availability are delayed for several months)
	• Assess and address issues (if appropriate) for:
	– Palliative care issues
	– Diet and nutrition issues
	– Stress management
	– Quality of life (physical, mental-emotional, social, spiritual)
	• Refer to other members of oncology team (counselor, social worker, dietitian)
	• Refer to resources (support groups, prescription medication payment programs, indigent care programs)
	• Document and update patient's version of survivorship care plan
	• Follow-up appointment with healthcare provider to update clinic's version of survivorship care plan
Educate patient and/or family members on how to:	Educate the patient about Administer and interpret • Find services and resources for legal and cultural documents and processes

– Prepare for the test	• What is being done for each type of treatment	• QOL assessment tools
– During the test	• Side effects from treatment and how to address	• Symptom distress tools
– Following the test	• When to call the healthcare provider	• Refer to counseling
• Explain to the patient how to interpret the staging information	• How to take medications correctly	
	• What can and cannot be combined with medications (herbs, alcohol)	
	• Financial support for each treatment	
	• Referral to clinical trials	
	• Maintaining QOL during treatments	
	• Physical activity throughout treatment to reduce long and late side effects	
	• Evaluation of outcomes	
		• Help the patient and family members with informed decision-making
		• Symptom management

level–appropriate media and printed materials, booths at community or cancer awareness events, or other public events. These outreach efforts allow navigators the opportunity to promote the value of early detection and prevention along with cancer resources and services available in the local area and how to access the resources.

Navigation programs involved in community outreach must be tailored to meet the needs of the community based upon or identified through a comprehensive community needs assessment. The community needs assessment provides a description of the community served, a list of the top priorities seen in the community, and identifies health disparities and gaps. In looking at the community and working with patient populations, navigators identify barriers to care as well as interventions to these barriers and methods to link individuals to resources. Navigators must also be able to develop collaborative relationships with community partners and provide education to the community on the importance of cancer prevention and early detection for improving survival.

In the community, navigators have the opportunity to educate people on cancer prevention. Cancer prevention may target people who are healthy and at normal risk for developing cancer; extend to populations at intermediate risk resulting from environmental and lifestyle factors, genetic predisposition, and precancerous lesions; as well as including previous cancer patients at risk for developing secondary cancers. Education on cancer prevention should address healthy behaviors such as diet, exercise, sun exposure, and smoking cessation as well as following cancer screening and vaccination guidelines to reduce the risk of cancer developing. Manifesting effective communication skills, such as motivational interviewing, helps the navigator to assess the readiness, literacy ability, and to help individuals identify personal goals and stages of change related to adopting a new, healthier behavior.

5.7.3   Screening

Early detection and cancer screening are the next phase of the cancer care continuum. Cancer screening and early detection have been linked to improved outcomes for patients with cancer. Cancer screenings may be performed through a variety of settings and strategies. Screening programs may be conducted at community outreach health fairs, cancer awareness events, or other public events. Screening services may be provided at local health departments, local hospitals, or even in mobile vans that travel to rural communities. No matter the setting, navigation is essential for individuals with abnormal findings. Navigators need to develop collaborative relationships with community partners to ensure that screening participants with abnormal findings have a medical home. Navigation has been shown to decrease the time to diagnosis and increase the number of individuals completing diagnostic procedures.

To be effective, navigators must have core knowledge of the early signs of cancer and the current screening guidelines, as well as the available community and state resources for screening and diagnostics. It is important for the navigator to be familiar with screening services within the community as to the services they provide, funding programs available to support the cost of screenings, and available resources to provide treatment. Navigators should discuss cancer screening guidelines with individuals and recommend the test most appropriate to increase awareness and promote long-term health.

During this phase of the care continuum, navigators continue to assess, address, and remove barriers to cancer screenings such as transportation, medical coverage, availability, cultural reasons, lack of understanding/medical knowledge, and fear. Navigators should strive to find proactive solutions to each barrier to screening. For instance, many people cannot afford to take time off work to get screening tests performed. It would be pertinent for the navigator to identify facilities that can provide early morning hours or late hours that would not interfere with an individual's work schedule. For those individuals that have misinformation or are unaware of the cancer screening test, it is imperative for the navigator to provide education on the testing. Education and communication by the navigator can be proactive in addressing cultural barriers as well as anxiety and fear. Every effort should be made to educate and reduce the barriers to screening.

5.7.4 Diagnosis

A cancer diagnosis is made through a combination of tests, procedures, and consultations, which can be very overwhelming to patients and their families. As a member of the multidisciplinary team, the navigator works as an advocate, care provider, educator, counselor, and facilitator to ensure that every patient receives comprehensive, timely, and quality healthcare services. During the diagnostic phase, navigators can begin an assessment of patients' coping and psychosocial skills, provide emotional support, and refer to psychosocial services if necessary. Assessing and addressing issues of distress and barriers regarding their diagnosis allow patients to focus on being able to make informed decisions and to be an active participant in their care. The Commission on Cancer specifies that patients must be screened for distress at least once during a pivotal visit when patients are at greatest risk for distress, such as upon diagnosis, a pre- or post-op surgical visit, consultation with an oncologist, initiation of chemotherapy or radiation therapy, and transition into either survivorship or hospice care. Periods of increased vulnerability for distress among cancer patients may also include finding a suspicious symptom, during diagnostic workup, awaiting treatment, changing treatment modality, end of treatment, discharge from the hospital following treatment, medical follow-up and surveillance, treatment failure, recurrence/progression, advanced cancer, and end of life [31].

During this phase, as navigators are building trusting relationships with patients and their families/caregivers, this is an opportune time for navigators to discuss with patients their life goals. It is important for navigators to ask their patient:

- How much do you want to know about your cancer?
- Tell me what you currently know about your cancer.
- Who do you want to include in discussions about your cancer and its treatment options?

- Do you want to have information written down by me regarding your cancer?
- Tell me what is important to you.
- Tell me what you are hoping for.
- Now tell me your understanding of your clinical situation.

Navigators need to have candid conversations with the patient about his/her life goals so that whenever possible, these life goals can be preserved rather than sacrificed to the cancer and/or its treatment. A patient's life goals should be documented in the patient's medical record to help ensure that the oncology team is aware of these goals and that they incorporate them into the treatment decision-making process.

With an understanding of a patient's goals and an assessment of their health literacy and understanding of their illness, the navigator can begin to provide patient-centered education on the disease process, the staging workup, treatment options, and clinical trials. During the education process, a key role of the navigator is to validate patients' understanding regarding their diagnosis and treatment options. Navigators play a key role in clinical trial recruitment as they collaborate with clinical research nurses and physicians to identify patients who may be appropriate for a specific trial, advocate for patient enrollment, educate patients on the clinical trial process and assess patient's understanding, and address any barriers to patient participation. It is imperative for navigators to have an understanding of clinical research trials with respect to the historical background, elements of good clinical practice ethics and guidelines for the protection of human research participants, informed consent, and the various types and phases of clinical trials. It is critical to ensure that appropriate information is provided to patients in order for them to effectively participate in the decision-making process.

While providing patient-centered, personalized care, the navigator facilitates coordination and scheduling of appointments/procedures and facilitates communication between the multidisciplinary team and the referring physician. Navigators can make appropriate referrals to other providers on the teams and ancillary services such as dietitian, genetic counseling, rehabilitative services (i.e., lymphedema and speech/swallowing), fertility preservation, and palliative care.

As a member of the multidisciplinary team and the patient's advocate, navigators play an important role in the coordination of multidisciplinary clinics and/or tumor board conferences. As a participating member of the tumor board, the navigator plays a role in expediting the patient's care based upon knowledge of NCCN guidelines and evidence-based practice as well as advocating for the individual patient's needs, beliefs, values, and preferences. Navigators interact and communicate closely with various clinical and nonclinical specialists, including medical and radiation oncologists, surgeons, radiologists, pathologists, geneticists, pharmacists, clinical trial research staff, as well as rehabilitation specialists such as physical, occupational, and lymphedema therapists, dietitians, social workers, and financial counselors. The multidisciplinary team approach in cancer care enhances safe, efficient, effective, timely, and quality patient-centered care.

5.7.5 Treatment

The continuum of care for cancer patients following diagnosis includes the transition to treatment, survivorship, and/or end-of-life care. Care transition refers to the movement that patients make between healthcare practitioners and settings as their condition and care needs change during the course of their disease, including treatment, survivorship care, palliative care, and hospice care. Poor coordination of care during these periods of transition can lead to poor patient quality of life, increased utilization of emergency department services and hospital readmission rates, duplicated tests, and medication errors, which lead to increased healthcare costs and suboptimal overall patient outcomes. Navigators play pivotal roles in recognizing the stages of care transition, identifying patients at highest risk for gaps in care and providing logistical support, empowering patients by education about anticipated events throughout the trajectory of care, and facilitating communication among providers and between patients and providers to result in better coordination of care overall. Navigators must recognize that patients' needs evolve as care progresses along the continuum, warranting the need for continued reassessment [32]. Navigators must be familiar and knowledgeable to prepare patients for transitions in care in accordance with patients' preferences and goals of care.

To provide coordination of care during the treatment phase of cancer care, navigators should be knowledgeable about the assessment and management of common treatment-related side effects and late effects such as chemotherapy-induced nausea and vomiting, malnutrition, cancer pain, lymphedema, and fatigue. Side effects and late effects can have a profound impact on a patient's quality of life and well-being. Navigators can assist by identifying cancer patients at risk for side effects and late effects through screening, assessment, and identifying barriers; educating patients and families on coping skills, self-care skills, and symptom management; and coordinating referral to specialists of the multidisciplinary team, palliative care, and community resources to help patients improve their functional status.

In providing patient education, it is imperative for the navigator to assess a patient's health literacy in regard to ability to obtain, process, communicate, understand, and act upon health information. Navigators should understand the components of literacy including print (reading and writing), oral (speaking and listening), and numeracy (using numbers to make meaning) and be able to assess the patient's preferred method of learning: written (print material summarizing key points), verbal (face-to-face conversation), and/or pictorial (visual interpretation when presenting statistical information). In educating patients, it is important for navigators to provide the information using simple/plain language, in an organized fashion, and to allow for teach back to demonstrate patient understanding. Basic patient education during the treatment phase should include the type and role of the treatment modality, scheduling/number of treatments/dosing schedule, side effects of the treatment, strategies to prevent and/or manage side effects, how and when to report side effects to the healthcare team/clinic, intimacy/safe sex and handling of bodily fluids, safe handling of oral chemotherapy/targeted therapy, and the importance of nutrition, hydration, and activity during treatment. Education sessions should allow time for patients and their families/caregivers to ask questions, to have their questions addressed, to provide teach back to demonstrate their understanding, and to obtain informed consent.

In the phases of diagnosis and treatment, healthcare providers can sometimes lose sight of the importance of maintaining patients' quality of life. As patient advocates, navigators are in a position to help refer the patient to palliative care for symptom management and cancer rehabilitation to supplement their care. Palliative care, as specialized medical care for individuals with serious illnesses, is focused on providing relief from symptoms, pain, and the stress of illness with the goal to improve quality of life for both the patient and the family. The integration of palliative care into standard oncology care allows for the prioritizing of patient pain and symptom management, emphasizes communication with patients and families, and establishes coordination of care [33].

Ideally, rather than allowing the patient to become deconditioned from the cancer and its treatment, the navigator can intercede, as early as the time of diagnosis and across the care continuum, and promote ways to maintain the patient's function and activity level thus diminishing the impact of the side effect of deconditioning and preserving and/or restoring the patient's quality of life. Navigators can be proactive in identifying impairments and referring patients appropriately for cancer rehabilitation services to treat these impairments such as exercise therapy, pain management, physical and occupational therapy, lymphedema, and speech/swallowing therapy. Navigation through a complex oncology care continuum, including cancer rehabilitation, is of utmost importance for the best possible outcomes for patients with regard to both quantity and quality of life.

5.7.6 Survivorship

There are currently more than 14 million cancer survivors in the United States, a number that is expected to grow exponentially due to an aging population and improved methods for early detection and cancer treatment. The number of cancer survivors is projected to reach 18 million by 2020. The National Coalition for Cancer Survivorship defines a cancer survivor as an individual affected with cancer from the time of diagnosis through the remainder of his or her life [34].

After the completion of active treatment, whether surgery, chemotherapy, or radiation therapy, patients may feel a sense of abandonment by the oncology team as they transition to the phase of survivorship. Cancer survivors have physical, social, psychological, and spiritual needs. There is increasing evidence indicating that cancer survivors experience a reduced health-related quality of life attributed to physical impairment and psychological issues. Many cancer survivors experience persistent physical symptoms and late/long-term effects of treatment. Commonly reported persistent symptoms of cancer survivors of all types of cancer include fatigue, sleep-wake disturbance, pain, peripheral neuropathy, difficulty concentrating and remembering, and decreased physical functioning. Cancer survivors may also experience persistent physical symptoms and late effects related to the type of cancer and treatment such as menopausal symptoms, bowel dysfunction, changes in sexuality and sexual function, and cardiac toxicity. They may experience anxiety and fear of recurrence.

In the Institute of Medicine (IOM) report "From Cancer Patient to Cancer Survivor: Lost in Transition," the importance of addressing the ongoing physical and psychosocial challenges of cancer survivors was emphasized to encourage the multidisciplinary approach to survivorship as a distinct phase of the cancer continuum. The IOM report noted four major components of cancer survivorship care as (1) prevention of new and recurrent cancers and other late effects; (2) surveillance for cancer spread, recurrence, or second cancers and assessment of late psychosocial and physical effects; (3) intervention for consequences of cancer and treatment; and (4) coordination of care between primary care providers and specialists to ensure that all of the survivor's health needs are met [35].

Navigators have an essential role in ensuring that quality survivorship care begins at diagnosis and continues throughout the balance of patients' lives. In order to be able to address the needs of cancer survivors and to provide patient-centered survivorship care, it is imperative for navigators to understand the issues that cancer survivors face. In "Seasons of Survival," Mullen described a model for cancer survivorship in which survivorship begins at diagnosis and requires early identification and intervention to positively impact quality of life and patient outcomes [36]. He identified the seasons of survival as acute, extended, permanent, and expanded additional seasons to transition, chronic survivorship, and end of life. The acute or early phase of survival encompasses the period from diagnosis through the end of active/initial treatment. During this period, patients often focus on two main concerns of cancer recurrence and the ongoing effects of treatment. Throughout this season, patients commonly experience anxiety and fear related to the impact of the cancer diagnosis on their life and future. Extended survival is the period when the acute phase of care is completed and the patient enters surveillance with watchful waiting and possible intermittent therapy. This season is often associated with fear of recurrence and dealing with long-term effects from treatments.

Permanent survival is the period when the activity of the disease or the likelihood of recurrence is sufficiently small that the cancer can now be considered permanently arrested. This is the season in which patients are considered cancer-free but suffer from late or long-term effects of treatment. During this period, survivors can also be faced with psychosocial problems such as finding or keeping employment, health insurance coverage, financial issues, and social isolation. The season of transition recognizes that a survivor evolves from a cancer patient to survivor and must create a "new normal" or transition back into a precancer lifestyle. Several factors can affect a cancer survivor's ability to adjust to the new situation. These factors can be disease-related, treatment/rehabilitation-related, and survivor-related such as the individual's personality, coping skills, belief and culture system, and available support system. Chronic survivorship includes those who, as a result of the advances in cancer treatments, are living with chronic or metastatic disease. Throughout the seasons of survival, it is imperative for healthcare providers and navigators to continually offer the components of survivorship care in the forms of prevention through health and wellness promotion, surveillance for recurrence and screening for new cancers, intervention for management of lasting physical and psychosocial effects, and coordination of care to cancer survivors.

Maintaining the quality of life of a cancer survivor is a key component of survivorship care. The quality of life for a cancer survivor includes their physical well-being by control or relief of acute symptoms and late effects and the maintenance of function, psychological well-being with the ability to cope with illness, social well-being with the ability to deal with the impact of cancer on their roles and relationships, and spiritual well-being with the ability to maintain hope and derive meaning from the cancer experience. Navigators, through their contact and relationships with cancer patients and survivors, are instrumental in assessing quality of life. Navigators have a crucial role to play in education, assessment, and referral to resources to improve a survivor's function and quality of life.

Referral to rehabilitation and survivorship care plans are two components of survivorship care in which navigators play a key role in improving cancer survivors' function and quality of life. The goal of cancer treatment includes preventing as much deconditioning and maintaining function in activities of daily living as possible during acute cancer treatments and thereby requiring less reconditioning after treatment is completed. With their understanding and assessment of late and long-term side effects, navigators can be proactive in identifying impairments and referring patients appropriately for services to treat these impairments such as exercise therapy, pain management, physical and occupational therapy, lymphedema, and speech/swallowing therapy. Navigation through a complex oncology care continuum, including cancer rehabilitation, is of utmost importance for the best possible outcomes for patients with regard to both quantity and quality of life.

Planning for survivorship care through the use of end-of-treatment summaries and survivorship care plans has been recognized by the IOM as an important part of the continuum of cancer care. In 2012, the American College of Surgeons Commission on Cancer (CoC) added "Standard 3.3 Survivorship Care Plan" as part of the requirements for accreditation. The treatment summary and survivorship care plan provide guidance for primary care physicians, the oncology team, and other healthcare providers in the coordination and continuity of care for cancer survivors. The essential items in the survivorship care plan, as recommended by the IOM, include a follow-up care and management schedule, the providers responsible for follow-up, a list of symptoms of recurrence, and tests warranted for surveillance. In congruence with the IOM's four goals of survivorship care (prevention, surveillance, intervention, and coordination), survivorship care plans should provide:

- A summary of an individual's cancer diagnosis and treatment information (the treatment summary)
- An overview of both physical and psychosocial effects of diagnosis and treatment
- A detailed follow-up plan that outlines surveillance for recurrence and potential late effects as well as recommendations for health promotion strategies
- Referrals and resources for physical, psychosocial, and practical needs

The goal of the survivorship care plan is to help the survivor live a higher quality and longer quantity of life. The care plan serves as a guide for the survivor and the primary care provider for the essential screenings and recommended lifestyle changes, identifies potential late and long-term effects of cancer and treatment, and assists in identifying and accessing needed resources. With the growing shortage of oncology specialists in the United States, cancer survivors are no longer able to be followed long term by their treatment team and need to transition back to the care of their primary care physician. The navigator can be especially helpful in assisting with the transition process by educating patients on the transition process and with developing and implementing the survivorship care plan.

5.7.7   End of Life

End of life distinguishes the time when cancer therapy is no longer effective and the disease progresses. The coordination of care is transitioned to hospice care. Navigators also play an integral role in the transition of care to hospice care, which is a specialized branch of palliative care provided to patients who have a life expectancy of 6 months or less and who are no longer receiving cancer-specific treatment because their disease is deemed incurable. In the United States, the average length of time a patient receives hospice care is only 5 days, and approximately 21% of metastatic patients will succumb to their disease while hospitalized in an intensive care unit. These numbers can be correlated with poor or inadequate communication regarding advanced disease and end of life between the patient and the treating oncologists. Navigators should advocate the use of hospice services by recognizing seasons of survival, changes in a patient's quality of life, and understanding that patients may have end-of-life tasks to complete. Statistics have shown that patients who enroll in hospice care at home sooner actually live longer with better quality of life than those who continue treatment until too ill to be given anymore.

During the transition to hospice/end-of-life care, navigators should continue to assess for and identify barriers such as challenges with the healthcare system, financial concerns, and health literacy needs. Serving as the patient's advocate, navigators can help support the patient and family by providing resources for planning legally, financially, and emotionally for end of life and making sure that the patient's voice is heard as to their goals for quality of life and a good death.

5.8   Case Study: Phases of the Continuum

On a Saturday morning in November, Natalie, a thoracic oncology nurse navigator for a university-based medical center, participated in a community health awareness event. Natalie met with members of the community for outreach education/prevention to discuss the hazards of tobacco, resources for smoking cessation, and low-dose CT lung cancer screening. During the event, Natalie met B.B., a woman aged 56 years with a smoking history of 31 pack-years. She quit smoking 8 years ago and is asymptomatic but concerned about developing lung cancer.

The institution provides low-dose helical CT lung cancer screenings based on the results of the National Lung Screening Trial, a lung cancer screening study that demonstrated a reduction in lung cancer mortality with the detection of early stage tumors. It was shown that high-risk patients—those with a strong smoking history—who received a low-dose spiral CT screening had a 15%–20% lower mortality from lung cancer compared with patients screened with a chest x-ray [37]. Based on these data, the US Preventive Services Task Force and the American Lung Association recommend screening for current and former smokers based on specific guidelines [37].

After obtaining the high-risk medical history of B.B., Natalie educated her on the lung screening guidelines recommended for current (>30 pack-year smoker) and former (<15 years since quitting) smokers who are apparently healthy and between the ages of 55 and 74 years, including an annual screening with low-dose CT. B.B. wished to pursue the low-dose CT screening. Across all aspects of the cancer care continuum (screening, treatment, follow-up), nurse navigators provide instrumental and emotional support, address barriers to patient care, coordinate referrals, and strengthen patient-provider relationships. The nurse navigator assisted B.B. in the scheduling and completion of the low-dose helical CT screening.

B.B.'s CT scan results indicated a 5-mm lung nodule. Based on the institution and the Fleischner Society guidelines for recommended follow-up, B.B. should have an initial follow-up CT at 6–12 months and then at 18–24 months if there is no change [38]. When lung nodules do not require immediate diagnostics, the surveillance program of the institution is implemented. The abnormality was communicated to the patient's primary care physician, and the follow-up surveillance guidelines are coordinated by the nurse navigator and primary care physician.

Unfortunately, 24 months later, surveillance imaging noted progression in the size of the lung nodule. CT-guided biopsy was performed with pathology identifying adenocarcinoma non-small cell. The thoracic nurse navigator, Natalie, arranged for B.B. to be seen in the multidisciplinary thoracic clinic where she met with a surgeon, medical oncologist, radiation oncologist, nurse navigator, and social worker. During her consultations with the surgeon and oncologists, treatment options were discussed. Pretreatment staging workup of pulmonary function testing, bronchoscopy, and PET/CT was performed.

Based upon test results, B.B. is deemed well enough for surgery and elects to proceed with surgery. B.B. meets with Natalie to discuss next steps and address barriers to care. Natalie educates B.B. on the recommended surgical procedure and postoperative care. In the past 24 months, B.B.'s socioeconomic situation changed as well in that she is now unemployed and temporarily living with her daughter and two small grandchildren. Natalie refers B.B. to the financial assistance (FA) counselor and assists her in preparing the documents she will need to bring with her (bank statements, income tax records, denials from Medicaid applicable, etc.). The nurse navigator also referred B.B. to national financial assistance resources of Cancer *Care* and Chronic Disease Fund and pharmaceutical drug assistance programs for free drug/drug replacement programs. The social worker also helps B.B. with decisions about employment and disability.

B.B. undergoes video-assisted thoracotomy with lower lobectomy and mediastinal lymph node dissection as the primary course of treatment. The surgical pathology identified a 3.7-cm moderately differentiated adenocarcinoma with focal pleural involvement, clear surgical margins, and two positive lymph nodes. B.B.'s case is presented in Tumor Board Conference. As the patient's advocate, Natalie shares with the board that B.B. continues to utilize supplemental oxygen most of the time since her surgery and has experienced some persistent chest wall pain. Natalie also shares that B.B. has been granted financial assistance from the hospital system for her treatment. Per NCCN guidelines for Stage IIIA T2N2M0, the multidisciplinary team recommends adjuvant chemotherapy followed by radiation therapy. The sequential rather than concurrent treatment will allow B.B. more time for her to recover from the surgery.

B.B. meets with the medical oncologist and nurse navigator to further discuss the plan for six cycles of cisplatin/pemetrexed chemotherapy. In meeting with B.B. for her chemotherapy education session, Natalie provides the information using simple/plain language, in an organized fashion, and to allow for teach back to demonstrate patient understanding. Natalie refers B.B. to the center's pulmonary rehab program to assist her to regain and maintain pulmonary function following surgery. During the course of chemotherapy, Natalie continues to follow B.B. assessing and assisting with symptom management and barriers.

Upon completion of chemotherapy, Natalie meets with B.B. and the radiation oncologist to initiate the transition to adjuvant radiation therapy. Natalie educates B.B. on the short- and long-term side effects and management of the side effects. As the transition to radiation therapy is another pivotal touchpoint, during the radiation therapy education session, Natalie utilizes the NCCN Distress Thermometer for a psychosocial assessment. On the distress thermometer, B.B. reported difficulty with emotional problems in regard to treatment decisions and feeling "sadness," "fear," and "worry." In her discussion with the oncology social worker and the nurse navigator, B.B. expressed her concern about her disease and her treatment affecting her ability to care for herself and loss of "normal life." B.B. was encouraged to participate in the cancer center's Coping Skills program facilitated by the oncology social worker to help cancer patients develop skills to cope with the emotional and physical impact of cancer.

Following the completion of radiation therapy, Natalie meets with B.B. for her end-of-treatment visit. During the visit, Natalie and B.B. discuss her treatment summary and survivorship care plan providing an overview of both physical and psychosocial effects of diagnosis and treatment and the plan for follow-up medical management. Natalie educates B.B. on possible late and long-term effects that someone with non-small cell lung cancer and treatment may experience. Natalie and B.B. discuss the psychosocial issues that cancer survivors may experience as well as health promotion strategies. Natalie refers B.B. to the survivorship programs offered at the cancer center.

Nine months following completion of chemoradiation therapy, B.B. reports to her medical oncologist that she is experiencing discomfort to her left flank region. PET/CT imaging indicates a mass to the adrenal gland suspicious for metastatic disease.

The mass is biopsied confirming stage IV metastatic disease, and molecular testing confirms PD-L1 positivity with the absence of EGFR, ALK, and ROS1 indicators. Natalie meets with B.B. to educate her on the recommendation for further treatment with an immunotherapy agent, pembrolizumab. During the meeting, Natalie encourages B.B. to discuss her goals of treatment and her wishes for quality of life.

After 6 months of immunotherapy, B.B. experiences difficulty with immune-related side effects which decrease her quality of life. B.B. wishes to discontinue treatment. Natalie meets with B.B. and her daughter to discuss the transition to end-of-life hospice care. They discuss the role of hospice care and the services that can be provided. Natalie discusses with B.B. and encourages her to begin leaving her legacy for her daughter and granddaughters by writing cards, recording videos, and recording audiotapes of B.B. reading bedtime stories.

Navigators help individuals overcome barriers to care and navigate through the screening/diagnostic, treatment, survivorship, and end-of-life care continuum. Navigators need to have an awareness of the healthcare system, available community resources, and act as members of the multidisciplinary team in order to address an individual's identified barriers and needs as well as the coordination of care along the continuum. The role of the navigator along the continuum of care is bidimensional in nature with a patient-centered (empowerment with education and knowledge) and health system (multidisciplinary) orientation to deliver timely, seamless care. Within the multidisciplinary team, the navigator works as an advocate, care provider, educator, counselor, and facilitator to ensure that every patient receives comprehensive, timely, and quality healthcare services.

References

1. Hendred S. Patient's barriers to receipt of cancer care, and factors associated with needing more assistance from a patient navigator. J Natl Med Assoc. 2011;103(8):701–10.
2. Coleman E. (n.d.). The care transitions program health care services for improving quality and safety during care hands-offs. http://caretransitions.org/definitions.asp. Accessed 12 Aug 2017.
3. Lattimer C. When it comes to transitions in patient care, effective communication can make all the difference. J Am Soc Aging. 2011;35:69–72.
4. Bridges W. Transitions making sense of life's changes. 2nd ed. New York: DaCapo Press; 2004. https://rossinagil.files.wordpress.com/2015/01/william-bridges-1.jpg.
5. Rancour P. Using archetypes and transitions theory to help patients move from active treatment to survivorship. Clin J Oncol Nurs. 2008;12:935–40.
6. Coleman E, Smith J, Frank J, Min S, Parry C, Kramer A. Preparing patients and caregivers to participate in care delivered across settings: the care transitions intervention. J Am Geriatr Soc. 2004;52:1817–25.
7. National Transitions of Care Coalition. Who we serve. www.ntocc.org?Home/WHOWESERVE. aspx. 2008. Accessed 12 Aug 2017.
8. National Transitions of Care Coalition. Improving transitions of care, findings and considerations of care coalition. September 2010. www.ntocc.org/home/healthcareprofessionals/wws_hcp_tools.aspx. Accessed 12 Aug 2017.
9. Ventura T, Brown D, Archibald T, Goroski A, Brock J. Improving care transitions and reducing hospital readmissions: establishing the evidence for community based implementation strategies through the care transitions theme. Remington Report. 2010; 24–30.

10. Oncology Nursing Society, The Association of Oncology Social Workers, and the National Association of Social Workers joint position on the role of oncology nursing and oncology social work in patient navigation. 2010. http://www.ons.org/publications/positions/navigation. Accessed 12 Aug 2017.
11. Patient-centered cancer treatment planning: improving the quality of oncology care [Workshop Summary]. Washington, DC: The National Academies Press; 2011.
12. Case M. Oncology nurse navigator: ensuring safe passage. J Oncol Nurs. 2011;15:33–40.
13. C-Change. Cancer patient navigation. 2005. www.cancerpatientnavigation.org/resources.html. Accessed 12 Aug 2017.
14. Institute of Medicine. Delivering High-Quality Cancer Care: Charting a New Course for a System in Crisis. Washington, DC: The National Academies Press; 2013. As adapted from National Cancer Institute. The Cancer Control Continuum. Adapted from David B. Abrams, Brown University School of Medicine.
15. Wagner EH. Chronic disease management: what will it take to improve care for chronic illness? Eff Clin Pract. 1998;1(1):2–4.
16. Gentry S. Overview of professional roles and responsibilities. J Oncol Navig Surviv. 2016;7(6):28–31.
17. Bellomo C. The effects of navigator intervention on the community of care and patient satisfaction of patients with cancer. J Oncol Navig Surviv. 2014;5(6):16–20.
18. Merriam-Webster. (n.d.). Accessed 13 Aug 2017 from http://www.merriam-webster.com/disctionary.
19. American College of Surgeons. 2016. Accessed 13 Aug 2017 https://www.facs.org/quality-programs/cancer/coc/standards.
20. Calhoun, E, & Esparza, A. eds. (2017). Patient navigation overcoming barriers to care. New York: Springer. https://link.springer.com/chapter/10.1007%2F978-1-4939-6979-1_1.
21. Oncology Nursing Society. 2013. Accessed 13 Aug 2017 https://www.ons.org/sites/default/files/ONNCompetencies_rev.pdf.
22. Role delineation in oncology navigation. J Oncol Navig Surviv. 2017;8(8):374–5.
23. Fillion L, Cook S, Veillette AM, et al. Professional navigation framework: elaboration and validation in a Canadian context. Oncol Nurs Forum. 2012;39:E58–69.
24. Cascella S, Kerren J. Mujer a mujer/woman to woman: using a unique venue for culturally appropriate outreach and navigation in an underserved area to increase screening. J Oncol Navig Surviv. 2012;3(2):20–6.
25. Koh C, Nelson JM, Cook PF. Evaluation of a patient navigation program. Clin J Oncol Nurs. 2011;15:41–8.
26. Lagrosa D. Breast patient navigation program hopes to reduce disparities among Hispanic/Latina women. J Oncol Navig Surviv. 2011;2(3):20–1.
27. Arias J. Patient navigation: blending imaging and oncology in breast cancer. J Oncol Navig Surviv. 2012;3(1):16–21.
28. Eley RM, Rogers-Clark C, Murray K. The value of a breast care nurse in supporting rural and remote cancer patients in Queensland. Cancer Nurs. 2008;31(6):E10–8.
29. Wilcox B, Bruce SD. Patient navigation: a "win-win" for all involved. Oncol Nurs Forum. 2010;37:21–5.
30. Doll R, Barrroetavena MC, Ellwood AL, et al. The cancer care navigator: toward a conceptual framework for a new role in oncology. Oncol Exch. 2007;6(4):28–33.
31. American College of Surgeons Commission on Cancer Standards 2015. Cancer program standards 2012, version 1.2.1: ensuring patient-centered care (educational standards). 2014. https://www.facs.org/quality-programs/cancer/coc/standards.
32. Wagner EH, Bowles EJA, Greene SM, et al. The quality of cancer patient experience: perspectives of patients, family members, providers, and experts. Qual Saf Health Care. 2010;19:484–9.
33. Goldsmith J, Ferrell B, Wittenberg-Lyles E, et al. Palliative care communication in oncology nursing. Clin J Oncol Nurs. 2013;17:163–7.

34. National Coalition for Cancer Survivorship. Our mission. http://www.canceradvocacy.or/about-us/our-mission. Accessed 2 Aug 2017.
35. Hewitt M, Greenfield S, Stovall E, editors. From cancer patient to cancer survivor: lost in transition. National Cancer Policy Board. Institute of Medicine. Washington, DC: National Academies Press. http://www.nap.edu/catalog/11458html. Published 2006. Accessed 2 Aug 2017.
36. Mullen F. Seasons of survival: reflections of a physician with cancer. N Engl J Med. 1985;313(4):270–3.
37. National Cancer Institute. National lung screening trial: questions and answers. www.cancer.gov/types/lung/research/nlst-qa. Updated November 12, 2014. Accessed 6 Aug 2017.
38. Fleischner Society. Fleischner society recommendations for follow-up of small lung nodules detected incidentally on CT (patients ≥35 years of age). http://snmmi.files.cms-plus.com/docs/PET_COE/off_the_wall/Fleis.pdf. Accessed 6 Aug 2017.

Community Outreach

6

Linda Fleisher, Emily Gentry, Evelyn Gonzalez,
and Andrea Tillman

6.1 The Value of Community Outreach

There are multiple factors that negatively impact the access and use of healthcare services, and the idea of "build it, they will come" is unfortunately a misnomer. If the goal is to reduce the burden of cancer and serve all communities, then outreach efforts to navigate the public to reduce their risk, get screened, diagnose cancer at its earliest stage, access the optimal quality cancer care, and maintain or improve the quality of life of cancer survivors are essential. Moreover, the most successful outreach efforts are built upon a deep understanding of the diverse communities surrounding diverse healthcare organizations and emerge from enduring relationships that are based on mutual trust and the provision of services that are of value to the community. Effective programs also have strong partnerships with other organizations in the community, recognizing that it takes "a village" to understand and address the myriad of challenges faced by the public to prevent cancer occurrences, detect cancer at its earliest stage possible, and support the physical and emotional needs of cancer patients and long-term survivors.

Within the cancer context, our "audiences" are composed of those at risk, those with symptoms, those in the midst of treatment, and those who are cancer survivors who have completed acute treatment. Therefore, it is important to think of outreach not solely as education-focused, prevention-focused, or detection-focused but rather

L. Fleisher, PhD, MPH (✉)
The Children's Hospital of Philadelphia, Research Institute & Fox Chase Cancer Center,
Population Science, Philadelphia, PA, USA
e-mail: FleisherL@email.chop.edu

E. Gentry, RN, BSN, OCN
Sarah Cannon Cancer Institute at Medical City Healthcare, Irving, TX, USA

E. Gonzalez, MA · A. Tillman, BS
Office of Community Outreach, Fox Chase Cancer Center, Philadelphia, PA, USA

© Springer International Publishing AG, part of Springer Nature 2018   111
L. D. Shockney (ed.), *Team-Based Oncology Care: The Pivotal Role of Oncology Navigation*, https://doi.org/10.1007/978-3-319-69038-4_6

focused on the continuum of care, recognizing that the needs of the public and cancer patients often are met outside of the traditional hospital setting. It is important to recognize that "the community" is the fundamental context for cancer patients and where many of the needed services are located. It is in this intersection of the community and the healthcare system where outreach is critically needed to overcome the barriers to access and utilization.

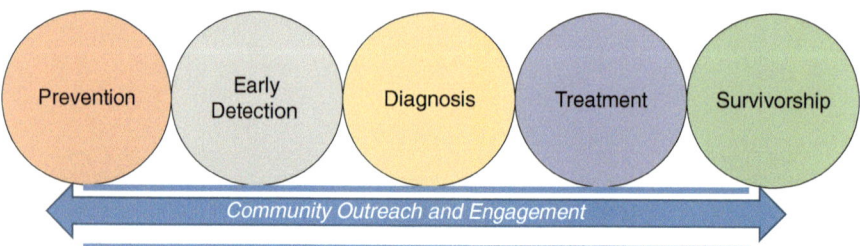

This chapter will highlight the value of effective community outreach and patient navigation, as well as an in-depth exploration of the foundation of effective outreach, including conducting a community needs assessment, building partnerships, and developing cancer-related services utilizing traditional and innovative approaches. It provides resources to guide a community assessment and describes key characteristics of successful community partnership and outreach. The case study provides an in-depth example of a long-standing community outreach program at a comprehensive cancer center, designed based on a comprehensive community assessment linking education and screening through navigation. It also highlights the potential for utilizing emerging communication technology (text messaging) as an adjunct to navigation.

6.2   Key Elements of Community Outreach and Patient Navigation

The integration of community outreach and patient navigation is a winning combination to help consumers and patients manage the complexities of cancer screening, treatment, and survivorship. It is important to build these efforts on the body of experience and research that has been accumulated over many years. Outreach in communities is not new and certainly does not have to be complicated. Effective outreach requires knowing the community and being reliable, trusted, creative, and very determined. Outreach should be targeted (based on insights gleaned from a community assessment) to address barriers and crafted to communicate a message that can be heard and understood. In addition, an evaluation process needs to be incorporated into the planning phase in order to be certain the outreach program goals will be successfully achieved. Outreach also involves serving as an accessible, credible, and reliable source of information equipping people in the community to participate in prevention, treatment, or survivorship efforts. When this information is provided in concert with trusted organizations and individuals in the community, it becomes even more powerful. Outreach involves serving as a guide to help patients and families through systems that are often complex and foreign.

Community Outreach Key Elements of Success
- Meet people where they are.
- Be respectful.
- Listen to your community.
- Build trust and relationships.
- Get the word out in a non-stigmatizing manner.
- Offer service and information in a variety of locations (including home visits) and at nontraditional times, especially after work hours.
- Make written information friendly and easy to understand.
- Provide information in the primary language of those who will use the service.
- Follow up, follow up, and follow up!

Patient navigation is an emerging profession, and navigation programs have been initiated across the United States, Canada, and other parts of the world. While the definitions and tasks may differ, common themes across programs have emerged. These patient navigation roles equally apply in the community setting, although the type of issues being addressed or the services being provided may focus more on one aspect of care—prevention, screening, and/or survivorship. Even for patients in treatment, connections to community services and programs are often critical to helping patients cope with their disease and treatment.

Patient Navigation Roles
- Providing intensive, personal assistance for patients
- Identifying and addressing patients' barriers to seeking or receiving care
- Moving patients along the cancer care continuum in a more timely manner
- Connecting patients to community and medical resources

6.3   Understanding the Community Profile and Performing a Community Needs Assessment [1, 2]

A key step in developing community outreach is to understand the community's cancer profile. This is accomplished through a community needs assessment. Simply put, a community needs assessment is an analysis of various data points that exist both inside and outside of a healthcare organization. These data sources include state and national tumor registries, information about health and wellness behaviors, sociodemographic data, cancer incidence statistics, and much more. All of this information will be examined to highlight issues such as barriers to care, targets for clinical practice improvement, gaps in care compliance, and targets for educational and community outreach.

6.3.1 Turning the Cancer Registry into a Resource

One option for gathering community cancer data would be to pull information from the hospital's cancer registry database, as well as reviewing state-level data. This data review should highlight not only incidences of specific cancers that are prevalent in the community, but the database will also provide information regarding treatment trends, treatment compliance, and other key metrics. Armed with these data, the navigation team can collaborate with other parties, both within and outside of the healthcare enterprise, to develop programs or educational materials and/or partnerships that could help address gaps in education or solve treatment-related issues as well as quality performance improvement projects.

6.3.2 Assessing and Evaluating Internal (Healthcare Organization) and External (Community) Resources for Data

Beyond the cancer registry, the healthcare organization is often home to other resources that can inform outreach efforts. These resources might include:

- IRS-required community needs assessment (see box)
- Marketing department
- Preexisting community outreach
- Population health data
- Business development activities

Beginning in 2012, as part of the Affordable Care Act, the IRS required that hospital organizations conduct a community health needs assessment (CHNA) and respond to the needs identified in order to satisfy 501(c)(3) nonprofit status. Implementation strategies to address the identified needs are documented as a community benefit. The CHNA must be completed every 3 years and must have input from community members. Historically, hospitals generally counted charity care as their community benefit; however, the program has evolved to include population health strategies. *Every nonprofit hospital is required to conduct a community needs assessment for their IRS-approved nonprofit status. Before you start, check with your organization about their community needs assessment. This is usually found on the public website and is often conducted by marketing, government affairs, or community outreach departments. This could save you significant time and resources and would allow you to design your program to meet the needs of your organization* [3].

Beyond the walls of the institution, community and governmental agencies may be home to a wide array of data sources that could focus and fuel outreach:

- Voluntary organizations, such as the American Cancer Society, conducting community assessments
- Local government and public health organizations, such as the local and state health departments
- United Way 211 Community Resource Hotline [4]
- Cancer Control P.L.A.N.E.T. for state profiles [5]

All of these data resources are worth exploring in order to gather data that could help highlight areas that deserve more attention from the navigation team as they develop the program or refine it. Data also must be current; reviewing statistics that are outdated will not help in creating an outreach program that addresses the community's current needs.

6.3.3 Structuring the Community Needs Assessment

More specifically, for accredited cancer centers, the Commission on Cancer (in 2015) developed specific and relevant guidance regarding the foundation for patient navigation and its connection with community needs assessments. Healthcare organization and supporting service line personnel must respond to the data revealed by the community needs assessment with programs and outreach that match and meet the identified challenges and patient and community priorities.

Standard   3.1   (www.facs.org/publications/newsletters/coc-source/special-source/standard3132)

Patient Navigation Process

A patient navigation process, *driven by a community needs assessment (conducted every 3 years)*, is established to address healthcare disparities and barriers to care for patients. Resources to address identified barriers may be provided either on site or by referral to community-based or national organizations. The navigation process is evaluated, documented, and reported to the cancer committee annually.

The patient navigation process is modified or enhanced each year to address at least one barrier identified by the community needs assessment.

A properly designed needs assessment will highlight risks for cancers and barriers or disparities that interfere with prevention, screening, and care. Prevention and screening needs are identified based on statistics of cancer incidence and mortality and socioeconomic factors. Barriers and disparities encountered by patients and the community can be identified by surveying various data sources. These sources may include surveys and interviews with staff members, social workers, chaplains, physicians, community organization representatives, patient/community focus groups, and other stakeholders. The assessment should consider cancer statistics and incidences in the community and seek to find channels to reach all the relevant audiences. Other sources for review could include state and county cancer data including both state and facility tumor registry data, accreditation reports, and American Cancer Society annual reports. Reviewing data from these sources allows the healthcare team to investigate and validate barriers to treatment.

Examples of data points include:

1. Patient age
2. Race/ethnicity
3. Income
4. Education
5. Insurance status
6. Travel distance to facility
7. Time to first treatment
8. Cancer risk indicators
9. Cancer-specific needs
10. Healthcare barriers and disparities

6.4 Leveraging the Community Needs Assessment into a Community Outreach Program

Once the community needs assessment identifies the specific actual and potential needs of the community, the healthcare organization can align its outreach programs accordingly. For example, does the community have high lung cancer rates? What outreach strategies can be used to increase the use of community-based smoking cessation services and lung cancer screening programs? Who are the various stakeholders and community partners that might be important to address community awareness, transportation services, language translation, service providers, and funding?

6.4.1 Pinpointing Barriers

One important purpose of the community needs assessment is the identification of barriers. Obvious barriers are the financial burdens of care. Other barriers could be language difficulties that inhibit communication or understanding of the diagnosis, transportation issues that disrupt inpatient and/or outpatient care schedules, myths about cancer and its treatment, and many others.

With the barriers identified, the next step in the community outreach agenda is to rally all possible resources that can be engaged to support improvements in care. For example, the community assessment data provide information that could be shared with community and governmental leaders. These conversations might stimulate the development of new city transportation routes to ameliorate transportation barriers, open channels for communications with foundations that could provide financial resources for underserved populations, or open doors to agencies that might assist with language or education issues. The assessment data also will equip and empower the cancer community with a perspective on which issues can be addressed over the short term and which will require more long-term focus. It provides a means of prioritizing solutions.

6.4.2   Translating the Community Needs Assessment in Community Action

The community needs assessment should fuel specific types of community outreach, based on the deficiencies the assessment highlights related to prevention, screening and treatment availability, access, compliance, education, etc. In addition to the data from the community assessment, the involvement of the community in the planning and implementation of these outreach activities and programs will provide additional insights and credibility that can feed the ongoing development of action plans. The formation of a community advisory panel and involvement of community members as educators and navigators are essential to ensure that the activities and programs that are developed by the healthcare organization are culturally appropriate and tailored and address the more complex issues in each community. The involvement of the community is the foundation of community action, which is essential for long-term sustainability.

6.4.3   Planning and Evaluation

Developing an outreach plan with specific activities and resource needs can serve as a guide to implementation and evaluation. This plan can become the road map for your outreach activities. Community outreach can include a wide variety of services, including:

- *Educate and elevate community knowledge of the importance of cancer screening.* Educational programming in the community can be conducted through partnerships with religious, social service, and recreational organizations. These programs can include speakers from the community and should be provided in a variety of languages with a culturally relevant approach
- *Bring cancer screening directly into the community through mobile programs and local partnerships.* Mobile services, including breast, prostate, and cancer screening, can be provided in the community or by setting up screening in

community health centers. Patient navigators are essential to identifying community leaders who might help organize or schedule mobile programs and help promote the importance of follow-up care.

- *Increase access to screening through transportation, low-cost screening option, and assistance with insurance.* Although community members may see the value of cancer screening, they may not have the financial resources or appropriate insurance to cover the cost of screening, diagnostic follow-up, or treatment. Patient navigators can assist community members in accessing free screening and with applications for state/national government-sponsored insurance or financial assistance programs.
- *Promote healthy lifestyle behaviors to reduce cancer risk.* For example, host nutrition seminars to discuss the connection between cancer and diet, or cancer and sedentary lifestyles, at community centers, churches, or other places where adults and families gather. The need for this tactic could be highlighted by needs assessment data.
- *Empower the community by providing reliable, easily accessible, and understandable information.* Educational information needs to be tailored to the community, meaning materials must be easy to read, translated into the dominant area languages, and accessible in print and electronic mediums. Many community outreach programs support the credentialing of community outreach staff as medical translators, and some healthcare organizations provide materials that are specifically designed to reach patient populations with limited literacy skills.

The program plan can also guide the monitoring of the program as well as serve as the foundation for the program evaluation. According to the Institute of Medicine, only by implementing a program to continuously monitor care and outcomes can we properly assess the quality of care that is offered, properly define barriers to high-quality care, and continuously improve care [6]. Building measurement tools into the assessment process and navigation process is crucial.

The community needs assessment might support deeper involvement with other community-focused groups. The particular resource group will vary based on the type of cancer the healthcare organization wishes to target. Women's service organizations, for example, have proved to be valuable resources in building programs that support audiences who may be affected by breast and ovarian cancer.

6.5   The Role of Navigation Across the Continuum of Care

Patient navigators are an essential component of an effective outreach program, like community educators, and have a strong connection to members of the community and a deep understanding and appreciation for the challenges that patients face, particularly those with more limited resources and support. Navigators often live in the community or are well acquainted with the community and can actively seek out individuals who are in need of care. They often encourage community members to attend cancer screening and education events, arrange for transportation, and assist with identifying free or low-cost screening services. For patients in treatment, they commonly work closely with social work to identify and address practical barriers (e.g., transportation, child care) as well as guide patients through their cancer journey. They may connect them to community support groups or adjunct services. And it doesn't stop there. Navigators are critical to cancer survivorship as well.

Effective survivorship programs that reach into the community are connected to key elements of the cancer care continuum.

6.6   Connecting the Survivor Back to the Community

A best practice for reintegration of the survivor into the community would first begin with the delivery of the survivorship care plan to the patient. The survivorship care plan summarizes their cancer treatment experience, including the names and contact information for their healthcare team members; an overview of their cancer treatment(s), such as surgery, radiation, chemotherapy, clinical trials, etc.; as well as future surveillance recommendations and educational information regarding healthy lifestyle guidelines [7]. The patient, patient's primary care physician, and the survivorship navigator should all receive a copy of the document. At Sarah Cannon Institute, in the Medical City Healthcare Division, disease-site navigators transition patients to a survivorship navigation team consisting of a nurse and a social worker [8]. This team reviews the patient's understanding of the survivorship care plan, including self-management practices, for example, instruction regarding ongoing oral therapy.

Additionally, they provide ongoing emotional support and connect the patient to community resources that may be needed. Emotional support is a significant portion of the survivorship navigator's practice. The authors' professional experience indicates a patient can take up to 2 years to deal with the emotional toll of a cancer diagnosis and treatment. Cancer can be socially isolating and emotionally disruptive. Survivorship navigators must be skilled in helping patients overcome these issues in order for the patients to successfully reintegrate with the life they want.

Another key step to connecting the patient back to the community is working to help the survivor access resources that will help the survivor with daily circumstances that may still prove challenging. For example, there are community nonprofits that offer home cleaning services to cancer patients. Survivorship programs must be intentional in forging relationships with community partners that will fill the tangible needs that survivors will encounter. Other examples of needs that can be incorporated into the survivorship navigation program might include support with returning to work, child care so that survivors can attend follow-up appointments, gas cards and bus cards for transportation needs, counseling, and exercise classes. Community organizations offering these benefits exist in many cities, and survivorship navigators must engage these partners to support their patients.

From a medical perspective, the survivorship navigator must also help survivors access ongoing clinical services, such as behavioral health counseling, child life services for the children of survivors, and oncology rehabilitation services to better the survivor's quality of life. Furthermore, it is good practice to invite survivors to community screening events to enhance their awareness of health maintenance and surveillance issues.

To build an effective survivorship navigation program, healthcare administrators can survey patients and support groups to identify felt needs beyond those referenced here and evaluate options in the community to support the survivorship navigation program. Where community support options do not exist, the healthcare provider can champion those opportunities with community leaders.

6.6.1 Survivors and Social Media: Connecting to a Virtual Community

Many cancer survivors find relief and solace in communicating with other survivors. Survivorship navigators can help patients connect with other survivors by making their patients aware of chat groups, blogs, online meeting rooms, and other social medical channels that link survivors. These social medical channels are national and local in scope, and most survivors do not distinguish between local and national online support networks when assessing their emotional value.

6.6.2 Survivors Helping Survivors: Connecting Shared Journeys

Survivors are often eager to help other cancer patients. It has proved to be a useful part of the healing journey for cancer patients. Survivorship navigators must ensure that patients understand the available opportunities to connect survivors with other survivors, as well as other patients undergoing treatment. Events such as the American Cancer Society Relay for Life, Us TOO, Komen Foundation, etc., all provide venues for survivors to help and encourage other survivors. Helping survivors participate in these close-knit communities promotes emotional healing.

6.7 Community Navigation Case Study – Fox Chase Cancer Center Outreach

6.7.1 Overview

Patient navigation at Fox Chase Cancer Center, one of the 45 National Cancer Institute–designated Comprehensive Cancer Centers, spans the continuum from navigation through our outreach and community screening programs to the clinical domain with nurse navigators in almost every service line of the cancer center. This mixed model of community health educators and nurses provides a continuum of care for all of our patients and especially those who are underserved. The patient navigation programs were designed in tandem based on previous experience of the program leaders in patient navigation and current research and best practice approaches. Although funding, goals and metrics, leadership, and organizational reporting are distinct, the two programs are connected through collaborative program leadership. This case study focuses on the development of the community navigation to increase follow-up and the development and piloting of a text messaging reminder intervention to reduce no-show rates for the community-based mobile mammography service.

6.7.2 Community Outreach

The Office of Community Outreach (OCO) at Fox Chase, which is the primary outreach and education arm for the Center oversees the Community Education and Mobile Screening Programs. This office has long-standing relationships within the community with various healthcare and community-based organizations, and has provided cancer education and screening for over 25 years. Like many other healthcare organization's cancer outreach programs, the OCO works collaboratively with multiple departments in the health center and works externally through diverse partner organizations to address key health gaps that have been identified by the community needs assessment. For example, the OCO provides free bilingual cancer education, has secured funding to expand cancer screening to medically underserved communities, develops plain language materials to address low literacy levels, and provides cultural competence training to staff to enhance their ability to work with a diverse patient mix.

Through the speaker's bureau program, OCO outreach staff members have directly reached over 8500 individuals with cancer education materials and 10,000+ people via resource tables at community health fairs and expos. These community engagement efforts enable staff to disseminate evidence-based information that promotes healthy lifestyles and behavioral changes. Without the ongoing support of externally based community organizations, the OCO's success would be limited. Pre- and post-test evaluations show increases in knowledge, changes in attitudes, and an increased likelihood to participate in cancer research among targeted community populations.

6.7.3 Mobile Mammography

The Mobile Mammography Program is jointly managed by Fox Chase's Office of Community Outreach and Radiology Department, which screens close to 4000 women serving a diverse population in the greater Philadelphia area through corporate and community partnerships. To foster the collaboration, a shared database is used to schedule and track all participants. Although all women and their providers were sent the mammogram results, there was not much information if women who had abnormal findings actually received follow-up care, either at Fox Chase or other facilities. A pilot project to conduct a follow-up call to a sample of women who had abnormal findings showed that almost 25% had not sought follow-up care, with women from underserved communities having the highest rates.

6.7.4 Mobile Mammography Navigation Services

Based on this assessment, we developed a pilot program from November 2010 to December 2012 to provide navigation services to underserved women, which included a follow-up telephone call and support to access follow-up care, including assistance with obtaining insurance if needed, transportation, language translation, and general psychosocial support. Almost 100 (N = 95) underserved women with abnormal mammograms were navigated. All had insurance-related barriers and over half (n = 56) have had language barriers. About 1 in 10 had transportation issues, and only three reported fear as a barrier to follow-up. All of these women chose to have their diagnostic follow-up at Fox Chase, and two were diagnosed with cancer. The community navigation often meets the women at the center and introduces them to the nurse navigator to facilitate coordination of services. For example, the navigator could assist in obtaining prior films/results, obtaining a prescription for follow-up services, and scheduling an appointment at Fox Chase. Additionally, the community navigator will ascertain if special needs exist, such as translation services or assistance with transportation to Fox Chase. If so, she or he will work with a network of partners and resources to assure that the individual is able to return to Fox Chase and have a positive experience once here. Unless asked not to, she or he will also meet the individual at Fox Chase to escort them to their scheduled appointment. Should an individual cancel or not show up for an appointment, the community navigator will contact them to offer additional help as needed. The navigator also assists people with insurance issues or concerns. If the person in question is uninsured or has insurance not accepted by Fox Chase, the navigator will try to identify options. These can range from help applying for medical assistance to referral to another facility that does accept the insurance if desired by the individual to working with Patient Financial Services to obtain charity care. Based on this pilot, these navigation services have now become part of routine service of the Mobile Mammography Program.

6.7.5 Mobile Mammography Text Messaging Pilot

With the mobile mammography screening navigation in place, we also were committed to ensuring that all women scheduled for an appointment show up to be screened. Women who do not show up for a scheduled appointment put their own health at risk, deny an available appointment to another woman, and diminish the efficacy of the program. In 2011, the no-show rate was 12% in the corporate setting and 15% in the community setting.

As a quality improvement project (with IRB review and approval), we developed a text messaging reminder pilot with funds from the Verizon Foundation in 2014.

The objectives of this quality improvement project are (1) to decrease the mobile mammography unit no-show rate by sending text message appointment reminders to patients and (2) to assess the efficacy of the text message reminders at addressing the no-show rate by collecting satisfaction survey data from patients that received the texts and that came to their scheduled appointment. The goal is to improve service delivery on the mobile mammography van, with a specific focus on increasing service delivery to medically underserved populations.

Our first step was to verify the use of cell phone use among our clients and also determine the health literacy level for the text messages. We found in surveying a convenience sample of clients (N = 50) who use the service that almost 90% used cell phones, and 83% in the community setting indicated that they sometimes to always need help filling out medical forms. We developed text messages in both English and Spanish and included linguistically salient message-based formative research conducted with our clients. The program included up to three text message appointment reminders during the weeks before scheduled appointments to 200 patients with cell phones, 100 screened at participating community sites and 100 screened at participating corporate sites. At the end of the pilot, we found the overall no-show rate for the community sites as 5.3% and 8.5% for the corporate sites, a drop from the before pilot rates.

Some of the lessons learned from this pilot using text messaging as an additional outreach strategy to support a community mammography program may be of value to others. One of the major challenges we faced was determining how many languages we need for the text messages. Our community had a significant Latino population, and therefore, we considered a Spanish language option. However, these messages need to be translated by a certified medical translation service, which added cost and time. In addition, our contacts at Hispanic clinics told us that their patients will not answer the phone most times if they don't know the number, and text messages are better because they can see it without worry as long as their phone has this capability. Integrating the text messages into an existing scheduling process was another lesson learned. If appointments are scheduled in a computerized system, it would be easier to add text messages to the routine. If you schedule by hand, you will have to text by hand as well. It takes time to copy and paste or type multiple messages multiple times. Finding the appropriate number of text messages to send is very important. Anecdotal feedback from those who participated indicated that "we had the perfect number sent (2 to 3)." We also found out that it was important to space out the text messages and to include relevant information such as the items they needed to bring (e.g., prescription, previous films), so there was time to obtain them and the actual time of the appointment closer to the actual date.

Text message reminders have the potential to increase the number of women screened for breast cancer and improve the efficiency of the program by decreasing no-show rates. The rise of cell phone use, particularly among minority and low-income individuals who have had higher no-show rates in the past, demonstrates a new method for addressing cancer screening disparities. Text message reminders (either in addition to or in place of phone call reminders) may be adopted as standard practice to supplement navigation services for community mammography screening.

Conclusion

Developing collaborative partnerships within the community is key to successful community outreach programs. There will not be enough manpower or material resources available at the healthcare organization level to sustain an effective community outreach effort. The best programs empower navigators to know how to partner with community organizations (schools, churches, social gatherings). Navigators must be creative and innovative as they seek community partners. For example, effective outreach sometimes needs a nontraditional approach, and this may involve partnerships with atypical community groups, such as partnering with a motorcycle club to distribute information on prostate cancer or a local male radio personality providing a testimonial as an opener for a local entertainment venue.

Community outreach focuses on prevention, early detection, and also successfully transitioning cancer patients after completion of their acute treatment back into the community for their long-term survivorship care.

In conclusion, the community needs assessment can and should help shape the navigation process, as well as program development, community outreach strategies, and evaluation across the cancer continuum from prevention to survivorship.

References

1. National Library of Medicine. www.nlm.nih.gov/hsrinfo/community_benefit.html.
2. Association for Community Health Improvement. www.healthycommunities.org.
3. www.chausa.org/communitybenefit/resources/defining-community-benefit.
4. www.uwgc.org/211.
5. https://cancercontrolplanet.cancer.gov.
6. Institute of Medicine. Crossing the quality Chasm. 2001. www.nationalacademies.org/hmd/Reports/2001/Crossing-the-Quality-Chasm-A-New-Health-System-for-the-21st-Century.aspx.
7. Commission on Cancer Program Standards. 2016. www.facs.org/quality-programs/cancer/coc/standards.
8. Boyd J, Narvarte K. Survivorship Navigation. Presentation delivered to Seventh Annual Conference of the Academy of Oncology Nurse & Patient Navigators, Las Vegas, NV, 2016, November.

Diagnosis and Preparing Patients for Their Oncology Consultations

7

Margaret Rummel, Paula Sanborn, and Penny Daugherty

7.1 Introduction

When a patient is diagnosed with cancer, it is an overwhelming experience. There are a multitude of appointments, tests, consults, and treatments that the patient and family experience to achieve the best outcome. This chapter, through case study examples, highlights the role of the oncology nurse navigator (ONN) in helping patients navigate the complex healthcare system and decrease barriers to care. The role of the ONN is multidimensional. They are often the point of contact for the patient and family throughout the cancer continuum. ONNs serve as an advocate for patients and families providing education on their disease, including treatment options, side effect management, and resources. They facilitate multidisciplinary communication, provide support, and help connect patients with community resources.

The objectives of this chapter are the following:

- Demonstrate the role of the ONN in helping patients prepare for their oncology journey and the importance of a multidisciplinary approach to care.
- Identify the barriers that ONNs face when assisting patients throughout the cancer continuum and solutions to overcome those barriers.
- Learn about the challenges and opportunities that ONNs face in navigating oncology in patient's exceptional situations.

M. Rummel, BSN, MHA, OCN, ONN-CG (✉)
Abramson Cancer Center, Philadelphia, PA, USA
e-mail: margaret.rummel@uphs.upenn.edu

P. Sanborn, BSN, CPHON, CPN, ONN-CG
Nationwide Children's Hospital, Columbus, OH, USA
e-mail: Paula.Sanborn@nationwidechildrens.org

P. Daugherty, RN, MS, OCN, ONN-CG
Northside Hospital Cancer Institute, Atlanta, GA, USA
e-mail: penny.daugherty@northside.com

© Springer International Publishing AG, part of Springer Nature 2018
L. D. Shockney (ed.), *Team-Based Oncology Care: The Pivotal Role of Oncology Navigation*, https://doi.org/10.1007/978-3-319-69038-4_7

- Show the value of navigation to the healthcare organization, thereby demonstrating the bidimensional value that navigators bring to the institution as well as the patient.

This chapter consists of three case studies highlighting the role of the ONN in providing multidisciplinary care throughout the cancer continuum.

7.2 Conclusion

Navigation is recognized as a fundamental component of patient-centered care. In 2012, the Commission on Cancer (CoC) recognized the importance of navigation in achieving patient-centered care and requires that all CoC-accredited cancer centers have a navigation process in place for the cancer patients they see and treat. These case studies demonstrate the value of navigation in three different settings. This chapter illustrates the value of navigation both to patients and to the healthcare organization and the important role that navigation plays in the cancer continuum, as well as the contribution to providing patient-centered care.

Case Study 1

An Adventure Out of the Oncology Nurse Navigator Comfort Zone

Penny Daugherty

Objectives

- To illustrate the dynamic role of the oncology nurse navigator (ONN) beginning at diagnosis and enlarging to encompass caregivers, the community, and the hospital system
- To reveal the fragility of all involved in the many nuances of the continuum of the cancer experience
- To include education of the hospital system offering a template for what we as ONNs in all disease sites can achieve
- To provide an introduction into the ambience of a lesbian family as well as the commonalities that we all hold as intimate needs

Introduction
This case study chronicles the experience of a 49-year-old lesbian woman who was diagnosed with triple-negative breast cancer (TNBC). She was in a 30-year committed relationship, which included two teenage children. It highlights the role of the oncology nurse navigator (ONN) whose site-specific specialty was gynecologic

oncology patients but was requested to provide navigation by an administrator at her facility. The ONN is a seasoned (39 years) oncology nurse who had experience with breast cancer patients in her former, longtime role as a research coordinator, so she viewed this request as an opportunity to enlarge her current boundaries. She requested and received support and assistance from the lead breast ONN at the hospital.

Background Situation

Chelsea is a 49-year-old woman who came to the cancer center for her annual screening mammogram as she'd done for the previous 5 years. As an Ashkenazi Jewish woman, she was familiar with the commonly known risk of both ovarian and breast cancer, but she was mildly annoyed at having to take time away from her work as a corporate attorney for a very large Atlanta company. Her life partner of 30 years, Lee, was also of Ashkenazi Jewish descent and had urged her to be a positive role model for their two teenage children.

As she would later relate to the ONN, she came to the breast cancer center for her mammogram irritated at the 30-minute waiting time and was even more exasperated when after the mammogram she was told there were some "suspicious spots" noted and an ultrasound was needed, another absence from her professional life. The ultrasound revealed the same mass, and so the next step was a biopsy, and the results confirmed the presence of cancer.

The ONN called her later the same day as the biopsy results had been shared with her, and Chelsea would later say that all she remembered of that conversation was "I am your nurse navigator and going forward, we will work everything out together. I promise."

The ONN explained to Chelsea that the biopsy identified her cancer as grade 3 invasive ductal carcinoma that was negative for estrogen receptors (ER), progesterone receptors (PgR or PR), and human epidermal growth factor 2 (HER2). Initially, Chelsea was pleased at all the "negative" receptors and asking if this meant less treatment. The ONN tried to give Chelsea a detailed definition of "triple-negative breast cancer (TNBC)" but sensing the anxiety in Chelsea's voice, as well as her inability to repeat information, she asked to set up a face-to-face appointment with someone in her family who could help process the information. Chelsea replied she could bring her partner. The ONN noticed that the patient's face sheet indicated that she identified herself as married and it indicated her *husband's* name was Lee; the ONN asked Chelsea if she was referring to Lee, and Chelsea replied affirmatively. The ONN agreed to a time the following morning and Chelsea introduced Lee (who was a woman) as her husband. To get some background and to understand the sudden structure change to their relationship, the ONN asked them both to share a little about their life. They jointly talked about having been together since college and in the past 2 years had formalized their marriage in Florida (where it was a legal activity). They talked about wanting to have a family after they'd both completed college and how they had chosen a friend as a sperm donor, planning to eventually have two children and, in fact, had twins, a boy and a girl, presently 16 years old.

The ONN went on to re-verbalize the definition of TNBC and also the rationale for testing for breast cancer susceptibility gene (BRCA) germline mutations as well as utilizing next-generation sequencing (NGS), also known as massively paralleled sequencing, which has enabled a detailed characterization of the molecular under-pinnings of breast cancer, which has identified recurrent gene mutations or copy number aberrations (CNAs) among the different subtypes, and some of them are currently followed as potential therapeutic targets [1]. She gave them further details about treatment sequencing, explaining that given a choice of potential treatments for Chelsea, neoadjuvant (prior to surgery) chemotherapy might be selected [2]. She also briefly mentioned the importance of genetic testing and counseling but shared with her that due to the absence of individual BRCA mutations in her family, there was the possibility of false negatives and false positives [2]. This would be followed up later, but the ONN was cognizant of the stress-induced shortened attention span that both Chelsea and Lee were exhibiting as they repeatedly asked the ONN to repeat her words.

The ONN went on to explain that she would be making appointments with the breast surgeon and also a reconstructive plastic surgeon the same day. She also arranged an appointment with a medical oncologist who specialized in breast can-cer. The hospital, as an accredited National Cancer Institute Community Oncology Research Program (NCORP) facility, is a Commission on Cancer (CoC)-accredited breast cancer treatment center, so all services were available on the main campus, with the goal of offering comprehensive care to all patients with cancer, including imaging, diagnostics, radiation, surgery, state-of-the-art clinical trials, and chemo-therapy. The ONN also suggested that both Lee and Chelsea seek out the integrative modalities offered at the Cancer Support Community (CSC) such as meditation, Reiki, tai chi, and yoga—all of which would serve to ease stress and promote relaxation.

The ONN observed that Lee and Chelsea held each other's hands very tightly during this conversation, and she reached over and lightly covered both their hands with hers and told them, "We will do this together and I will be with you every step of the way." Chelsea and Lee would later say that they mutually embraced this con-versation and felt that their ONN was "going to guide us safely to the other side of this terrifying experience for our whole family."

The ONN went to all appointments with Chelsea and Lee and sat with them after each appointment to answer any questions that came up. She gave them a hospital-provided binder that included information about all available services as well as a weekly diary for patients/caregivers to take notes. The ONN would review their notes with them each week in the infusion suite, and they were instructed to call her as needed with any questions and/or concerns. The ONN also suggested to Lee that she keep a journal as well since she was supporting Chelsea and needed the support of her own thoughts [3].

It was decided that dose-dense doxorubicin coupled with cyclophosphamide fol-lowed by weekly paclitaxel and followed by surgery would be the course of treat-ment for Chelsea. This would be tailored around Chelsea's work schedule and Lee, who had her own business, would be the designated driver to chemotherapy ses-sions. The ONN provided both verbal and written information regarding the possible side effects of this chemotherapy regimen such as nausea and vomiting, lowering of blood counts (and the resultant possibility of infection), neuropathy, and alopecia, and advised them both to maintain close contact with her to assist in dealing with side effects. She also set up Chelsea with the hospital's American Cancer Society navigator to proactively plan for a wig, as Chelsea had expressed concern about meeting with clients after losing her hair.

The ONN discussed the children's emotional needs and suggested a program at the local Cancer Support Community (CSC) as well as a very active breast cancer support group, also at the CSC. Chelsea and Lee took the contact information to follow up with, and the ONN also reached out to the CSC program coordinators and gave them a synopsis of Chelsea and Lee and their family. The CSC Executive Program Director was a lesbian, in a similar relationship, and as a licensed clinical social worker (LCSW) a mental healthcare professional who provides psychological counseling, as well as many of the practical aspects generally related to social workers. She offered to meet with and counsel Chelsea and Lee. The ONN mentioned this to Chelsea who was very interested in going forward, so a contact was initiated. At first Lee was very resistant to "exposing her personal life" to a stranger, but the ONN spoke with the CSC Executive Program Director who endorsed and encouraged the ONN to share her lifestyle commonalities with Lee as a means of encouragement, which she did. After knowing this, Lee expressed that she was "much more comfortable" with the meeting and felt it was beneficial to their relationship and also for their children, since she expressed that they were all experiencing a great deal of stress and fear. The ONN felt that this was a positive step at emotional pre-habilitation for this family [4].

After several meetings with the CSC Executive Program Director, the ONN asked both Chelsea and Lee for their feedback, and they both verbalized that this was a positive experience for their family and had reduced some of the stress in their personal relationship.

The ONN began to attend the weekly Breast Multidisciplinary Conference to enhance her current knowledge of breast cancer treatment as well as demonstrate to the breast cancer physicians that she was functionally involved in the navigation needs of Chelsea and her family.

When the ONN visited Chelsea and Lee at the infusion suite during treatment, some of the nurses expressed to her that they were unsure how to dialog with same-sex couples, especially regarding questions related to intimacy. The ONN appealed to the Operations Director of Oncology and offered to do a PowerPoint presentation to all the nurses on intimacy, and he agreed. The ONN queried all patients who were in same-sex relationships to get their feedback about issues they felt were important, neglected, and/or ignored. She also reached out to the lesbian, gay, bisexual, transgender, and queer or questioning (LGBTQ) community, soliciting their feedback about their unmet needs, and was astounded at the expressed gratitude that this education would be provided to nurses.

When the PowerPoint was completed, he provided an opportunity for the ONN to present this education to all the oncology nurses, which she did, complete with handouts including extensive references, positioning diagrams, demonstrations of sexual devices, various emollients, and a list of certified sex therapists in the metropolitan area. This list was compiled with the assistance of Ann Katz, PhD, author of many of invaluable sexuality books [5, 6].

The ONN also benefited from the work of Mandi Pratt-Chapman, MA, Director of The George Washington University (GW) Cancer Institute, and her extensive education regarding the needs of the LGBTQ community [7].

Many of the nurses provided feedback that this had been enlightening and demystifying enough to them that they felt that they could begin a therapeutic channel of communication with their patients. They would later report newly successful conversations they'd been able to have with patients.

That initial in-service became an integral component in the education of all new nurses in an extensive internship provided by the hospital, and feedback has been overwhelmingly positive to this inclusion.

This education related to the needs of the LGBTQ community has also become an inclusive and mandatory component of the core competencies for navigators at the hospital, including the viewing of selected presentations from AONN+ as well as National ONS Congress podium sessions [8, 9].

The ONN was asked by Chelsea how she could regain some sense of control and purpose to her life as she went through treatment. She inquired about diet and lifestyle changes in terms of exercise. The ONN gave Chelsea information about the special diet for TNBC, which was researched extensively by several medical oncologists working with breast cancer, most notably Dr. Ruth O'Reagan at the University of Wisconsin [10]. The ONN gave Chelsea the names of Dr. O'Reagan and Dr. Vince Cryns to research since she had noted that Chelsea expressed eagerness to participate in her care by researching and understanding the details of each facet of care. Chelsea told the ONN that thoroughly researching everything was her "M.O. after years of law school."

Chelsea researched the low methionine diet and reported to the ONN that she was going to begin a new diet strategy based upon her newly found knowledge that there is evidence that cancer cells grow less robustly and sometimes undergo cell death (known as apoptosis) when deprived of methionine, which is an essential amino acid.

The ONN connected Chelsea and Lee with the hospital-certified oncology dietitian, and they worked out a viable, nutritionally sound diet that was plant-based, eliminated red meat and was also instrumental in helping Chelsea lose the 15 lbs she had gained during her chemotherapy treatments.

Chelsea had also researched the positive connection between exercise and fighting cancer, and the ONN gave her some scientific articles that supported this, which encouraged Chelsea to join the hospital-sponsored gym on campus, and she began a committed regimen of aerobic and cardio exercise, which she did 5–6 days a week, exercising an hour a day. She told the ONN that in the beginning it was very hard to make this commitment, but Lee and her two teenage children joined her in the rigorous routine, and it had measurably lessened the stress they had all been experiencing. Chelsea also said she felt a sense of control over her life and also a sense of purpose that she felt had been "slipping away" since the beginning—with the diagnosis, the treatment, and the fatigue she experienced—which for her had been very frightening because she considered herself a high-energy person prior to her diagnosis [11].

At this point, Chelsea is in remission. She is aware of the high possibility of recurrence with TNBC, but she has embraced her "new and improved" lifestyle, and she and Lee regularly attend the TNBC support group at the CSC, as well as participating in the integrative modalities offered there, Reiki and meditation, and her children have also invested themselves in these activities.

Challenges

Not all stories have a happy ending, and most stories are told when there is an ending, recurrence, metastasis, or death. This is a dynamic story—as all our stories are, and the learning experience for this ONN was to work within each moment each individual need and, when faced with a deficit in staff knowledge and understanding about the discreet needs of individuals in the LGBTQ community, to provide empathetic education to practitioners so that they might enlarge their scope of awareness in order to provide the most efficacious care to all who depend on us to guide them through each treatment and help diminish the stress to them and to their loved ones.

Opportunities

As navigators, we have a myriad of opportunities to educate and guide our patients and those who love and care for them through their cancer experience, actualization, and treatment. As we "connect the dots" for patients, we have a valuable potential role in navigating our colleagues through education—to expand their boundaries of empathy and successful care for multicultural families. When a need is identified, whether it be patient-centric or staff deficit, the potential is ever present for us to be leaders in education in our multidisciplinary team.

Implications for Stakeholders

We are all stakeholders as we interact with each other and know that we each are interchangeable, given an emergent and unexpected set of circumstances, so we, as navigators, have the privilege as well as the responsibility to visualize and implement every moment of our lives as a best practice to take to and share with each other. This is the commitment we embrace when we humbly and proudly identify ourselves as navigators, and so we must intrinsically seek opportunities to be the mainstay of education wherever it is needed so that all are served in the circle of care, empathy, and compassion.

Case Study 2

Pediatric Osteosarcoma Patient

Paula Sanborn

Objectives

- To highlight the important role of the oncology nurse navigator (ONN) in pediatric cancer care
- To understand the challenges of navigating a pediatric patient through the cancer continuum
- To describe the new pediatric osteosarcoma intake process and referral bundle to multidisciplinary team specialties to improve patient outcomes and quality of life

Introduction

This case study narrates the story of an 8-year-old girl presenting with osteosarcoma. Piper will be cared for at a designated comprehensive cancer center by the National Institutes of Health (NIH) and a member institution of the Children's Oncology Group (COG) where she will be treated by the sarcoma team, which includes a pediatric sarcoma specialist (pediatric oncologist), a pediatric sarcoma advanced practice nurse, the sarcoma nurse navigator, a social worker, a pediatric surgical oncologist, and a pediatric orthopedic oncologist.

Background

Piper had a history of 3 months of right leg pain and achiness with slight knee swelling that went away with cold therapy. Piper had visited her pediatrician for the complaint of pain three times over the past 3 months, and her mom was instructed to give her ibuprofen at night for a diagnosis of growing pains. Piper injured her leg in a soccer game that initiated increased right knee swelling and pain that awakened her at 3:00 am. Piper's mom noted increased swelling of the right thigh and immediately took her to a small tertiary hospital close to their home. An x-ray of her right femur and right knee was obtained and revealed an aggressive heterogeneous sclerotic and lucent lesion with moth-like appearance, measuring 10 cm within the right distal femoral diaphysis and metaphysis. The emergency physician contacted the children's hospital Physician Consult Transfer Center (PCTC) that is available 24 hours a day for consulting services, and was connected with the oncologist on call. The oncologist on call instructed the physician to discharge Piper if her pain was well controlled and instructed them to not allow her to ambulate until she is evaluated by an orthopedic surgeon, and they would be contacted in the morning with a follow-up plan to see an orthopedic surgeon. The oncologist on call contacted the ONN via email with patient information and x-ray reports. The ONN obtained patient information through Piper's electronic health record (EHR), obtained the images of the femur and knee x-rays, and reviewed them with the orthopedic oncology surgeon and pediatric sarcoma oncologist. An MRI of the right femur and a CT of the chest are ordered, and an appointment with the orthopedic oncology surgeon is scheduled for the next morning following NCCN guidelines for staging of the osteosarcoma patient [12].

The sarcoma ONN contacts the family, introduces herself, explains her role as their partner in their upcoming journey and that she will meet them in the radiology department prior to Piper's tests, and gives the family her contact information to call with questions or concerns. She explains the MRI and chest CT and their implications and gives them directions to the radiology department and the orthopedic oncology surgeon's office. The ONN does an initial screen for transportation needs and notes the family does not have any at this time. Part of the intake process for the ONN is getting to know the family up front and making a connection to help guide them through the most difficult time in their lives when their child is diagnosed with cancer. During their conversations, Piper's mom is tearful and states they are all very scared, and that they have two other children to whom they don't even know where to begin to explain to them about Piper's condition. The ONN reviewed with mom that the hospital has a psychosocial team that will help them tell the siblings and Piper about her cancer in a developmentally appropriate way. Mom reports she is worried they have no insurance, she was recently laid off from her job, and she and dad have recently separated. Piper, mom, and her siblings have recently moved to a small apartment about 2 hours from the hospital, and dad has recently moved in with a new girlfriend. Childhood cancer is a family disease. It significantly affects the lives of the parents, their siblings, and the community [13]. The ONN lets mom know that we have a team of financial counselors and a social worker that will help with obtaining healthcare coverage for Piper. The ONN acts as a new resource for the patient and family. During their conversation on the phone, she listens, debriefs, offers support, and provides information until their first appointment with the orthopedic oncology surgeon and the pediatric oncologist [14].

The next morning, the pediatric ONN meets Piper and her parents in the radiology waiting room. Piper is tearful and holding on to her favorite blanket. The ONN greets Piper with a hug and sits on the floor next to her chair and asks her about her favorite blanket. Piper states that her grandmother had made her the blanket when she was a baby, but her grandma was gone now because she had died with cancer in her lungs. The ONN helps Piper and her parents go back to have her chest CT completed, where mom and dad were visible during the testing and could calm and talk Piper through the procedure. When Piper arrived to MRI, she was greeted by a child life specialist who asked Piper to color at a small table with other children while she waited. Piper handed over her blanket to her mom and sat with the child life specialist.

The child life specialist then went back to MRI with Piper and helped her pick out a favorite movie she could watch while her MRI was completed, explaining everything to Piper as they prepared her for the MRI. The child life specialist stayed in the MRI environment with Piper to talk with her and keep her calm. Piper's mom and dad were also able to talk with Piper throughout the MRI to help keep her still during the exam. Child life staff members are certified professionals who are prepared at the bachelor's and master's level in child life, child development, and other related fields. The child life specialists are a part of the healthcare team, and they contribute to minimizing fears and stresses experienced by children, adolescents, and families as related to healthcare experiences. They support the patient's emotional, social, and cognitive growth in the context of his or her family, culture, or developmental age. They provide age-appropriate and safe play environments, recreational events, and activities that help to enhance a patient's understanding of medical procedures and diagnosis using age-appropriate techniques [13].

The ONN meets the family at their appointment with the orthopedic oncology surgeon and the pediatric oncologist. The MRI is reviewed with the family, and the orthopedic oncologist discusses possibilities of cancer, including the diagnosis of osteosarcoma versus Ewing sarcoma due to the nature of the aggressive lesion seen on the MRI. A PET scan to complete the staging workup following NCCN guidelines is scheduled for the next morning prior to a biopsy of the tumor [12, 14]. The family requested to go home for the night and return instead of being admitted, so they can call extended family. The orthopedic oncology team arranges for the biopsy, and the ONN contacts the family with instructions and directions. The ONN contacts the research team with the possible new diagnosis of Ewing sarcoma or osteosarcoma for possible clinical trial options for Piper. The biopsy of a possible malignant bone sarcoma is the final most important planning procedure prior to initiation of treatment [14]. Piper's biopsy confirms her diagnosis of high-grade osteosarcoma. The ONN meets with the family in the surgery waiting consultation room with the orthopedic surgeon and the pediatric oncologist to relay the diagnosis of cancer to Piper's mom and dad.

The oncologist reviews with Piper's parents that her chest CT was negative for lung disease, and her PET CT scan only showed activity in her right leg; therefore Piper's disease is considered localized. The pediatric oncologist explains osteosarcoma to Piper's parents and discusses with them that pediatric bone tumors are rare but are the most common neoplasm in children with the most common of these bone tumors being osteosarcoma, with approximately 400 patients identified each year.

Bone cancers represent 5% of all cancers in children 5–9 years old, 11% in children 10–14 years old, and 8% in children 15–19 years old, and that osteosarcoma most commonly occurs in the long bones of the lower limbs [14]. Piper's mom tells the oncologist that her mother and sister have both died of cancer. Her mom died of lung cancer last year and her sister of breast cancer when she was 30. Mom expresses concern that it may be hereditary. The oncologist explains that in rare cases, osteosarcoma may be associated with predisposition syndromes such as Li-Fraumeni syndrome (p53 tumor suppressor germline mutation), Rothmund-Thomson syndrome (RECQL4 gene mutation), radiation exposure, hereditary retinoblastoma (mutation in the RB1 gene), osteochondroma, fibrous dysplasia, chronic osteomyelitis, Werner syndrome (loss of function mutation in WRN gene resulting in premature aging), and Bloom syndrome [14, 15]. The oncologist explains to Piper's parents that a genetic workup by a geneticist will be completed to include a cancer-focused patient and family history.

The pediatric oncologist goes on to explain the standard therapy to treat Piper's osteosarcoma combines chemotherapy and surgery that consists of a limb-sparing surgery or amputation. She goes on to explain the role of chemotherapy in stopping the cancer cells that may be proliferating systemically in Piper's body and the need to stop these cancer cells from continuing to divide out of control and spread to other parts of her body. The chemotherapy includes up-front intensive treatments including cisplatin, doxorubicin, and methotrexate for 10 weeks. This will hopefully provide preoperative shrinkage and consolidation of the primary tumor, and facilitates the resection of the tumor and limb-sparing procedure [14]. After recovery from surgery (usually 2 weeks), chemotherapy with cisplatin, doxorubicin, and methotrexate is continued for another 18 weeks and that treatment should begin within the next few days. She explains that clinical studies have shown that patients need to have both tumor resection and chemotherapy to have good outcomes [14]. Piper will need a few more tests prior to starting her chemotherapy and will have a port placed to receive her chemotherapy.

After the oncologist and surgeon leave, the ONN sits with Piper's mom and dad. Piper's mom is distraught and states she feels "numb." The physical and emotional care information that the family receives at the initial appointments can become very overwhelming. It's the role of the ONN to assess absorption of information given at this initial appointment and continually update and reteach families about their child's disease and treatment options [14]. The ONN discusses the chemotherapy Piper will receive and the plan for Piper to get a port placed. The ONN has brought two teaching notebooks and reviews with mom and dad what a port looks like and how it's accessed [16].

She explains the side effects of doxorubicin and the possible short-term or long-term effects of cardiomyopathy, and that Piper will need a baseline EKG and echocardiogram prior to her first dose, and then she will be monitored throughout her treatment regimen for any changes in her heart function [17]. The ONN also explains the chemotherapy drug cisplatin, and that it can cause changes in Piper's hearing and that she will need a baseline audiogram prior to receiving her first dose, and will have subsequent retesting throughout therapy to evaluate for hearing loss [18]. The ONN lets Piper's parents know that she will arrange for her audiogram, EKG and echocardiogram, and admission for a port placement and initiation of chemotherapy.

As the pediatric ONN goes back to the surgery recovery area with mom and dad, Piper is awake and crying. She asks her mom and dad immediately upon approaching if she is going to die. Developmentally, she understands the word cancer as death because it is associated with the loss of her grandma and aunt. The ONN and Piper's parents explain to her that her cancer is different and there are medications she can receive to help kill the cancer. School-age children are capable of conceptual thinking in combination with concrete images. Through memory, they can navigate information about self, the problem, and an end goal. Before the age of formal operations, children at Piper's age are not capable of abstract thought [13]. Because most of the information about cancer and its treatment are abstract and foreign to children, the pediatric ONN must give explanations that are related to their world of experience and in simple concrete terms [13]. Discussing the chemotherapy as the medicine to make the cancer go away is concrete and to the point for Piper.

When Piper returns for port placement and admission for chemotherapy, the ONN contacts the oncology child life specialist and asks her to go to the preop area to see Piper and show her what a port looks like with "chemo duck." Chemo duck is a stuffed animal that has a port along with a dressing and tubing that can be flushed. Chemo duck has a book that talks about why he needs his port and how it gets accessed for his chemotherapy. Upon arrival to the preop area, Piper's mom states that she told Piper her hair would fall out and she was concerned about what that would look like. The oncology child life specialist quickly ran back to her office and returned with Ella, a friend of Barbie who is fighting cancer, is bald, and has a few different wigs from which to choose. Piper is excited to open the box and immediately talks about which color wig Ella will wear. Play enhances the educational opportunities for children of all ages [19].

After arrival to the floor, the pediatric ONN meets with Piper and her parents, answering questions or concerns prior to her chemotherapy initiation. The ONN strives to initiate family-centered care regardless of Piper's parents being divorced. She gives them both teaching notebooks and materials, and ensures that they both receive the information. The foundation of family-centered care is the understanding that the family is the true expert in the care of their child and the primary source of strength and support [20].

The pediatric ONN ensures consults are sent through the "new patient bundle," which includes a fertility consult (to be completed prior to chemotherapy initiation), social work, psychology, palliative care team, recreation therapy specialist, child life specialist, art therapy, music therapy, massage therapy, pastoral care, genetics, and the school liaison.

The social worker evaluates for financial barriers and helps Piper's parents apply for healthcare assistance and community resources. She helps mom and dad problem solve childcare as a team due to their recent divorce. Security was called in the surgery holding area when dad's new girlfriend showed up. Guidelines for visitation were discussed and documented for dad's girlfriend. The pediatric ONN and social worker collaborated with mom and dad to discuss boundaries of the girlfriend's visitation to limit additional stress to Piper and the rest of the family.

Piper and her family met with the pediatric psychologist to assess for emotional functioning individually and as a family unit. Piper expressed concerns about the fighting and not wanting her parents to fight more since she was sick. Piper felt it was her fault that her parents were fighting. Piper practiced biofeedback to help her learn to calm herself when she felt anxious or upset about her parents or her cancer. The psychologist also met with Piper's parents and her siblings to help in their adjustment of their new journey into the world of pediatric cancer. Piper's siblings are both afraid that Piper is going to die. The ONN engages them in helping to hold Piper's hand during access or counting during the cleaning of her hub prior to medications [21]. By engaging them in Piper's care, they find a way to cope and help their sister.

Piper's mom is also worried about Piper not being able to attend school. The ONN assures mom that a consult was initiated to the STAR program. The STAR program has a schoolteacher on the oncology floor to help patients stay on top of their schoolwork. The school liaison meets with mom and Piper and explains that she will communicate all information to Piper's school and work on getting her a tutor. The ONN encourages mom to contact the school to find out if her teacher will allow Piper to Skype into the classroom weekly to stay connected to her peers. The school liaison will also arrange to visit Piper's school and explain to the children in Piper's classroom that Piper has cancer, and she will leave a bear and backpack on Piper's chair in the classroom while she is absent and going through treatment.

On the second day of Piper's admission, the ONN found Piper in the playroom, playing games with other pediatric cancer patients and the recreation therapist.

Piper is engaged and laughing. She reports she was feeling a "little yucky" this morning, but she didn't want to miss play group. Piper has experienced art therapy where she said she got to "hang out" with Mary, the art therapist. During her art therapy session with the art therapist, Piper not only created an art project, but she ended up expressing her fears and concerns about being made fun of when she loses her hair [19]. Piper also enjoys music therapy when she gets to learn to play the drums or guitar. She verbalized it makes her laugh when her dad covers his ears, and that making loud music is fun. Music and art therapy are effective in promoting socialization by increasing interaction, verbalization, independence, and cooperation. It can enhance the patient's relationship with hospital staff in developing a sense of trust and decrease isolation during the hospital stay [22, 23]. To help control Piper's nausea and vomiting, massage therapy has been consulted. Massage therapy helps control chemotherapy-induced nausea and vomiting [24]. It also helps patients relax. The ONN also gives Piper's mom and dad a tour of the parent resource center where they can go to relax, exercise, get a haircut, and even get a free massage twice a week.

The sarcoma team collaborates with the palliative care physician and a physical therapist who meets the osteosarcoma patients at initial diagnosis to start preparing them for their upcoming surgeries, while the palliative care physician works with the oncology team to manage Piper's side effects [25, 26]. These members of the team will stay with the patient from diagnosis through their surgical intervention and after therapy to help them regain their precancer state.

Palliative care helps prepare the patient for their upcoming limb-sparing surgery or amputation by prescribing gabapentin 2–3 weeks prior to their surgery and then escalates doses during the acute phase [25]. Piper's mom had also requested a referral to integrative medicine to review other therapies they could use. The pediatric institution does not have an integrative medicine practice, and when the ONN contacted the collaborating adult hospital, they would not take Piper as a patient due to her age. The ONN contacted the palliative care physician and nutritionist to see mom jointly to discuss aspects of nutrition and other modalities of care. The physical therapist works with the patient and family, regaining strength and as much functionality as possible prior to surgery. The same physical therapist sees them the day after their surgery to start working on rehabilitation with a goal to achieve their highest functional status to permit them to return to their role in society and hence enjoy dignity and improved quality of life [26].

Piper and her family have a lot of questions about the limb-sparing surgery, including limb salvage, rotationplasty, and amputation. With the consent of Piper and her family, the ONN arranges for patients and their parents who were treated for osteosarcoma and had a limb salvage, rotationplasty, or amputation to meet Piper and her family. After meeting these three families, Piper decided she wanted to have the rotationplasty surgical procedure. This procedure involves resection of the lesion in accordance with good cancer surgery guidelines, and then a rotationplasty of the Van Nes type is performed. The ankle then functions as a knee joint, and the final result is a below-knee amputation rather than a high above-knee amputation with functional results [27]. After Piper decides on the rotationplasty surgery, the ONN arranges for her to meet another 10-year-old osteosarcoma survivor who has the rotationplasty and is very active and plays basketball and softball.

During Piper's first hospital stay, her bedside nurse contacted the ONN to let her know that Piper was refusing to take her oral medications. Mom also reported she had never really had to take pills prior to her diagnosis, so she was not surprised. The ONN contacts the child life specialist and requests they work on pill swallowing with Piper during her admission. The child life specialist has a "Mario" game of pill swallowing where the candy pills are of varying sizes, and at each level, Piper gets a prize. Prior to discharge Piper was at level 3 of the 5 levels, and was very excited for her next return to the hospital to work on getting to level 5 of the pill swallowing game.

The ONN met with both mom and dad and completed discharge education including signs and symptoms of anemia, neutropenia, and thrombocytopenia; who and when to call with questions, concerns, or fevers greater than 100.5 around the clock; mouth care regimen; tips for controlling nausea or vomiting; and treatment for constipation. The ONN also reviewed the treatment calendar and upcoming schema. The ONN picked up the prescriptions from the pharmacy and had the parents write both the generic and brand name on the medication bottles; then she reviewed each medication's dosage, purpose, schedule, and side effects. She had both parents repeat back the medication list. Lastly, the ONN had both parents practice taking Piper's temperature with a Tempa•Dot. Parents of newly diagnosed pediatric cancer patients require specialized education in order to care for their child with a newly diagnosed cancer [28]. *The Children's Oncology Group Family Handbook for Children with Cancer* is utilized as the teaching guide for newly diagnosed pediatric cancer patients [16]. It is essential that families understand the basics of their child's disease, what to expect from their chemotherapy and biotherapy, how to recognize adverse side effects, what is considered an emergency, and how to seek help [14].

Upon discharge, the ONN takes Piper and her family to the outpatient Hematology/Oncology Clinic and the Outpatient Hematology/Oncology Infusion Center for a tour. The ONN reviews what to expect during her next clinic visit and chemotherapy admission. Piper becomes anxious and begins to cry when discussing having her port accessed. The ONN takes Piper to the treatment room and allows her to place lidocaine cream on both her "chemo duck" and Ella, Barbie's friend with cancer. Prior to Piper's first return to the clinic, the ONN contacts the child life specialist and Piper's psychologist and lets them know when Piper is coming, so they can be present to help support and distract Piper during her first port access. The ONN communicates patient information through all team members to provide seamless care for the patient and family. This enhanced communication among healthcare providers builds relationships within the team and directly enhances the patient experience [14].

At Piper's first clinic visit to have a physical exam and labs drawn, the ONN reviewed Piper's lab results with mom and dad, including how to calculate the absolute neutrophil count (ANC). She discussed the possibility of needing blood or platelet transfusions between her chemotherapy admissions. Piper's mom verbalized to the ONN that she is concerned about the distance they will be driving, but she does not want to have Piper treated anywhere else. The ONN discusses the possibility of mom taking Piper to an outside cancer clinic in their area for transfusions only. The ONN collaborates with a local outpatient clinic and arranges for orders for transfusion to be sent to the clinic. When Piper required blood or platelet transfusions, she was able to stay closer to home and not travel 2 hours to the pediatric institution. The social worker also provided transportation resources, including gas cards and mileage reimbursement to the family.

Challenges

This case study presented many challenges for the pediatric ONN. The pediatric patient can be difficult to navigate due to their developmental stage and their inability to understand information and treatments. Fear of the unknown can lead to anxiety and ultimately poor outcomes. The family's marital discord was a challenge in trying to keep communication open and effective when caring for Piper. The distance to the pediatric center was over 2 hours and posed a problem for the family in an emergency or when she required weekly transfusions. Not having an integrative medicine practice within the pediatric hospital and the adult hospital not willing to see Piper due to her age were a challenge in meeting the family's request for integrated care. Keeping communication effective with the orthopedic oncology team in preparing Piper and her family for upcoming surgery and keeping their team upto-date in her progress with chemotherapy can be challenging.

Opportunities

Piper and her family presented many opportunities for the pediatric ONN. Utilizing the entire psychosocial support team to help Piper and her family adjust to treatments, port access, taking oral medications, dealing with chemotherapy-induced nausea outside the realm of medication, and utilizing the wonderful world of play, art, and music helped Piper adjust to her cancer diagnosis. Collaborating with the palliative care physician and nutritionist to jointly see Piper's mom to discuss integrative medicine avenues when there was no integrative medicine available was a benchmark event for the ONN. Finding an adult oncology infusion center that was willing to administer Piper's transfusions as needed was a huge undertaking and collaborative approach to helping overcome the difficulty of the long drive to the pediatric center. The ONN invites the orthopedic oncology surgeon and his staff to all weekly sarcoma team meetings and sarcoma tumor boards, and she attends the Orthopedic Oncology Clinic when sarcoma patients are being seen to improve communication between the teams. The physical therapist and the palliative care physician also attend this clinic to create a multidisciplinary clinic for the patient and family.

Implications for Stakeholders

As oncology nurse navigators in the pediatric or adult cancer journey, we are all given the opportunity to make a difference in both the patient and their family's lives. In our day-to-day interactions, we have the best opportunities to include dignity, respect, collaboration, and information sharing. The value of our position is that we are committed to making the cancer journey for our patients and families a journey filled with purposeful intentions and a patient experience that is filled with our full attention and engagement. We are the "git 'er done" people in our workplace, and we own it. Patients and families value our coordination in care and truly getting to know the patient that in downstream revenue, we are able to triage and manage patients effectively and efficiently and decrease ED visits and missed appointments. "It takes a village" is a great alternative expression for the ONN role. We are not number one. We are just "the one" within a community of the multidisciplinary team who collaborates, communicates, and advocates for our patients tirelessly to make their journey as personal and patient centered as possible.

Case Study 3

When the Patient Is Your Friend

Margaret Rummel

Objectives

- To highlight the important role of oncology nurse navigators (ONNs) in the care of patients with colon cancer
- To understand the challenges ONNs face when navigating patients between an academic cancer center and local oncology providers
- To describe the boundaries that ONNs must keep when navigating patients who are friends

Introduction

This case study is the story of a 74-year-old male with newly diagnosed colon cancer who received treatment at two local cancer centers as well as an academic medical center (AMC). It will focus on the challenges faced with being treated at three institutions and the importance the ONN played in his care. The patient was a close friend of the ONN, which posed challenges when the ONN was asked to give advice as a friend and outside her scope of practice.

Background

AV presented to his local physician with bowel changes. He described narrow malodorous stools and occasional blood in his stool for the past few weeks. He stated he had noticed the bowel changes over the past 6 months. He had no other symptoms such as weight loss or fatigue. He put off going to the physician as he was helping to care for an elderly parent and just did not put it high on his priority list. His last colonoscopy was 11 years ago and showed diverticulosis. AV is a very healthy and active gentleman with an excellent performance status. Family history includes a brother with leukemia in a complete remission and his 98-year-old father with a history of skin cancer. His mother died in her 80s of an unknown cancer. There is no family history of colon cancer or polyps. Past medical history includes rotator cuff repair, hernia repair, diverticulosis, and melanoma in situ removed from his abdomen in 2015. AV is married with a wife and two children. He owns a videography business.

He was worked up locally and his colonoscopy showed a mass at the rectosigmoid junction. The biopsy showed adenocarcinoma. It was at this point that AV reached out to his friend who is an ONN at a large AMC to help obtain a second opinion. The ONN knew that this would be a challenging case as AV and his family had been friends for over 30 years and were like family. The ONN offered to connect AV with the GI navigator who would be better suited to meet his needs, but he was adamant that he only wanted his friend to help him. The ONN knew this would be difficult, and she would rely on her GI colleagues for direction since she rarely navigated GI cancers.

The ONN spoke with AV and obtained a history and asked that he send his records for review. AV's goal was to be seen by a multidisciplinary team to discuss all his treatment options, including clinical trials. He had many questions regarding his diagnosis. His ONN provided education about adenocarcinoma and explained that adenocarcinoma is a cancer that develops in the lining of the colon or rectum. It starts in the cells that form glands making mucus to lubricate the inside of the colon and rectum. This is the most common type of colon and rectum cancer [29]. AV seemed satisfied with this answer, and his ONN told him she would provide more information when she met with him.

The ONN arranged for a multidisciplinary consult with GI surgery, medical oncology, and radiation oncology all in the same day. AV lives over 2 hours away and it was important to have all appointments on the same day, so he could make an informed decision about his treatment.

The ONN met AV and his family and went with him to his consults at his request. He had a sigmoidoscopy at his GI surgery consult, and the pathophysiology of his disease was discussed. He needed additional testing for staging to determine if his disease had spread locally or was systemic. An MRI and CT scan of the abdomen and pelvis was ordered as well as lab work. The physician explained that if the tumor was locally advanced, then the standard of care was neoadjuvant chemoradiation prior to surgery. If the disease was metastatic, then the treatment would be chemotherapy. There was also a possibility that if the tumor was in a specific location above the peritoneal reflection, then it would be treated as colon cancer and surgically resected prior to other treatments. At his consult he asked about a genetic predisposition for his colon cancer. The physician and ONN explained that based on his history, there was no indication that his cancer was hereditary and that he did not need genetic testing.

His ONN reinforced the above plan of care and provided additional education regarding his testing. The ONN scheduled his tests and reviewed the schedule and test preparation with AV. The tests would be done at the AMC, as the multidisciplinary team felt it was better to have all his initial testing done at one facility with experts in all areas that just focus on GI cancers. AV was in agreement with the plan.

Next he met with radiation oncology. The radiation oncologist discussed the role of radiation therapy in his care and that he would need staging results to further determine an individualized plan of care as discussed with his surgeon. The ONN provided basic education on radiation therapy but would discuss further once staging was complete and the type of radiation therapy was determined. AV expressed a desire that if radiation therapy was needed, he be treated closer to home. The ONN offered to help facilitate this once his testing was completed and the stage of his disease was known.

AV met with the medical oncologist who reinforced the discussion that occurred at the other two consults but also discussed chemotherapy options with AV. Again, based on staging he will most likely need chemotherapy. The exact plan was deferred until staging was completed.

The ONN met with AV and his family and reviewed the next steps in his care. AV also asked about the possibility of getting chemotherapy locally if needed. The ONN stated she could also help with this once his case was reviewed at tumor board and the final plan was determined. AV left with a plan and all his current questions answered. The ONN kept in touch with AV to be sure things were moving according to plan.

AV's staging workup was completed, and his case was presented at the GI multidisciplinary tumor board. He had a T3N1 (stage III disease); his chest CT showed small pulmonary nodules, and his MRI of the abdomen/pelvis showed extramural tumor extension and regional lymph node involvement in the presacral region. Tumor board recommendations were for chemotherapy followed by chemoradiation and then surgery [30]. AV was called with the test results, and his ONN then called to discuss his goals of care and to confirm where he would like to get treated. The ONN had an extensive discussion with AV and addressed his many questions. AV wanted to be treated closer to home, so they discussed options for the many local facilities he could go to. AV decided that he would be treated at the local cancer center that was affiliated with the AMC. It was close to his home, and the affiliation could help make the transition of care seamless. The ONN sensed some uncertainty from AV. She asked some more questions and that was when he asked, "What would you do if you were me? Tell me honestly as my friend, would you go through with this?"

The ONN paused and said that each person has to make the decision that they feel most comfortable with and that she would support him through the informed decision-making process but not tell him what she would do if she were in his position. She explained that the teams' recommendations were based on evidence-based practice and that it was the standard of care for his disease stage. AV asked how the team decided on the best treatment options for him. She explained that the NCCN guidelines provide the best evidence at the current time based on research and clinical data. She explained that these are regularly updated to reflect changes in clinical practice [31]. She answered his many questions and encouraged him to further discuss with his family and care team before moving forward to be sure he was comfortable with his decision.

AV's wife called the next day and asked more questions. She also asked what the ONN would do. The ONN gave the same answer to AV's wife as she did to AV the previous day. His wife articulated the difficulty with making this decision and said that it felt like they are on an "emotional roller coaster" as AV and his wife are also caring for an elderly parent as well as helping their two adult children. The ONN provided support and encouraged them to take advantage of resources at the cancer center where he will be treated, assuming he agrees to treatment. AV and his family were very anxious, and the ONN had the impression that AV and his wife felt that their friendship would provide them with 24-hour access for questions/concerns, and she was right. AV called or emailed the ONN many times during the next few days including off hours, with multiple questions. He was upset when he did not get an immediate response. The challenge for the ONN was to be supportive and helpful but to set limits and maintain professional boundaries, which were a difficult proposition. It was important for the ONN to establish healthy boundaries with AV and his family. She had a frank and difficult discussion with AV and his wife to establish the expectations of the relationship and explained that it was important for AV and his family to take ownership of his care with the support of the ONN [31]. It was important to the ONN that she not over-navigate AV as this would enable an unhealthy relationship. Sometimes as an ONN it is just easier to do things for the patient but that does not foster a therapeutic relationship or empower the patient to advocate for himself. AV needed to step up to the challenge [32].

During the discussion, the ONN outlined the boundaries on when to call or email and the expected time frame for a response. She provided the hours for AV to call as well as the on-call number for questions/concerns after hours. She also provided a list of colon cancer resources for AV should he need them. AV called the next day and decided on chemotherapy locally as the first step in his journey. His ONN connected with the GI ONN at the affiliated facility and was able to set him up with a medical oncologist who would administer the recommended FOLFOX (oxaliplatin with fluorouracil [5-FU] and folinic acid) chemotherapy regimen every 2 weeks for 4 cycles [31]. She provided education regarding his chemotherapy plan and discussed that he would be getting a port in his chest to receive his chemotherapy. She provided port teaching, and AV was happy with this plan as he did not want to get repeated peripheral sticks for his chemotherapy. This would be done locally. The ONN discussed his case with the GI ONN and did a handoff regarding his care. The two ONNs would continue to work collaboratively as AV's journey was far from over, and they shared how to manage his anxiety so that the teams were being consistent in the messages AV would receive. His AMC ONN called to confirm the plan and provided information about the medical oncology appointment. She then did a warm handoff to his GI ONN at the affiliated facility. She assured him she was not abandoning him as he was upset that she would not be "navigating" him. She explained to him that she would still be his ONN but that for the next 8 weeks his GI ONN would be better positioned to answer his questions and assist him as his treatment was local.

AV received four cycles of FOLFOX and returned to the AMC for his restaging scans as requested by his team. He saw the surgeon for a repeat sigmoidoscopy. The restaging scans and sigmoidoscopy showed an interval decrease in size of the rectosigmoid carcinoma with residual area of mural semi-annular thickening and decreased size of pelvic lymph nodes. There were no new sites of disease in the pelvis.

AV and his family met with the AMC ONN again at this appointment to move forward with the next step of the process, which was chemoradiation. The AMC ONN's discussion with AV was that he wanted to get his radiation (XRT) locally but at a facility other than where he was receiving his chemotherapy. His reasoning was that his wife heard very good things about the radiation physician, which influenced his decision on where to get his radiation therapy. The new challenge for his AMC ONN was to coordinate radiation treatment at a third facility that was not affiliated with either of the other two facilities, while he continued chemotherapy with his current oncologist. AV was agreeable with this plan and understood that he would be traveling daily for radiation at one location and then go to another location for his chemotherapy. The AMC ONN encouraged him to get his radiation at the local cancer center but he refused.

The AMC ONN contacted the ONN where AV wanted to receive XRT to help coordinate his radiation consult. Once again, she set the limits with AV and told him that his radiation ONN would be his point person for XRT-related questions and toxicities. His AMC ONN provided extensive education about what to expect at his radiation consult and reviewed the plan as she understood it. Basic patient educational materials were reviewed with AV, and his questions were answered. The plan was for him to receive 28 fractions of 3-D conformal radiation therapy along with concurrent chemotherapy. This type of radiation therapy shapes the radiation beams to match the shape of the tumor. It targets the cancer while sparing healthy tissue [33].

His plan was neoadjuvant chemoradiation with infusional 5-FU. He was scheduled back at his local cancer center to discuss next steps of concurrent chemotherapy to be done with his radiation. His AMC ONN provided education regarding his chemotherapy and expected toxicities such as nausea and vomiting, low blood counts, and risk of infection. This was important to reinforce with AV as he helps care for his elderly parent and is around his young granddaughter who goes to day care. She provided some written educational material and confirmed that his GI ONN and oncologist would review it in more detail when he met with them to start the second phase of treatment.

The AMC ONN coordinated with her ONN colleagues between the three facilities to be sure that AV had seamless transitions in care in the next steps of his journey. She wanted to be sure that all his ONNs were on the same page and that we were all communicating the same information. The three ONNs spoke often to keep the lines of communication open.

The AMC ONN kept in touch with AV, and he did very well throughout his chemoradiation. He continued to work out at the gym several times a week. His main complaint was that he was more fatigued than usual but he felt that his exercise helped him stay "centered." He also complained of some occasional diarrhea and peripheral neuropathy. The AMC ONN encouraged him to discuss these side effects with his oncologist.

He completed the second phase of treatment and returned to the AMC to discuss the final step in his treatment, which was surgery. He met with the surgeon and had a repeat sigmoidoscopy and scans. His scans showed no evidence of abnormal FDG uptake in the rectosigmoid colon and no evidence of FDG-avid locoregional or distant metastatic colon cancer. AV called his ONN at the AMC to share the results and to also ask questions about his upcoming surgery such as did he need surgery and if there were other options available. He admitted to his AMC ONN that he was scared about the side effects of surgery and the effect surgery would have on his quality of life (QOL). He verbalized that despite all he had been through, his QOL was very good for a 75-year-old man, and he was not sure he wanted surgery. The AMC ONN encouraged him to keep his next surgical appointment to review his options and then make an informed decision.

It was discussed with AV that the standard treatment of locally advanced rectal cancer with neoadjuvant therapy is usually followed by resection (low anterior resection in this case) [30]. In the event of a complete clinical response, he can consider a watch and wait strategy of close surveillance rather than oncologic resection, but that is not the standard of care. The risks and benefits of LAR including intraoperative and postoperative complications were discussed with AV. He was very concerned about change in bowel habits as well as the possibility of a colostomy. After an extensive discussion about the risks, benefits, and alternatives, AV decided to proceed with surveillance only. He asked about clinical trials, but he did not meet the eligibility for any current trials. He stated he understood the risks of waiting including development of local invasion and metastatic disease. It was explained to him that if he should have a recurrence, there is a chance he will need a more invasive operation. The AMC ONN confirmed the plan with AV as well and reviewed his recommended surveillance schedules [30]. At his 3-month follow-up, AV's scans showed no changes. He reports that he feels well and is spending quality time with his family and is continuing to work.

Challenges

This case study presented many challenges for the ONN. It was difficult navigating a friend whom the ONN felt took advantage of their friendship. It was hard to set boundaries, and he may have been better served by the GI navigator but he refused, leaving the ONN with the challenge of navigating and advocating for him to be sure he received the very best care. This was in spite of the fact that the ONN was not familiar with GI cancers. Other challenges included keeping the communication channels open between all three treatment facilities and giving AV consistent messages throughout his disease trajectory. His ONN supported him with his decision to not undergo surgery even though she knew that surgery was the standard of care.

Opportunities

This patient also presented many opportunities for the ONN. As a disease-specific navigator, it served to expand her knowledge and skill set with another disease site. It also allowed the ONN to build relationships with new navigators and to develop a list of colleagues whom she could call on in the future. The ONN learned the value of setting boundaries and expectations early in the patient relationship and providing consistent messages. This case study showed the value of navigation for oncology patients in helping to facilitate the best care possible throughout the disease trajectory in several different locations.

Implications for Stakeholders

ONNs are uniquely positioned in our role to coordinate care for our patients. ONNs are able to see the "big picture" of the plan and identify early on issues that may impede care. ONNs are the "lynch pin" to getting patients and families through treatment. Critical thinking skills are paramount to the ONN role, and creative thinking often helps keep patients on track as we think outside the box. We practice patient-centered care, and the relationships we develop with our patients and families are the core of our practice. We are able to keep patients on track as well as within the healthcare network, thus keeping downstream revenue within the system. The power of our role is the ability to get things done and build a vast network of colleagues that can help at a moment's notice.

References

1. Shah SP, Roth A, Goya R. The Clonal and mutational evolution spectrum of primary triple-negative breast cancers Nature [cited 2017 Mar 16]. 2012. http://www.nature.com/doifinder/10.1038/nature10933, https://doi.org/10.1038/nature10933.
2. Zardavas D, Phillips WA, Loi S. PIK3CA mutations in breast cancer: reconciling findings from preclinical and clinical data. Breast Cancer Res. 2014;16(1):201. https://doi.org/10.1186/bcr3605.
3. Herndon SC. Caregiver coping strategies: keeping a gratitude journal. Conquer Patient Voice. 2016;2(5):118–9.
4. Gentry SS. Navigation considerations when working with patients. Oncology nurse navigation delivering patient-centered care across the continuum, vol. 1. 1st ed. Pittsburgh, PA: Oncology Nursing Society; 2014. p. 94–5.
5. Katz A. Woman cancer sex. Hygeia Media. 2009.
6. Katz A. Providing care for the whole patient: sexuality and cancer. The Oncology Nurse APN/PA 9.2. 2016.
7. Pratt-Chapman MP. How you CW an be a champion to LGBTQ cancer patients. In: Paper presented at American Academy of Nurse and Patient Navigators; 2016.
8. www.ons.org/content/2016-congress-archived-session-same-only scarier-cancer-care-and-lgbt-community.

9. Ballard D, Hill JMF. The nurse's role in health literacy of patients with cancer. Clin J Oncol Nurs. 2016;20:232–4. https://doi.org/10.1188/16.CJON.232-234.
10. www.onclive.com/sap-partner/cancer-centers/carbone/carbone-cancer-center-clinical-trials-test-dietary-therapy-for-triplenegative-breast-cancer.
11. Thomas MA, Peters EA. Setting specific navigation. Oncology nurse navigation delivering patient-centered care across the continuum. Pittsburgh, PA: Oncology Nursing Society; 2014. p. 196.
12. O'Reilly R, et al. NCCN pediatric osteosarcoma practice guidelines. The National Comprehensive Cancer Network. Oncology (Williston Park). 1996;10(12):1799–806, 1812.
13. Baggott CR, Association of Pediatric Oncology Nurses (U.S.). Nursing care of children and adolescents with cancer, vol. xvi. 3rd ed. Philadelphia: Saunders; 2002. p. 717.
14. Cripe T, Yeager N. Malignant pediatric bone tumors—treatment & management. Cham: Springer; 2015.
15. Carnevale A, Lieberman E, Cardenas R. Li-Fraumeni syndrome in pediatric patients with soft tissue sarcoma or osteosarcoma. Arch Med Res. 1997;28(3):383–6.
16. Murphy K. Children's oncology group family handbook for children with cancer, 2nd ed. 2011. https://childrensoncologygroup.org/downloads/COG_Family_Handbook_2nd_Ed_English_HighRes.pdf. Accessed Jun 2017.
17. Dunn J. Case presentation of doxorubicin-induced cardiomyopathy: a short- and long-term side effect of pediatric cancer treatment. J Pediatr Oncol Nurs. 1991;8(2):84.
18. Ruiz L, et al. Auditory function in pediatric osteosarcoma patients treated with multiple doses of cis-diamminedichloroplatinum(II). Cancer Res. 1989;49(3):742–4.
19. Walker C. Use of art and play therapy in pediatric oncology. J Pediatr Oncol Nurs. 1989;6(4):121–6.
20. Pearson M. Caring for children and adolescents with osteosarcoma: a nursing perspective. Cancer Treat Res. 2009;152:385–94.
21. Scialla MA, Canter KS, Chen FF, et al. Implementing the psychosocial standards in pediatric cancer: current staffing and services available. Pediatr Blood Cancer. 2017;64(11). https://doi.org/10.1002/pbc.26634.
22. Walker CL. Use of art and play therapy in pediatric oncology. J Assoc Pediatr Oncol Nurses. 1988;5(1–2):34.
23. Standley JM, Hanser SB. Music therapy research and applications in pediatric oncology treatment. J Pediatr Oncol Nurs. 1995;12(1):3–8; discussion 9–10.
24. Mazlum S, Chaharsough NT, Banihashem A, Vashani HB. The effect of massage therapy on chemotherapy-induced nausea and vomiting in pediatric cancer. Iran J Nurs Midwifery Res. 2013;18(4):280–4.
25. Zhukovsky DS, Herzog CE, Kaur G, et al. The impact of palliative care consultation on symptom assessment, communication needs, and palliative interventions in pediatric patients with cancer. J Palliat Med. 2009;12(4):343–9.
26. Punzalan M, Hyden G. The role of physical therapy and occupational therapy in the rehabilitation of pediatric and adolescent patients with osteosarcoma. Cancer Treat Res. 2009;152:367–84.
27. Jacobs PA. Limb salvage and rotationplasty for osteosarcoma in children. Clin Orthop Relat Res. 1984;188:217–22.
28. Haugen MS, Landier W, Mandrell BN, et al. Educating families of children newly diagnosed with cancer: insights of a Delphi Panel of Expert Clinicians from the Children's Oncology roup. J Pediatr Oncol Nurs. 2016;33(6):405–13.
29. www.cancer.org/treatment/understanding-your-diagnosis/tests/understanding-your-pathology-report/colon-pathology/invasive-adenocarcinoma-of-the-colon.html. Accessed May 2017.
30. NCCN Guidelines: Colon Cancer: Version 3. https://www.nccn.org/professionals/physician_gls/pdf/rectal.pdf. Accessed June 2017.
31. NCCN Guidelines: Colon Cancer: Version 3. https://www.nccn.org/professionals/physician_gls/guidelines-development.asp. Accessed July 2017.
32. Blaseg KD, Daugherty P, Gamblin KA. Oncology nurse navigation: delivering patient centered care across the continuum. Oncology Nursing Society: Pittsburgh, PA; 2014. (Chapter 2)
33. www.oncolink.org/cancer-treatment/radiation/overview/radiation-therapy. Accessed June 2017.

The Role of the Navigator During a Patient's Cancer Treatment

8

Linda Burhansstipanov and Lillie D. Shockney

8.1 The Role of the Navigator During Cancer Treatment

The navigator commonly remains the constant multidisciplinary team member who is accompanying the patient, physically or virtually, throughout their cancer treatment process, as the patient moves from one phase of treatment to the next. There are diverse names to describe the navigation role, including community health workers, community navigators, patient navigators, social workers, and nurse navigators. Each of these navigators supports the patient in different and sometimes overlapping ways. For a review of the similar and distinct roles of diverse navigation types, see Willis et al.'s 2013 study delineating navigator roles [1]. In this chapter, the term "navigator" is inclusive of any individual whose primary role is to reduce barriers to care for cancer patients unless the more specific term is used to differentiate scope of practice considerations. The scenarios provided are to illustrate how navigators can support patients in critical ways throughout treatment. The reader should adapt scenarios according to available resources, with the general rule that community and patient navigator roles support practical and logistical patient needs, while nurse navigators provide nuanced clinical education, and social workers are experts in counseling and psychosocial support.

The major cancer treatment modalities are surgery, radiation therapy, and chemotherapy. For certain types of cancers, stem cell transplant or hormone therapy is appropriate. More recently, significant strides have been made in immunotherapy, targeted therapy, and precision medicine. Clinical trials test new therapies not yet proved to be efficacious, as well as alternative and supplemental therapies.

L. Burhansstipanov, MSPH, DrPH (✉)
Native American Cancer Research Corporation, Pine, CO, USA
e-mail: lindab@natamcancer.net

L. D. Shockney, RN, BS, MAS, ONN-CG
Johns Hopkins University School of Medicine, Baltimore, MD, USA

© Springer International Publishing AG, part of Springer Nature 2018
L. D. Shockney (ed.), *Team-Based Oncology Care: The Pivotal Role of Oncology Navigation*, https://doi.org/10.1007/978-3-319-69038-4_8

149

8.2   Education and Support During Consultations About Surgical Options

Commonly, the first phase of treatment may be surgery to remove the cancer and hopefully achieve clear margins around the tumor. Patients need to understand their surgical options, risks and benefits of each, and have any medical jargon that is confusing to them interpreted. The navigator can provide this type of education, as well as encourage the patient to be an active member in the decision-making about the surgical option finally chosen. The patient also needs the ability to ask questions so that they also understand what to expect to be an outcome of this phase of treatment. The navigator can help the patient identify pertinent questions. Table 8.1 [2, 3] summarizes some common questions to facilitate such an interactive discussion. The navigator can review the list with the patient and then highlight which, if any, of the questions and anticipated answers are most important.

8.2.1   Before Surgery Takes Place

The navigator will need to spend time with the patient and family caregiver to prepare the patient for surgery. This includes educating the patient about the type of surgery that will be done, how to prepare for the surgery day, what to do and not to do due to having surgery (e.g., nothing to eat after midnight, no blood thinner medications for a specified period of time preoperatively), and what to expect on the day of surgery, as well as for several days after surgery. The navigator may need to refer the patient to cancer prehabilitation for core strengthening, teaching skills related to prevention of risk of developing lymphedema postoperatively, or other rehabilitation needs. How long the patient may need to be out of work should be discussed as well, because the patient may not have adequate sick days at work as an employee benefit, which can result in his/her paycheck being less than whole; this could impact the patient's ability to pay their monthly bills. This can have a domino effect in that they then may also be short of funds to pay for new prescriptions, parking while seeing the doctors after surgery, and other additional expenses that can be incurred as a result of the surgical treatment. This is another reason why it is important for the navigator to continuously and consistently reassess the patient for barriers to care and provide resources to undo those barriers.

8.2.2   Following the Surgery

Any surgery requires follow-up care. For those hospitalized for a finite period of time, when ready for discharge, the inpatient oncology nurse taking care of the patient will provide specific discharge instructions to the patient and their family. These may be related to wound management drain care and measurement, physical activity, management of side effects, medications to be taken for pain control, recognition of signs of possible infection, and other factors associated with the patient postoperatively. Cancer rehabilitation may be needed to continue to work with the

Table 8.1 Examples of patient questions to ask the surgery team

- How many hours do I need to fast before the operation? What about my medications? Which ones can I take or not take before the surgery? Can I drink water?
- What time do I need to be at the hospital?
- What can I bring with me into the operating room (e.g., spiritual item)
- Where should my family wait? Can they stay with me until I have to go into the operating room? Who will talk with them? Can a translator be present if needed?
- Can I have a prayer or spiritual ceremony performed while I am in the hospital awaiting surgery?
- What type of surgery will be done?
- Is the surgery dangerous? What other kinds of treatment can be used instead of surgery?
- What are the risks and benefits?
- How many operations will need to be done? Why can't all be done at one time?
- Will I need to be in the hospital each time? How long will I need to be in the hospital each time? Can a family member stay with me in the hospital?
- How long will I need for recovery? How soon can I go back to work? What precautions will I need to take?
- Will I be in much pain? If I get nauseous with the standard pain medications, what alternatives are available to me?
- What type of anesthesia will be used? Does it include anti-nausea or pain control medication with it?
- Will I have drains, catheters, or intravenous lines?
- What will the scar look like? Where will it be? How big will it be?
- Will I go home with drains, and if so, for how long? Who will show my family how to help me with my drains?
- When can I resume driving?
- What are the side effects or after effects of the surgery?
- Will I need special care at home after the surgery?
- How soon following the surgery can I have the reconstruction or prosthesis surgery?
- What are the side effects and risks that I should consider related to reconstruction or prosthesis surgery?
- What can be done if the surgery is not successful?
- How soon does the surgery need to take place?
- What would happen to me if I decide to not have any surgery?
- Will I be able to work after my surgery, and if so, how soon after surgery?
- How soon after the surgery will you have pathology results to tell me if most or all of the cancer has been removed from my body?
- What else will be learned from the pathology results that will impact other treatment decisions going forward?
- Can I be cured of this cancer by doing this surgery?
- How soon after surgery will I meet with you in the clinic again?
- How soon after that visit will I see other doctors for additional phases of my treatment?

patient and their family caregiver during the hospitalization as well as postdischarge. Navigators can find resources for physical, financial, cultural, and emotional support. Navigators also commonly help ensure the patient has the postoperative appointment prescheduled with the surgeon before being discharged from the hospital. For those having ambulatory surgery, the same type of teaching and coordination of care support is provided.

8.3   Chemotherapy

Chemotherapy is used to cure cancer, slow cancer growth, control cancer, or ease cancer symptoms (also called palliative chemotherapy) by shrinking tumors that cause pain or to shrink the tumor before performing surgery or radiation therapy. Chemotherapy medications are administered to the patient using various modalities. The amount and type of chemotherapy the patient receives is based on the type of cancer cells (histology), stage of cancer, size of the tumor, and whether the cancer has spread (metastasized). It may be given alone or with other treatments, such as surgery, radiation therapy, or biologic therapy. The chemotherapy regimen selected is based on evidence-based research of what chemotherapy regimens will be the most appropriate for the patient. The patient should be engaged in the discussion with the medical oncologist about the treatment options.

8.3.1   Education and Support About Side Effects from Chemotherapy

Chemotherapy agents affect both the cancerous and the healthy cell DNA. The healthy cells that are particularly susceptible to chemotherapy are cells that multiply quickly such as the skin (including body, facial, and head hair), the digestive system (mucous membranes throughout the gastrointestinal tract, mouth through anus), and the bone marrow (which makes red and white blood cells that make the immune system). Chemotherapy side effects differ based on the medications and the patient's individual responses to the medications. Common side effects may include fatigue, sluggishness, tiredness, nausea, vomiting, loss of appetite, mouth sores, diarrhea, constipation, hair loss, skin rash, fever, skin darkening, sensitivity to sun, hot flashes, neuropathy, and neutropenia. Navigators can prepare the patient and family for ways to recognize these side effects as well as provide methods to diminish or even prevent them from happening. Most side effects are not permanent, but some can be. Clinical trials may be offered as part of the chemotherapy treatments the patient receives. If so, the patient will be in close contact with the research nurse, as well as with the navigator and medical oncology nurse practitioner.

Navigators also need to remind the patient and family that everyone reacts differently to chemotherapy. The patient may feel well with the first round of chemotherapy treatment and have a difficult time during the second round of therapy. If or when the patient has side effects, the navigator and patient must tell the appropriate provider involved with their chemotherapy. The oncologist may change the drugs the patient is receiving or the dosage of the drugs to lessen the side effects. But they cannot do this unless they know what problems the patient is experiencing.

Table 8.2 [2, 3] summarizes some common questions a patient may want to ask of their chemotherapy team. Navigators can review the list with the patient and

Table 8.2 Examples of patient questions to ask the chemotherapy team

• How can I get my body strong to help reduce the side effects of chemotherapy?
• What is the purpose of the chemotherapy?
• What side effects am I likely to have with this chemo?
• How can the side effects be lessened?
• How long will the side effects last?
• How do I know if the side effects are not normal, so I can contact the doctor?
• Can I just quit treatment whenever I want?
• What can I do about side effects that are permanent (like heart problems)?
• Will my health insurance pay for these medications? If not, who will?
• Where do I have my chemo treatments? In the clinic or the hospital?
• Are oral or pill-form chemo drugs less effective than intravenous (IV) methods?
• How do these chemo drugs affect my other medications (e.g., diabetes, heart, or arthritis drugs)?
• Why do some people who are taking the same medications as me not have as many side effects? Why do some people have more side effects?
• How can I describe the severity of my side effects to my providers so that they understand what I am going through?
• Do the side effects mean that the drugs are working?
• Can I drive myself to my chemotherapy appointments?
• How often will you see me while I am receiving my chemotherapy care?
• How many hours will I be at the chemotherapy infusion center?
• What should I bring with me to my chemotherapy appointments?
• What tests are done, when, and why?
• How soon will my chemotherapy start and when will it likely be completed?
• If I get really sick with a high fever, what will happen?
• What determines if you decide to reduce the dosage of the drugs?
• How do you determine that the chemotherapy drugs are still working?
• How do you determine if the drugs are still benefiting me if the dosage is reduced?
• Do I have to take any precautions after each treatment I receive?

then highlight which, if any, of the questions and anticipated answers are of interest.

8.3.2   During Chemotherapy [4]

The navigator should ensure that the patient has transportation to and from the chemotherapy appointments with the family or loved ones. Sometimes the patient feels a little nervous and other times feels sick. It may be safer to have someone other than the patient drive.

Patients may benefit from seeing the chemotherapy suite where the treatments will be given, even before they are due to start their treatments. This can reduce anxiety.

Chemotherapy is stressful for most people. The navigator can discuss strategies for relaxing or remaining calm during the sometimes very lengthy chemotherapy infusions. Some people like to do puzzles, others read, and many like to listen to music or audiobooks.

8.3.3   After the Chemotherapy

Patients may experience sudden thirst or nausea after chemotherapy. Staying hydrated even if the patient doesn't feel thirsty will be emphasized as very important to do. Having the patient know when side effects, if they were to occur, would start to manifest is needed for planning their time, including when they will need help at home. Patients can feel very anxious after the first treatment, because they don't know how their body will react. They also may worry that if their side effects are too severe, the oncologist may reduce the dosage. Such a reduction may raise the question as to the effectiveness of the medicine if they are receiving a lower dose than originally prescribed and is considered the standard of care. There usually is evidence-based research, however, to demonstrate to patients that they are still getting benefit from the chemotherapy, even at a lower strength.

8.3.4   Chemotherapy in the Form of Oral Oncolytics

As referenced earlier in this chapter, not all chemotherapy treatments are intravenously administered. There is a growing pipeline of oral oncolytics to make it more convenient for the patient to self-administer. This results in the provider and other oncology team members having no direct control over ensuring that the patient is taking the medications as prescribed. Oral adherence is critical to the treatment working effectively. Although it is great for patients to be on oral chemotherapy drugs due to convenience and the elimination of needing to come to a facility for an infusion, it places the patient in charge of ensuring that they are taking these medicines as prescribed. The patient may need additional teaching and tools (e.g., pill holders by time and day of the week) to help them stay on course for adherence. Because these medicines will likely be provided through an outpatient pharmacy, the patient's prescription coverage may not cover all of the expenses of the drugs. Checking into discounted drug programs through the pharmaceutical companies that manufacture these specific drugs is a task a navigator can do that can reduce the financial burden for the patient and aid in keeping the patient adherent to the drug as intended. The navigator therefore needs to provide the patient with educational information along with tools and resources to help keep the patient on track for self-administration of the right dosage at the right time in the right manner. For some patients, this may require a family caregiver assisting with this task and to be specifically trained on how to do this.

8.4   Radiation

Radiation therapy has been in use for over 100 years. High doses of radiation kill cells or keep them from growing and dividing (breaks up the DNA inside the cells). Since cancer cells grow at a faster rate than normal cells, radiation therapy can be very effective. According to the American Cancer Society, "Unlike chemotherapy, which usually exposes the whole body to cancer-fighting drugs, radiation therapy is usually a local treatment. In most cases, it's aimed at and affects only the part of the body being treated." [5] Radiation treatment is planned to damage cancer cells, with as little harm as possible to nearby healthy cells. Normal cells are also destroyed by radiation, which is why providers monitor the intensity carefully. About half of all people who are diagnosed with cancer undergo radiation.

Radiation therapy goes by different names: radiotherapy, brachytherapy (internal radiation), x-ray therapy, cobalt therapy, electron beam therapy, and/or irradiation. Most methods of radiation therapy don't reach all parts of the body, which means they're not helpful in treating cancer that has metastasized to many organ sites within the body. Still, radiation therapy can be used to treat many types of cancer either alone or in combination with other treatments.

The radiation oncology team consists of a radiation oncologist, a radiation physicist, a dosimetrist, a radiation therapy technologist, a nurse, and potentially dietitians, physical therapists, social workers, and dental specialists [5]. Navigators can serve as a liaison between the patient and the radiation specific team members. Again, the patient should be engaged with the radiation oncology team in discussions about the type of radiation, duration of treatment, and dosage that are optimal for the patient to receive.

8.4.1 Education and Support About Radiation Therapy and Side Effects

Common radiation side effects include fatigue, loss of appetite, skin problems (dry, itchy, sunburned, swelling, soreness), constipation, cough, fever, and pain. Most side effects from radiation therapy (e.g., itching, skin reddening, and skin burn) subside after a few weeks. Some side effects require immediate response from the provider, such as coughing, fever, or unusual pain. When side effects become too severe, radiation is stopped and the patient must have some time to recover and heal before continuing the treatment. This is known as a break in therapy. Side effects from radiation sometimes do not occur for several weeks. When they do occur, the patient or navigator must ensure that the healthcare provider knows about side effects experienced. The patient and/or navigator must discuss how to alleviate side effects. For example, lotions that normally help with dry skin, such as aloe lotions, can irritate radiation "burn" or dry skin. The most common side effect from radiation therapy is fatigue, which is cumulative and commonly lingers for a period of time after treatments are totally completed. Encouraging the patient to remain physically active can reduce this known and bothersome side effect.

Table 8.3 [2, 3] provides a list of questions the navigator might review with the patient to prioritize patient concerns.

Table 8.3 Examples of patient questions to ask the radiation oncology team

• What is radiation therapy? Do people die from radiation poisoning?
• Will this treatment *cause* cancer?
• What type of radiation treatment will I be getting? What's the difference between external beam radiation and internal (brachytherapy) radiation? Pros and cons of each? Do I have a choice?
• If or when I have questions about my radiation treatment, who should I ask?
• Can I continue to work during these treatments?
• Where is the best place to have the treatments?
• How long will it take for each treatment? For the whole series?
• Will I be able to drive myself to and from my treatments?
• What side effects can I expect? How long will they last? Can these side effects become chronic? Permanent? Are there possible long-term side effects?
• How do I manage side effects if they occur?
• What side effects should I report to the radiation oncologist?
• How much will this treatment cost? Is it covered by insurance?
• How much of a risk is involved? Will the radiation affect the surrounding areas of the body?
• Will I be having other kinds of treatment in addition to the radiation?
• Is my family safe from radiation while I am going through treatment?
• If I have radioactive seeds or some other solid type of radiation products internally, am I safe to hold family members? May my grandchildren sit on my lap safely?
• Are there any alternatives to radiation treatment?

8.4.2 Prior to Radiation Therapy

Because radiation usually interferes with the healing from surgery, the navigator must help the cancer patient understand that she/he may need to wait until the body heals from the surgery before beginning radiation therapy. Many patients are frightened of radiation, and their fears should be addressed before treatment.

> *Case study: A navigator in the southwest of the United States worked with a traditional Indian healer to help a patient prepare for how to deal with uncomfortable feelings during therapy. The patient was to be strapped down to help her stay in one position so that the radiation would go where it was supposed to go and not affect other parts of the body. Then the machine had to move to focus on a different angle of the tumor (or place where the tumor was removed). The sound and the closeness of the equipment were very frightening to the patient. The navigator continued to work with the patient after the healer had prepped her so that the patient was ready to hear loud sounds or the sudden movement of the equipment. "I got scared when the big machine came down on me 'cause I never experienced nothing like that in my life, so I got scared so I started praying in my own language and prayers. I asked the machine, whatever you are, believe and get me well. That's what I said to the machine, get me well" (Santo Domingo Pueblo patient).*

Navigators need to educate the patient about what to expect while receiving the radiation, as well as physical changes they may experience after the radiation. There should be specific education about the simulation visit, which is the first visit the patient will have to be fitted for a cast or for other methods to help the patient stay in one position. There are different techniques that are used to help the patient stay in a single position.

Patients must understand that the radiation oncologist will mark the area on the patient's skin where the radiation is to be directed. They will use India ink, another relatively permanent marker, or permanent tattooing of the skin. The navigator needs to remind the patient to avoid scrubbing off the mark. Patients should also be cautioned not to have the tattoo markings removed after treatment is completed because these markings may be needed in the future to alert healthcare professionals that the patient has received radiation in this area of their body. If parts of the patient's body, such as a woman's breast, are exposed, she needs to know who has the ability and authority to look through the observation window and see her unclothed, as well as what their purpose is in observing her.

Family members are sometimes concerned that the patient is radioactive following radiation therapy. The navigator can discuss this concern with the healthcare provider and clarify any safety issues. If very high dosages of radiation are used, the provider may recommend that the patient not hold infants or very small children for a short period of time. For most patients, the radiation is focused on a local area, and concerns are unwarranted.

8.4.3 During the Radiation Therapy

If the patient has side effects, the navigator should coordinate with the family and loved ones regarding transportation to and from the radiation appointments.

If the patient is receiving radiation at the healthcare facility, the navigator or any family member cannot be in the same room with the cancer patient while the treatment is being administered, because of exposure to unnecessary radiation. The navigator can stand outside the room in the window space and continue talking or praying with the patient. Some facilities provide speakers and earphones, so the patient and navigator can carry on a conversation while the patient remains still.

Some patients have severe reactions to radiation, which result in having to take additional medical prescription drugs, like cortisone (e.g., prednisone).

8.4.4 After the Radiation

Most patients still feel well after the first few treatments, and may require little assistance initially (e.g., help walking to the car). However, the patient can suddenly begin to experience side effects. The most common effects are feeling very fatigued and experiencing red, tender, dry skin on the area where the radiation is being focused. For skin problems, ask the healthcare provider for a lotion. For some patients, these side effects don't manifest until treatment is close to being completed.

Patients who are going through radiation therapy are often extra sensitive to sunlight and heat. They are likely to have no tolerance to heat. The navigator can encourage the patient to stay out of direct sunlight, to wear a hat that covers the head and face, and to wear double layers of long-sleeve shirts or a sunscreen type of shirt. And for 1 year after radiation therapy has been completed, the parts of the patient's body that were radiated should not be exposed to the sun.

8.5   Biologic Targeted Therapy

Targeted therapy is a type of cancer treatment that uses drugs or other substances to more precisely identify and attack molecules within the cancer cells [6]. Researchers have learned about some of the differences in cancer cells (or other cells near them) that help them grow and thrive [6]. This has led to the development of drugs that "target" these differences and block the growth progression and spread of cancer. These treatments are sometimes used alone but most frequently are used in combination with other treatments. Targeted cancer therapies are sometimes called "molecularly targeted drugs," "molecularly targeted therapies," "precision medicines," or similar names.

Targeted therapies, the focus of precision medicine, work unlike chemotherapy by acting on specific molecular targets that are associated with cancer [7]. Many targeted cancer therapies have been approved by the Food and Drug Administration (FDA) to treat specific types of cancer. Others are being studied in clinical trials (research studies with people), and many more are in preclinical testing (research studies with animals) [7].

8.5.1   Education and Support About Side Effects and Biologic Targeted Therapy

Navigators need to educate the patient and their family caregivers about biologic targeted therapies, how they work differently than chemotherapy drugs, and what side effects, if any, may occur. Some patients may receive this type of therapy for a long period of time, such as a year. In general, biologic targeted therapies are usually tolerated better than chemotherapy drugs. It is common, however, for patients, even after teaching, to still refer to all drugs as chemotherapy.

8.6   Hormonal Therapy

Endocrine glands secrete hormones directly into the bloodstream to affect the activity of other parts of the body (e.g., target site or organ). They serve as messengers, controlling and coordinating activities throughout the body [8]. Men and women produce hormones such as testosterone, estrogen, and progesterone and need these chemicals for efficient body functioning.

Hormone therapy is used when tumors have hormone receptor–positive cells (e.g., many types of breast cancer have estrogen receptor [ER]-positive cancers and/ or progesterone receptor [PR]-positive cancers; also, commonly prostate cancer patients are managed with hormonal therapy). Medications that block hormone receptors prohibit hormones from binding to the cancer cells and making them grow and divide. Thus, hormone therapy slows or stops the growth of cancer that relies on hormones to grow. Hormonal therapy may be used alone or in combination with other treatments. Hormone therapy is specifically designed to limit the body's ability to produce hormones and/or to interfere with how hormones behave in the body. Hormonal therapy also is used to ease cancer symptoms, particularly in men diagnosed with prostate cancer. Patients may be placed on hormonal therapy for 5–10 years to prevent distant recurrence of their cancer once other adjuvant therapies have been completed. Some patients with advanced metastatic hormone-positive cancers may be given these types of medications for however long the tumor continues to effectively respond to the treatment, thus keeping the cancer in control so that the patient's body can live in harmony with the disease that is now being treated as a chronic illness. Because hormonal therapies are less toxic to the body, they are a preferred treatment as a starting point for patients with advanced disease as well as for elderly patients who may not be good candidates for more aggressive therapies.

According to the National Cancer Institute [9], when used with other treatments, hormone therapy can make a tumor smaller before surgery or radiation therapy, lower risk of recurrence, or kill cancer that has returned or spread. Hormonal therapy can slow or stop the growth of cancers that rely on or use hormones to grow by blocking or interfering with hormones in the body.

Special attention should be given to transgender cancer patients on gender-affirming hormonal therapy. This therapy may be contraindicated during cancer treatment or may be completely safe. A discussion between the patient and the healthcare team about the risks and benefits of hormonal therapy for gender affirmation versus cancer treatment and potential contraindications may be facilitated by the navigator.

8.6.1   Education About Side Effects and Hormonal Therapy

Because hormones impact all of the body, and most hormonal therapy requires a reduction in the hormone, these therapies can have diverse side effects. When hormonal levels are lowered, most men and women experience weight gain, a lack of energy, and less interest in sex [10]. As with all treatments and side effects, each patient can react differently, and not all patients develop the same side effects. Some side effects also differ by the patient's gender. For example, and according to the National Cancer Institute, common side effects for men or women who receive hormone therapy include hot flashes, libido changes, and fatigue [11]. Navigators can work with patients to assess side effects, which may change in type and severity over time. When side effects interfere with daily functioning, the oncology care team should be contacted to address the side effects that are problematic. Navigators can help followup and monitor, as well as find resources, schedule appointments for referral, and educate the patient and family about what is happening and why these side effects are occurring. Navigators can also provide strategies to reduce side effects. Examples are getting a cool pillow to sleep on that can diminish night sweats. There should also be a candid discussion about the potential impact of hormonal therapy on the patient's sexuality and intimacy. Lower libido, vaginal dryness, and pain during intercourse are common side effects reported by women receiving these drugs. These side effects can directly impact their relationship with their spouse/partner. Therefore, it is critical that the spouse/partner also be educated about the purpose of the drug, its side effects, and how to help diminish the impact on their relationship. When partners are unaware, patients may discontinue taking the drug in order to be able to resume full sexual activity as they were experiencing prior to their diagnosis.

There are some types of antidepressants that can interfere with the absorption and metabolism of hormonal therapy drugs. The medical oncologist should review the drug list with the patient to ensure this is not an issue. The navigator should reiterate this information and remind the patient that if their primary care provider considers placing the patient on an antidepressant in the future, a conversation must take place between the oncology provider and the community provider first.

8.7 Immunotherapy

Immunotherapy is a type of cancer treatment that helps the body's system fight cancer. The immune system helps the body fight infections and other diseases, and includes white blood cells, and organs and tissues of the lymph system. One reason that cancer cells thrive is because they are able to hide from the body's immune system. Certain immunotherapies can mark cancer cells, so it is feasible for the immune system to find and destroy them. Other immunotherapies boost the natural ability of the immune system by boosting the T-cells (a type of white blood cell) to work more efficiently against cancer. Thus, immunotherapy stimulates the patient's immune system to attack cancer cells and give the immune system man-made immune system proteins [12]. Immunotherapy can include treatment vaccines, which work differently than regular vaccines. Immunotherapy is delivered intravenously, orally (pills or capsules), topically (cream that is rubbed onto the skin), and intravesically (goes directly into the bladder). The schedule for where and how the patient receives immunotherapy treatments depends on the type of cancer and how advanced it is, the type of immunotherapy the patient receives, and how the patient's body reacts to treatment [13]. The patient may have treatment daily, weekly, or monthly. Some immunotherapies are given in cycles. A cycle is a period of treatment followed by a period of rest. The rest period gives the body a chance to recover, respond to the immunotherapy, and build new, healthy cells [13]. The National Cancer Institute has more information on different types of immunotherapies [14]. This too is a growing area of treatment innovations.

8.7.1   Education About the Side Effects from Immunotherapy

Immunotherapy can cause side effects, which affect patients in different ways. The side effects and how they make the patient feel will depend on how healthy the patient was prior to beginning treatment, the patient's type of cancer, how advanced it is, the type of therapy the patient is receiving, and the dose. Doctors and nurses cannot know for certain how well the patient will feel during treatment [13].

The most common side effects from immunotherapy are skin reactions at the injection site. Other side effects include pain, swelling, soreness, redness, rash, fever, fatigue, headache, blood pressure changes, and other side effects [15]. Immunotherapies may also cause severe or even fatal allergic reactions. However, these reactions are rare.

Immunotherapies are rapidly expanding, and many new clinical trials are creating and comparing immunotherapy regimens. The navigator should stay abreast regarding which new immunotherapies are available, either as standard state-of-the-art care or through clinical trials. Although side effects are less common for immunotherapy than for most chemotherapy treatments, the navigator and other oncology team members need to continuously reassess side effects. When any side effects interfere with the patient's daily functioning, the navigator should use the expertise of the oncology care team for solutions. The navigator can help followup and monitor, as well as find resources, schedule appointments for referral, and help educate both the patient and family members about what is happening and how to reduce the side effects. Patients for the most part are very enthused about this new drug category because it is using the body's own immune system to fight their cancer.

8.8   Stem Cell Transplant (Formerly Called Bone Marrow Transplant)

Cancer stem cell treatments use adult stem cells rather than embryonic stem cells. Embryonic stem cells are "totipotent" or have unlimited capability to develop into any body organ, but embryonic stem cell collection raises many ethical issues and rarely is allowed in the United States. Adult stem cells are more limited and called "pluripotent," or capable of creating most tissues of an organism. Adult stem cell transplants are used to treat leukemia, multiple myeloma, and some types of lymphoma. "Hematopoietic" stem cells are inside the bone marrow. These cells have the ability to divide for indefinite periods in culture and to grow into specialized cells (bone marrow, blood cells). These stem cells are usually collected from the blood, which is less painful than collecting stem cells from the bone marrow as in the past.

The main types of stem cell transplants are "autologous" transplant (the stem cells come from the patient's own body) and "allogeneic" (the stem cells come from another person's stem cells whose bone marrow matches that of the patient). Both processes are very complex and require many months of preparation followed by many months of healing and recovery. The preferred approach is using the patient's own cells (autologous) if possible. The individual's stem cells are collected and stored, prior to depleting much of the immune system using chemotherapy drugs. Members of the healthcare team who work with stem cell transplant compare it to preparing for a marathon. The patient attempts to get as healthy as possible prior to starting the process. For example, a few of the steps for autologous stem cell treatment include:

1. Chemotherapy is given, usually by infusion in the vein, for up to 10 days (usually as an outpatient) to stimulate the production of bone marrow stem cells and promote their release into the blood.
2. Mobilization is a process in which certain drugs are used to cause the movement of stem cells from the bone marrow into the blood.
3. Collection and storage (about 8-hour process but can be up to 4 days) refer to the stem cells being collected and stored. They may be used later to replace the bone marrow during a stem cell transplant or for future treatments. Some cells are frozen for later use (cryopreservation).
4. Conditioning treatments use chemotherapy for up to 11 days to kill or suppress immune cells throughout the body.
5. Hematopoietic stem cell transplant (HSCT) requires an individual to be hospitalized and the stored stem cells infused into the bloodstream along with antibiotics to fight infections.
6. Recovery in the hospital is required from 10 days up to 4 weeks for most patients, depending on how well the patient is doing while the immune system begins to rebuild itself in a relatively sterile environment, free of infectious agents. The immune system gradually rebuilds itself within 3 to 6 months.

Stem cell transplants differ greatly, and the navigator must make certain that any information discussed between the patient and navigator is relevant to the specific type of transplant the patient is scheduled to have. This is a very demanding treatment on the patient and family, and the navigator must repeatedly assess their stress, anxiety, depression, and barriers (e.g., fear of losing job once the treatment has been completed).

8.8.1 Education About Side Effects from Stem Cell Transplants

There are many side effects throughout the transplant procedures, all of which require the navigator to explain and educate the patient and family. Because there are large dosages of chemotherapy medications, nausea and vomiting are common. The provider can prescribe anti-nausea medications, but none are effective 100% of the time [16]. Of note, these medications must be administered *prior* to the patient feeling nauseous to be most effective. Because the navigator may be frequently working with poor, uninsured and underinsured patients, the navigator may need to provide solutions for the patient to receive these drugs free of charge.

Mucositis is a common side effect, for which the navigator should provide methods on how to manage. Risk of infections is a serious side effect. Patients' family members and loved ones want to visit, but anyone who has been exposed to infection (cold, flu) within the previous week must remain outside the hospital room, and those who enter need to wear surgical masks. These infections may be viral, bacterial, or fungal. Some infections, like *Cytomegalovirus* (CMV), are present in most people's bodies prior to transplant, but because the immune system is wiped out for most stem cell patients, about 90% of patients (particularly those who have allogenic rather than autologous stem cell transplant) experience the infection following the transplant because they have an insufficient or no immune system. CMV is a common herpesvirus infection that for most healthy people has no symptoms. For those weakened due to the transplant, fever and fatigue are the more common symptoms. Unfortunately, there are no effective treatments, and the patient has to live through the flare-up until the infection subsides on its own. The navigator also needs to help family and loved ones understand that the patient cannot have flowers and plants around them because they carry bacteria and fungi [16]. Similarly, once home the patient needs to avoid contact with animal droppings (e.g., cleaning a cat litter box or bird cage, or mucking a horse stall).

Overall, the patient is supposed to avoid petting their pets for a few months or longer, depending on how well the patient is recovering.

Bleeding (e.g., nosebleeds) may occur, in large part from the conditioning treatment that while destroying cancer cells also kills platelets that help blood to clot. These nosebleeds usually subside within 3 weeks of completing the treatments.

Pneumonitis is a type of lung inflammation that's most common in the first 100 days after transplant. But some lung problems can happen much later—even 2 or more years after transplant [16]. Although the patient is tired and may not want to get up and walk around, such activity increases lung volume and helps reduce the risk of pneumonia and other respiratory conditions.

For those who have the allogeneic transplant using another person's stem cells, the issue of rejection is always a concern. Graft-versus-host disease (GVHD) can be life-threatening, and the navigator must help the patient return to the hospital immediately. This can happen very quickly, and about one third of allogeneic transplant recipients develop acute (10–90 days following transplant) GVHD. Symptoms are summarized in Table 8.4 [16].

The medical provider prescribes drugs to treat acute GVHD.

Chronic GVHD is more severe and can occur from 90 to 600 days following the stem cell transplant. Table 8.5 summarizes chronic GVHD side effects [16].

Depending on the degree of immediacy, the navigator can help the patient obtain timely appointments as needed.

Table 8.4 American Cancer Society acute GVHD side effects

- Rash
- Burning and redness of the skin on the palms and soles; can spread over the entire body
- Nausea
- Vomiting
- Stomach cramps
- Diarrhea (watery and sometimes bloody)
- Loss of appetite
- Yellowing of the skin and eyes (jaundice)
- Abdominal (belly) pain
- Weight loss

Table 8.5 American Cancer Society chronic GVHD side effects

- Rash on hands or soles of the feet (itchy and dry)
- Fever
- Decreased appetite
- Diarrhea
- Abdominal (belly) cramps
- Weight loss
- Yellowing of the skin and eyes (jaundice)
- Enlarged liver
- Bloated abdomen (belly)
- Pain in the upper right part of the abdomen (belly)
- Increased levels of liver enzymes in the blood (seen on blood tests)
- The skin feels tight
- Dry, burning eyes
- Dryness or painful sores in the mouth
- Burning sensations when eating acidic foods
- Bacterial infections
- Blockages in the smaller airways of the lungs

8.9   The Role of the Navigator on the Multidisciplinary Treatment Team

Cancer treatments require a diverse multidisciplinary group of medical providers (e.g., medical oncologists, nurses, surgeons, nurse navigators, radiation oncologists, etc.) and support (oncology social workers, navigators, pathologist, social workers, clergy, etc.). Although each specializes in a different aspect of the patient's care, they must work as a cohesive team in order for the patient to receive the full benefit from each individual. Coordination of care within a fragmented healthcare system today is more challenging than ever. This is another important component that navigators can provide not just to the patient but on behalf of the multidisciplinary team, serving as the continuous link across the continuum of care for the patient and providers as well as facilitating communication and promoting efficient delivery of care. Because it is rare today that all cancer consultations, tests, and treatments would happen within the same facility, helping to ensure the patient doesn't fall through the cracks has become another important role for the navigator to fulfill for the patient and the treatment team.

8.9.1   General Guidance for Patients Prior to Starting Any Cancer Treatment

Prior to treatment, the navigator can help the patient review sample questions and select which ones to ask the provider. These questions also may stimulate additional questions the patient or family members would like to have answered about the treatment [2, 17]. The navigator can encourage the patient to stay as healthy as possible, before, during, and following treatments. Examples of how navigators can support patients prior to treatment are included in Table 8.6. These examples are not all-inclusive but are merely examples to emphasize the diverse role navigators play in supporting patients diagnosed with cancer. Note that there may be different professionals serving the navigation role, depending on the barriers or challenges a patient faces.

Table 8.6 Examples of navigator interventions to support patients prior to beginning treatment

Patient barriers and challenges	Navigation interventions	Cautions and recommendations	Potential navigator types
Alcohol abuse	Navigators can find resources to help patients address alcohol disorders. Because chemotherapy and alcohol both target the liver, mitigation of alcohol consumption may help optimize patient outcomes		Social worker Patient navigator Nurse navigator
Completing paperwork, including documenting advance directives, wills, and last rites (for patients with advanced cancer) [18]	The navigator can make copies of the patient's records or a summary of the patient's information (e.g., insurance number, tribal enrollment number). Some patients may feel they have little or nothing to leave behind to surviving family and friends. However, most patients probably have family heirlooms, jewelry, artwork, regalia, or other items. It can be helpful to loved ones for the patient to document their wishes in writing. The navigator can assist the patient with completing paperwork if the patient is unable to complete it	A legal representative should be engaged to clarify legal language, and a notary will be needed to notarize the documents. When uncertain who to contact for legal guidance, the oncology social worker is likely to know	Patient navigator Nurse navigator Social worker

(continued)

Table 8.6 (continued)

Patient barriers and challenges	Navigation interventions	Cautions and recommendations	Potential navigator types
Employment issues	The patient often is still working when diagnosed with cancer. The navigator can work with the patient to identify employer leave options. The navigator should make copies of all documents to appeal any initial rejections	Employment protections include the Family and Medical Leave Act, Workers Compensation, Americans with Disabilities Act, and employer-sponsored paid or unpaid leave. If appeals are needed, the oncology social worker is a resource for other navigators	Patient navigator Nurse navigator Social worker
Emotional support	The navigator can encourage the patient to invite family over to visit before the patient goes to the hospital. Playing and talking with children and grandchildren may help the patient find internal strength to focus on treatment. Family may help the patient feel stronger. They may make the patient laugh and remind him/her how important it is to stay well to be able to teach and enjoy the next generation	Depending on the type of treatment, both adults and children who have illness symptoms (runny nose) may need to stay away from patients who are highly susceptible to infection following treatment (e.g., stem cell transplant)	Patient navigator Nurse navigator Social worker
Lodging	If the hospital is several hours from the home, the navigator can help the patient and family find affordable lodging. This is particularly important if the patient is scheduled to check in very early in the morning (e.g., 6:30 a.m.)	Many hospitals or their related charities can help pay for the hotel (see the financial resources under the "Tools" chapter)	Patient navigator Social worker
Life goals	The navigator should ask the patient about their life goals so that these can be incorporated into the treatment planning process whenever possible. These life goals (e.g., having a family, getting a promotion at work, studying to be a concert pianist) can then be preserved (e.g., by arranging for referral to fertility preservation team, radiation treatments scheduled before or after work, avoidance of chemotherapy agents that cause the side effect of peripheral neuropathy)	For patients with advanced, metastatic cancer, it is still important to know the patient's life goals and work with the patient to develop alternative ways to fulfill them in the future after the patient dies (e.g., having cards for young children when they reach specific milestones in their lives as teens and adults such as high school graduation, marriage, when the child has a first child)	Nurse navigator Social worker

(continued)

Table 8.6 (continued)

Patient barriers and challenges	Navigation interventions	Cautions and recommendations	Potential navigator types
Nutrition	Navigators can help find resources to support patient nutrition throughout treatment, such as food and supplements [19]	Navigators can help the patient discuss with the provider and members of the treatment team before starting a vitamin regimen	Patient navigator Social worker Nurse navigator
Physical activity support	Physical activity can help strengthen the patient before, during, and after treatment. Navigators can help patients find activities compatible with their lifestyles and interests	Be sure to check with the healthcare team before having the patient start an exercise regimen. Referral to a cancer rehabilitation program for prehabilitation and rehabilitation is ideal if accessible	Patient Navigator Social worker Nurse navigator
Spiritual support	Some patients may wish to renew spiritual activities. Navigators can support patients who prioritize spirituality. Referrals to clergy or other spiritual counseling resources are appropriate and may need to be brought in and out as the cancer progresses	There are times that the patient may be angry with God or a family member may express this, which may be the opposite of the feelings of the patient. This can trigger the need for family counseling by a spiritual advisor. Anger should be expected	Patient navigator Social worker Nurse navigator
Tobacco cessation	Tobacco interferes with cancer treatment success. Navigators can help patients find affordable cessation programs		Patient navigator Social worker Nurse navigator
Understanding insurance coverage	The navigator or a family member can contact the patient's insurance company (only if the patient was unable or unwilling to do so) to learn what is and is not covered by the health insurance policy. Oncology social workers and/or financial counselors can often find resources to help the patient get medications and treatments that may initially feel out of the patient's reach	The navigator needs to have HIPAA approval prior to contacting the insurance company on the patient's behalf	Patient navigator Social worker Financial counselor

8.10 General Guidelines About Educating Patients About the Importance of Adherence to Treatments

The navigator serves a critical role in supporting patient adherence to cancer treatment. To benefit most from cancer treatment, the patient needs to follow their healthcare team's recommendations. Patients may not understand all the information given to them by their oncology providers. The nurse navigator can help reiterate this medical information in ways to make it more understandable. The patient may need to take multiple medications, for example, but in different amounts and at different times of the day. This can be very confusing. Navigators can help the patient understand the purpose of the medications and create a reliable way for the patient to remember to take the medications as prescribed. For example, if the provider says to take a pill four times a day, it may not be clear if that means taking all four doses while awake through the day or if the medication is to be spaced out further and taken also during the night hours.

Maintaining their appointment schedule is also crucial. Patients need to understand why radiation is given daily, for example, and that appointments should not be missed. Without this type of vital patient education, there is risk that the patient may not receive their treatments in keeping with standards of care.

8.11 The Navigator's Role in Ensuring Access to Quality Cancer Care

Although quality cancer care is covered in a different chapter, it is worthwhile to restate here the importance of the navigator, whether patient navigator or nurse navigator, to serve as the patient advocate enabling the patient to get timely access to care without bias or cultural or racial discrimination. The following are examples of how barriers to care directly impact the patient's quality of care.

8.11.1 Case Study

Shirley, an American Indian woman from Texas (see Fig. 8.1), was involved with the Native American Cancer Research (NACR) Corporation Native Sister (patient navigation) program since 2003, when she was diagnosed with stage 4 breast cancer and given a 3-month prognosis. Shirley was denied care four times and attempted to obtain cancer care services three times prior to contacting NACR. The NACR staff (three Native Sisters) documented more than 200 hours helping her and her family from 2003 to 2005. The Texas Breast and Cervical Cancer Early Detection Program had to join the fight to help her obtain care. Her tribe is very poor, but provided her ~$500 in total. Shirley moved in with her daughter and family in Denver early in

Fig. 8.1 Shirley with her loving daughter Niko 2 days prior to her passing, June 25, 2007. *The Wall Street Journal*, July 2007

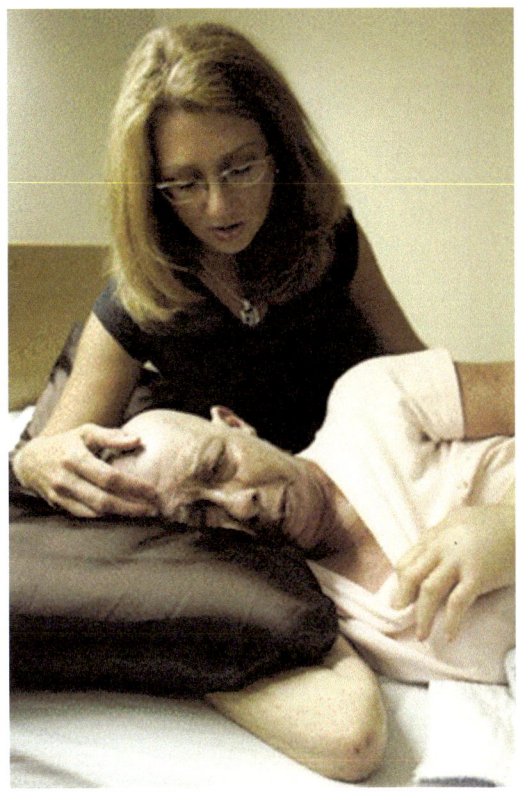

2004 with the help of NACR's Memorial Fund, which provides help to cancer patients and their families. Shirley started improving. Early in June 2007, NACR was contacted by a journalist from *The Wall Street Journal* who was doing a story on what happens to people who "fall between the cracks" of the National Breast and Cervical Cancer Early Detection Program. NACR contacted Niko, Shirley's daughter, to find out if she and her mother were interested in taking part. Niko said she was very interested and that her mom had moved back to Texas and was in a nursing home. The journalist flew to Texas to meet Shirley and Niko and interviewed them both. Shirley "walked on" (passed) on Monday, June 25, 2007. *The Wall Street Journal* used this photo taken on June 23, 2007, in their article. This very strong Native woman easily surpassed the 3-month prognosis with the help of the Native Sisters and her loving family. So when a patient is given a 3-month prognosis, how does the cancer program estimate how many navigators and hours will be needed? Obviously, this is a very difficult and dynamic question but also a very important one in determining value-based cancer care.

8.11.2 Barriers During Treatment

Access Barriers

- Individual
- Provider
- System
- Cultural
  - Case study clinical barriers are more subtle but equally condescending and disrespectful, such as the minority patient who waits for appointments and watches Caucasians being called for appointments when their scheduled times were much later than the minority patient's appointment. Other barriers are due to a lack of listening to the patient or asking relevant questions. A healthcare provider kept asking a two-spirited woman (lesbian) if her husband approved of her pursuing care that could affect her fertility. The woman already had four children and was in the same lesbian relationship for over 15 years. Cultural issues can become barriers unless there is a qualified community or cultural patient navigator available to help the patient. For example, a healthcare provider who was new to Alaska automatically recommended that Alaska Native patients receive the standard fecal occult blood test (FOBT) for colorectal cancer early detection. However, about 75% of Alaska Natives have *Helicobacter pylori* (*H. pylori*) infection [20], which has symptoms of blood in the stools. Almost all the patients the new provider saw were being referred for colonoscopies because the FOBT showed blood in the stools. The nurse navigator patiently explained to the provider that due to the excessive proportion of *H. pylori*, other colorectal cancer screening tests were recommended. Then the nurse provided the physician with the Centers for Disease Control and Prevention brochure on colorectal cancer among Alaska Natives (Fig. 8.2).

Assessment

- Individual—CoC standard for distress screening: Distress Thermometer as assessment tool at different time points
  - Practical challenges
    Resources for support
  - Physical distress
    Resources for support
  - Psychosocial distress
    Resources for support
- Provider: communication, bias

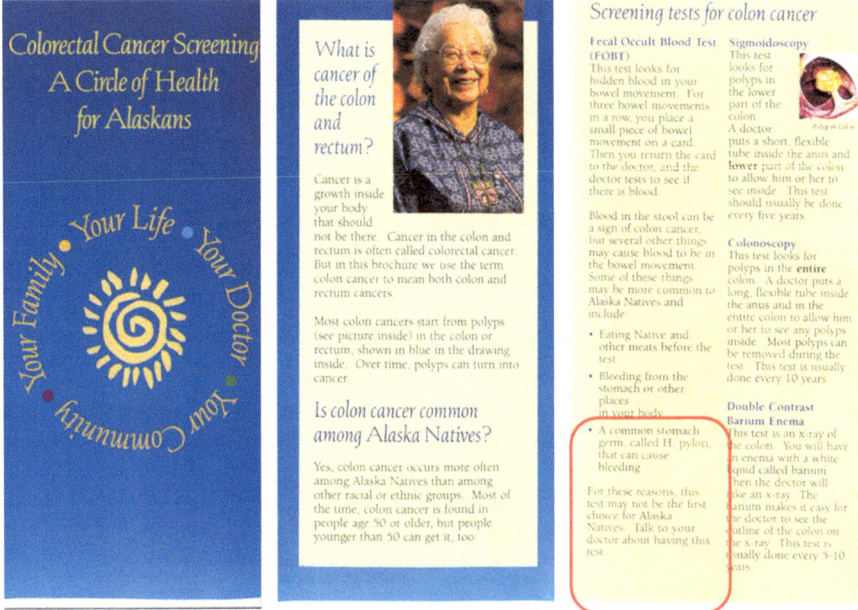

Fig. 8.2 Panel excerpts from CDC Alaska Native CRC brochure

- *Case study*: Clinical barriers sometimes are best identified by community patient navigators rather than staff internal to the clinical setting. For example, an American Indian woman for whom English was her second language was taking a long time (according to the nurse) in responding to the clinic's intake questions. The patient was frightened and needed the English translated into her primary language. She also wanted to think about how she should answer the nurse performing the intake, and then translate the response back into English. The nurse became frustrated, closed the curtain around the bed where the woman was sitting, and said in normal volume of voice, "She must be drunk. She's an Indian and they're all alcoholics. I can't finish this intake!" Obviously, the curtain did not provide any soundproofing, and the patient heard the response. She removed the hospital gown for examination, put on her clothes, and never returned to the facility. A single inept clinician can permanently damage the clinic-community trust and relationship. In this instance, the community patient navigator came to the woman's house and talked with her about the symptoms and concerns she had, never referring to the event that occurred at the hospital. The community patient navigator helped the woman pursue care through a different healthcare facility, 45 minutes farther away, but the staff were more respectful than at the initial clinic.
- System: navigator and other tools for assessments

8.12 Conclusion

Navigators are integral members of the multidisciplinary team. Because it is common for cancer treatment to involve multiple different modalities over time, it is vital that there be at least one member of the oncology team who remains in touch and supports the patient before, during, and following the completion of each phase of treatment. The navigator is the ideal team member for this role.

Patient and family education is a principal role for the navigator to perform; this education helps the patient to more confidently engage in the decision-making about the treatment they agree to receive. It also helps promote adherence to care.

There are myriad ways navigators support patients. Only a few were described in this chapter; however, others are described elsewhere within this book.

When someone is diagnosed with cancer, they commonly have many other things already going on in their life: work, family, and future life goals they are looking forward to achieving. The navigator can help educate the oncology team about these issues so that the patient is treated in a way that preserves their life goals and addresses personal and family issues, and thus receives patient-centered care.

8.13 Resources

Several websites provide information about cancer treatments, their side effects, recovery, survivorship, and quality of life. These include but are not limited to:

- The American Cancer Society (ACS). www.cancer.org
- The National Cancer Institute (NCI). www.cancer.gov
- The American Society of Clinical Oncology (ASCO). www.cancer.net and www.asco.org
- Cancer*Care*. www.cancercare.org
- National Center for Biotechnology Information (NCBI). www.ncbi.nlm.nih.gov
- The National Library of Medicine®. www.nlm.nih.gov/databases/databases_cancer.html
- Native American Cancer Research Corporation. www.NatAmCancer.org

8.14 Case Study: Chuck, Comanche Nation, and Colorectal Cancer Patient

8.14.1 Introduction

Chuck is an enrolled member of the Comanche Nation. He is 55 years old and of normal weight, has type II diabetes, and is a smoker and a recovered alcoholic (sober for 13 years). He was diagnosed with colorectal cancer. Chuck was treated for 3 months with bevacizumab (Avastin), irinotecan hydrochloride (includes

FOLFIRI, folinic acid, and 5-FU), and cetuximab, but his cancer had metastasized. He was successfully enrolled in the National Cancer Institute clinical trial NCT01079780. This trial was to determine whether giving cetuximab and irinotecan hydrochloride together was more effective with or without ramucirumab (Cyramza).

8.14.2 Background Situation

Chuck joined a cancer support group, but the distance made attending difficult, and the members were not Native. He started meeting with a few local Comanche Nation cancer survivors at one of their homes. Their support group is informal, but the three men help one another. They call the community patient navigator on the toll-free number in Denver when they need additional information. The community patient navigator contacts the nurse navigator when the information the three men need or want constitutes medical advice.

Chuck had a lot of fatigue, weakness, dizziness, nausea, vomiting, and severe headaches prior to joining the clinical trial. The headaches and dizziness were of issue because Chuck's work as a ranch hand was conducted on horseback and he fell a few times. Similarly, he had to stop work many times during the day in attempts to calm the nausea and to find a bush where he could vomit. Chuck was attempted to remain stoic throughout these symptoms, but the men in his support group insisted he get help. They called the community patient navigator and talked with him via conference call during one of their support group gatherings, and Lance said he would talk with Betty, the nurse navigator, to get her involved.

8.14.3 Clinical Challenge

The nurse navigator created a schedule to talk with Chuck's wife to confirm when and how he was taking his medication to keep his blood pressure in normal ranges. She did this the first 3 weeks that Chuck was enrolled in the clinical trial. He complained about the side effects during the trial and had difficulty recovering from a wound he incurred from a horse fall (he fell on a tree stump and had a deep cut on his shin that would not heal).

8.14.4 Clinical Solution

The nurse navigator talked with, the clinical trial nurse coordinator, and they worked on a wound management protocol. A volunteer nurse agreed to drive out to the ranch and show Chuck and his wife how to care for the wound. She traveled once each week to check on the healing for Chuck's wound because he could not miss any more work at the ranch.

8.14.5 Clinical Challenge

The clinical trial uses ramucirumab; common (10%–29% of users) side effects include high blood pressure, diarrhea, and headache. Chuck was enrolled in the trial in spite of his poorly managed high blood pressure. Of note, the dizziness and nausea side effects were lessened once Chuck was in the clinical trial. Chuck continued to have headaches but less severe than prior to the clinical trial.

8.14.6 Patient Challenge

However, Chuck continued to experience a lot of weakness and fatigue. He had difficulty grooming his horse prior to starting work on the ranch each day. His comments describing the weakness were "I had to sit down two to three times while brushing my horse. Then I had to carry my saddle from the tack room to set on a tie rail. Next, I'd need to move my horse to the tie bar so that I could lift the saddle, rotate around, and heave it onto my horse's back. Luckily, my horse stands real still because I'd have to lean against the tie rail or sit on the ground before I was able to cinch the girth. This whole process took about an hour, whereas it used to take 10 minutes before I was in cancer treatment. This meant I had to get to the ranch a lot earlier. After the saddle was cinched up, I'd have to rest before I got the bridle from the tack room and put it on my horse. I'd rest, lead him over to a mounting block, and get on. Then I'd have to just sit in the saddle and catch my breath…."

8.14.7 Community Solution

"…The Indian guys I work with would get on me about acting like a woman … all of it in fun until I finally told them I was in cancer treatment. Then my buddy Cal started grooming my horse and saddling him before I even got to the ranch. That was real nice."

8.14.8 Solutions by the Team

Chuck called the community patient navigator early in May and asked him how long the weakness and tiredness were going to last and if there was anything he could do to feel better. The community patient navigator explained that some fatigue could last as long as 2 years, occasionally even longer, but that it would gradually get better. In the meantime, the community patient navigator said he would contact the nurse navigator to get her medical advice and assistance for additional medications that may help. Because Chuck was in the clinical trial, the nurse navigator had to talk with the clinical trial nurse. The clinical trial nurse reached out to the dietitian for help with the fatigue and also contacted the clinical trial lead physician for a recommendation of medication to alleviate the fatigue symptoms. The nurse navigator talked with Chuck and scheduled a follow-up appointment with her, the dietitian, and the clinical trial nurse to work on strategies to address his issues. During the appointment, the dietitian helped Chuck and his wife understand the importance of high-iron and nutrient-rich foods and supplements. Both were willing to improve his diet but could not afford these foods. The nurse navigator called to find out if the oncology social worker was available and could help with a food supplement program. The appointment lasted 4 hours, but by the end, Chuck and his wife drove home with new prescription medication to lessen the fatigue symptoms, dietary supplements free of charge, and food discount coupons to use for shopping at the local market. His wife cooked, and Chuck ate the high-iron, nutritious foods.

8.14.9 Community Challenge and Solutions

By July, Chuck was not yet strong enough to dance in the pow wow, but his family and friends danced for him. The community patient navigator also came down to Comanche Nation and danced and prayed for Chuck. Following the pow wow, Chuck took part in three traditional Indian ceremonies with the help of his family and friends throughout the rest of the summer. Because the community patient navigator also was Comanche and involved with Chuck's care, he took part in one of the traditional ceremonies.

By the following year, Chuck was strong enough to dance again (only a few slower dances and widely spaced intervals in between dances). Chuck continues to work on the ranch and gradually returned to performing part-time construction jobs around the community (he could not do this work for 18 months following the completion of his chemotherapy). He is enjoying his family, friends, and community activities, and he talks openly about his cancer experience now, but only when asked. A common concept presented by Chuck when talking with others is the Creator gives us the strength to have this journey and helps us reorganize our priorities to enable us to become more involved in our families and our communities. The cancer and the treatments are very hard, but through our traditions and guidance of the Creator, we become well again.

8.14.10   Implications

Chuck's quality of life was greatly impacted by the side effects of his cancer treatment. Because of the help from the community patient navigator, nurse navigator, clinical trial nurse coordinator, the physician (to prescribe fatigue medications), the dietitian (to help Chuck and his wife with a high-iron and nutrient dietary plan), the oncology social worker (for inexpensive and free food supplements), the traditional Indian healer (for cleansing and spiritual ceremonies), and his local male support group, Chuck struggled through the side effects to gradually be strong enough to work on the ranch without help from his friends, take part in cultural activities (ceremonies and pow wow dancing and praying), and improve his relationships with his family and friends.

References

1. Willis LA, Reed E, Pratt-Chapman M, Kapp H, Hatcher E, Vaitones V, Collins S, Bires J, Washington E. Development of a framework for patient navigation: delineating roles across navigator types. J Oncol Navig Surviv. 2013;4:20–6.
2. Morra M, Potts E. Choices. New York: Avon Books; 1994.
3. www.NatAmCancer.org.
4. http://natamcancer.org/page80.html.
5. www.cancer.org/content/cancer/en/treatment/treatments-and-side-effects/treatment-types/radiation/basics.html.
6. www.cancer.org/content/cancer/en/search.html?q=targeted+therapies.
7. www.cancer.gov/about-cancer/treatment/types/targeted-therapies/targeted-therapies-fact-sheet.
8. www.merckmanuals.com/home/hormonal-and-metabolic-disorders/biology-of-the-endocrine-system/endocrine-function.
9. www.cancer.gov/about-cancer/treatment/types/hormone-therapy.
10. www.webmd.com/women/rm-quiz-secret-life-of-hormones.
11. www.cancer.gov/about-cancer/treatment/types/hormone-therapy#HTCCSE.
12. www.cancer.org/treatment/treatments-and-side-effects/treatment-types/immunotherapy/what-is-immunotherapy.html.
13. www.cancer.gov/about-cancer/treatment/types/immunotherapy.
14. National Cancer Institute. Immunotherapy. 2017. www.cancer.gov/research/areas/treatment/immunotherapy-using-immune-system.
15. National Cancer Institute. Immunotherapy. 2017. www.cancer.gov/about-cancer/treatment/types/immunotherapy.
16. www.cancer.org/treatment/treatments-and-side-effects/treatment-types/stem-cell-transplant/transplant-side-effects.html.
17. http://natamcancer.org/page51.html.
18. http://natamcancer.org/page49.html.
19. www.webmd.com/diet/features/cancer-supplements#1.
20. Parkinson AJ, Gold BD, Bulkow L, Wainwright RB, Swaminathan B, Khanna B, Peterson KM, Fitzgerald MA. High prevalence of Helicobacter pylori in the Alaska Native Population and Association with low serum ferritin levels in young adults. Clin Diagn Lab Immunol. 2000;7(6):885–8.

Transition to Survivorship

9

Pamela Goetz and Jennifer R. Klemp

9.1 Defining Survivorship Care

The terms "survivorship" and "survivorship care" are intrinsically linked with the label "cancer survivor." According to the National Coalition for Cancer Survivorship (NCCS), which defined the term, a person is a survivor from the point of a cancer diagnosis through the balance of life [1].

As the oldest survivor-led cancer advocacy organization, NCCS sought to change the image of a person with cancer from "victim" to "survivor." To help change this perception, NCCS identified the skills needed to navigate a cancer diagnosis and developed patient resources to teach these skills. Finding information, communicating, decision-making, problem-solving, negotiating, and advocating for one's rights are the six essential elements that patients can utilize to incorporate their preferences and goals into their care and in some way, gain some control as they face a life-threatening illness. Although often challenging to achieve, when patients are able to identify as, and are recognized as, the central member of their care team, they become more adherent to treatment, have less decisional regret, and have greater satisfaction with their care. This is the ultimate form of patient engagement. Patient engagement during treatment can result in more effective symptom management, improved adherence to recommended treatment, and improved outcomes. Patient engagement in survivorship care supports the survivor in managing

P. Goetz, BA, OPN-CG (✉)
Oncology Survivorship Navigator, Center for Patient and Family Services, Sibley Memorial Hospital, Johns Hopkins Medicine, Washington, DC, USA
e-mail: pgoetz4@jhmi.edu

J. R. Klemp, PhD, MPH, MA
Associate Professor of Medicine, Division of Clinical Oncology Director, Cancer Survivorship Cancer Risk and Genetic Counseling, The University of Kansas Cancer Center, Westwood, KS, USA
e-mail: jklemp@kumc.edu

© Springer International Publishing AG, part of Springer Nature 2018
L. D. Shockney (ed.), *Team-Based Oncology Care: The Pivotal Role of Oncology Navigation*, https://doi.org/10.1007/978-3-319-69038-4_9

posttreatment care, in identifying late effects of treatment, and/or with ongoing maintenance therapy. An engaged patient does not play a passive role in treatment, but is actively involved in planning the care and in behaviors leading to improved outcomes.

Nurse and patient (lay) navigators serve an important role within a cancer care team, during diagnosis, treatment, and survivorship care. They provide care coordination; assess patients' medical, psychological, and practical needs; address barriers to care; provide education; and refer to and coordinate access to services and specialists. Because cancer care is complicated and patients require multiple treatment modalities with providers often in more than one location or geography, the navigator serves as a quarterback, guiding the patient along the path of care. The navigator is responsible for supporting physician-directed care by assessing patient needs, including side effect management, emotional or spiritual distress, transportation needs, and insurance or financial issues, just to name a few. Patients experience many of these challenges beyond active treatment, and so the role of the navigator continues into the phase of cancer survivorship care.

9.2   Trajectory and Changing Patient Needs

Cancer survivorship includes several phases. Acute survivorship is the period from diagnosis through active treatment. Extended survivorship occurs in the period just after primary treatment ends and is referred to as the transition from active treatment. Permanent or long-term survivorship is the last phase that extends through the balance of life. In 1985, cancer survivor and physician Fitzhugh Mullan, MD, wrote an article published in *The New England Journal of Medicine* entitled "Seasons of survival: reflections of a physician with cancer" where he discussed the concepts of cure, survival, and how the stages of survival affect patients physically and emotionally [2]. In his essay, Dr. Mullan suggested that survivorship is not one condition, but many. He described how, as he was going through the acute survivorship stage, he faced the physical and mental challenges of the disease and treatment, and the particular joys of being a new father. Surviving cancer was not just managing the disease, but also living his life. As a strategy for addressing the distinct needs of cancer survivors, Dr. Mullan argued for dedicated research focused on survivorship. He also recommended that patients speak up to raise awareness about their experiences and to engage in building a cancer survivorship network.

Cancer presents patients with multiple challenges during treatment and along the path to recovery, which demands adaptation and personalization. A cancer diagnosis most often comes without warning and thrusts the patient into a life-threatening situation. The patient faces a new reality that requires a new vocabulary, learning about the disease, decision-making about providers and treatments, and anticipating how this may affect work, family, finances, and personal life. The period before treatment starts can be confusing and scary as the patient undergoes biopsies, imaging, and other predictive and prognostic testing [3]. Once treatment starts, the busy schedule of medical appointments serves to organize and focus the patient from one treatment modality to the next.

For patients treated with curative intent, primary treatment will include evidence-based cancer care or participation in a clinical trial that may consist of surgery, radiation therapy, and adjuvant or neo-adjuvant chemotherapy, sometimes with adjuvant treatment prescribed to reduce risk of recurrence. Patients with advanced cancer have ongoing cancer survivorship needs, where the cancer is treated as a chronic illness with ongoing monitoring and/or treatment and often the option of participation in a clinical trial. During the acute phase of care, patients focus on making decisions about providers and treatment, overcoming barriers to care (transportation, financial costs, insurance coverage, etc.), problem-solving around work and family responsibilities, and managing the side effects of treatment. And as Dr. Mullan pointed out, the cancer experience takes place in the context of other aspects of a person's life, which may be providing additional stressors or support and joy.

Navigators are key to supporting patients during the acute stage of survivorship. Nurse and patient (lay) navigators can provide support to improve quality of life and to coordinate care for patients regardless of the stage of disease. During the acute stage, navigators provide education, assess medical and psychological needs, coordinate care, make appropriate referrals, and connect patients with resources. Providers and other staff are focused on their scope of practice and their role within the cancer care team. The navigator advocates and guides the patient and their caregivers through the various treatment modalities and views the overall trajectory. Navigators can assist with patient goal setting and advocate with the care team for the inclusion of patient preferences in the cancer and supportive care plan. In this role, the navigator can provide useful information and perspective about the patient to the team in tumor boards, clinical rounds, disease working groups, and the outpatient clinic. Documentation of their actions and communication with the patient are critical elements of the patient's medical record. The following describes the role of navigation during the acute phase of survivorship.

9.3   Navigation During Acute Phase of Survivorship

- Provide education to the patient and their caregivers
  - Define complicated medical terms and ensure an understanding of the diagnosis.
  - Educate patients about the treatment plan, required providers, imaging, prognostic and predictive testing, etc.
  - Guide patients from one treatment modality to the next.
- Remove barriers of access to care
  - Facilitate/coordinate appointments.
  - Address insurance questions and link with financial support programs.
  - Address finances, employment, concerns surrounding disability, and other insurance questions.
  - Assess and facilitate supportive care needs including referrals to social work, psycho-oncology, psychiatry, and support groups.
  - Assess and facilitate transportation and logistics.

- View the patient as a whole person, including assessment, management, and referral
  - Engage the patient to define life and treatment goals, preferences, and realistic hopes for the future.
  - Identify cultural and/or sexual identity preferences.
  - Assess health literacy.
  - Identify patients who would benefit from pre-habilitation and cancer rehabilitation.
  - Assess and refer to oncology dietitian.
  - Assess and refer to palliative care for side effect management and care across the balance of life.
  - Administer or facilitate distress screening and make appropriate referrals.
  - Refer to integrative health and mind-body programs such as resilience training, acupuncture, yoga, meditation, Reiki, and expressive art therapies.

9.3.1 Transition of Care: Distress Screening

As patients transition along their cancer care trajectory, there are several "tools" that are helpful, and also part of national accreditation standards, that foster risk stratification of patient/caregiver needs.

9.3.2 Distress Screening or Completing a Comprehensive Needs Assessment

Assessment of physical, psychosocial, practical/financial, and existential needs is considered an essential part of cancer care. As outlined by the Institute of Medicine (IOM) of the National Academy of Sciences [4] and the National Comprehensive Cancer Network (NCCN) Guidelines, [5] there are numerous sources of psychosocial distress associated with cancer and its treatment. These sources of distress may include a lack of information or skills necessary to manage their cancer; emotional problems, such as anxiety and depression; a lack of transportation or other resources; and disruptions to work, school, and family, and are believed to contribute to poor adherence to prescribed treatments and a slower return to health. The main goal of screening is to maximize access to medical and supportive care for patients and their caregivers. Provider engagement in the screening process helps to identify current issues or risk factors and barriers that may prevent or hinder access to care. The cancer care team should identify, monitor, document, and manage distress across all phases of survivorship. It is considered best practice to address the psychosocial health needs of cancer patients and survivors, and to provide adequate psychosocial health services. However, cancer care teams do not consistently identify, manage, or refer patients and survivors to services that could address their physical and psychosocial needs. A comprehensive distress screening or needs assessment not only assists in the identification of unmet needs, but can foster communication between the cancer care team and the patient/survivor [6]. There are numerous examples of screeners available and one of the most commonly referenced is the NCCN Distress Thermometer and Problem List [7]. The patient will rank their level of distress over the past week on a 10-point scale, from "No Distress" to "Extreme Distress." This tool is a single snapshot of distress that requires context. The supplemental Problem List allows patients to indicate problems they have experienced in the past week and elaborates on the level of overall distress. It is important to complete a baseline assessment and then to readminister the screener at defined time points, especially at times of transition, when anxiety and uncertainty may be heightened. In addition, it is important that whatever tools are utilized that documentation be completed in the electronic health record, a "circle of care" be documented indicating if the issue was managed, a referral was made, or the patient declined follow-up. Furthermore, if a domain or need is assessed, the team must have a follow-up option in place for the patient/survivor. It is poor practice to identify a patient/survivor need and not have an evidence based management strategy or adequate referral source as a next step. To manage both patient/survivor and care team needs, a screening process should be defined and a workflow mapped out at various stages of the cancer control continuum.

9.4   Extended Survivorship (Transition from Active Treatment)

With improvements in early detection and advances in treatment, patients are living longer through and beyond cancer. As of January 1, 2016, the American Cancer Society reported that there are nearly 15.5 million cancer survivors living with or through their disease in the United States, with estimates of 20 million by 2026 [3]. Based on current data, 67% of all cancer patients will live 5 years after diagnosis [8]. Surviving cancer and its treatment leaves patients with ongoing medical and psychological care needs. With the increasing number of cancer survivors, research on this distinct phase of survivorship has increased, offering insights on the patient experience and evidence on best practices in care delivery. In 2005, the Institute of Medicine published the consensus report, "From Cancer Patient to Cancer Survivor: Lost in Translation" [9], noting the increasing number of cancer survivors and lack of awareness about the impact that cancer and its treatment have on the medical, functional, and psychosocial aspects of their lives. The report defined quality health-care and made recommendations on how to improve survivors' quality of life through best practices and policies.

The report's key recommendation was that healthcare professionals should provide a survivorship care plan (SCP) to patients completing treatment. A survivorship care plan is a document that describes the patient's diagnosis, including pathology, genetic/genomic testing, and the cancer care team, and a complete treatment summary (surgery, chemotherapy, immunotherapy, hormone therapy, and radiation) and spells out follow-up guidelines, based on late effects of treatment and well-person care, including imaging, testing, follow-up appointments, and referrals. The survivorship care plan also makes lifestyle behavior recommendations to reduce risk of recurrence and prevent of second cancers.

Typically, a member of the cancer care team, specifically an advanced practice provider, a physician (oncologist, physician, radiation oncologist), or a certified navigator, reviews the survivorship care plan with the patient, discusses management of any late and long-term effects of cancer treatment (see Table 9.1), and outlines the evidence-based follow-up plan for surveillance. The IOM (Institute of Medicine) recommends that a copy of the survivorship care plan is shared with the survivor and the primary care provider to facilitate coordination of care regarding cancer surveillance and the patient's other healthcare needs. There are many SCP

Table 9.1 Late and long-term effects of cancer

Treatment type	Late and long-term effects
Chemotherapy/immunotherapy	Cardiotoxicity/heart problems
	Cataracts/vision changes
	Cognitive impairment
	Endocrine dysfunction
	Early menopause/menopausal symptoms
	Fatigue
	Increased risk of recurrence and second cancers
	Infertility
	Liver problems
	Lung problems
	Mouth/jaw problems
	Nerve damage
	Osteoporosis
	Pain
	Rash
	Reduced lung capacity
Radiation therapy	Cataracts
	Cavities and tooth decay
	Fatigue
	Heart and vascular problems
	Hypothyroidism
	Increased risk of other cancers
	Infertility
	Intestinal problems
	Lung disease
	Lymphedema
	Memory problems
	Osteoporosis
	Pain
	Skin changes
Surgery	Disfigurement/body image issues
	Fatigue
	Lymphedema
	Mobility problems
	Pain

examples and templates available and most accreditation standards are fulfilled by including the data elements included in the ASCO SCP templates [10]. It is important that these elements be incorporated into the electronic health record. Unfortunately, to date, there is little evidence demonstrating the value of a survivorship care plan but active research is underway.

9.5 Navigation During the Transitional Phase of Survivorship

The specific type of cancer and stage of disease drive the goals of care and define whether treatment will be delivered with curative intent or for controlling what is considered a chronic disease. Regardless of the treatment goal, survivorship care needs are ongoing, including medical monitoring, as well as addressing practical and psychosocial concerns. In addition, incorporating prevention and lifestyle behaviors to decrease risk of recurrence or disease progression often become a priority for survivors.

Once the active treatment phase of survivorship is completed or patient is in maintenance therapy, many patients experience mixed emotions. While finishing treatment is something to welcome and celebrate, many individuals report that they also feel lost, anxious, or traumatized. The process of treatment provided a defined path, with frequent and regular contact with healthcare providers. Once treatment is complete or visits become less frequent, the path ahead may be unclear. Family members, friends, and employers may assume that life can resume as usual, but the survivor may not be ready or able to do that. The survivor may have lingering effects of cancer treatment and questions about how to manage their healthcare needs moving forward, how to manage fear of recurrence, what signs or symptoms of a new or recurring cancer to look for, how to find meaning from the cancer experience, and perhaps how their life priorities may have changed.

With growing evidence that cancer survivors have ongoing needs after adjuvant treatment and emerging guidelines supported by national accreditation standards surrounding best practices, cancer centers recognize their obligation to offer survivorship programs and services. Navigators continue to have a key role in guiding survivors in their care, and this continues through this transition phase and into long-term survivorship. Depending on how navigation is structured within an organization, a navigator may fill a variety of roles across the phases of survivorship care. A navigator may meet patients when diagnosed and follow them throughout their treatment and into survivorship. Other navigators may work with the patient during a single phase of treatment (i.e., only in surgery or medical oncology) or phase of care (active treatment, survivorship, palliative care). The navigator can provide context regarding the patient's life and treatment goals, as well as details about the cancer experience, including medical and psychosocial impacts, family history and risk factors, and other health conditions that are relevant to the survivorship care plan and to providing survivorship care.

Whether conducting a distress screening or meeting with the patient at their final treatment, the navigator can assess a patient's need for medical, practical, or psychosocial support and provide necessary referrals. The navigator may also take the opportunity to guide the patient to information and resources at the cancer center and in the community, web-based resources, or clinical trials that can support the patient in making healthy lifestyle changes.

9.6   Patient Navigation During the Intermediate Phase of Survivorship

- Facilitate a comprehensive survivorship care plan (SCP)
  - Inform the survivor about the goals of an SCP.
  - Collect needed records to complete the SCP.
  - Make an appointment or deliver an SCP.
  - Ensure documentation reporting the completion and delivery of an SCP.
- Provide education and coordination of care
  - Educate and coordinate evidence-based follow-up care with providers, imaging, and other testing.
  - Encourage adherence to follow-up guidelines, specific to healthcare utilization, maintenance therapy, etc.
  - Inform survivors about resources for improving their lifestyle.
- Assess survivors' current medical concerns
  - Refer and schedule with specialists and providers.
- Address needs and risks of the patient as a whole person, through assessments and referrals
  - Administer or facilitate distress screening.
  - Refer to palliative care for side effect management.
  - Refer to cancer rehabilitation.
  - Refer to oncology dietitian.
  - Refer for cancer genetics.
  - Refer to supportive care: social work, psychology, psychiatry, and support groups.
  - Refer to a financial counselor.
  - Refer to spiritual care.
  - Refer to integrative health and mind-body programs such as acupuncture, yoga, meditation, Reiki, and expressive art therapies.

9.7   National Accreditation Standards and Recommendations

9.7.1   Institute of Medicine

The Institute of Medicine (IOM) identified four domains of survivorship care that are needed to comprehensively address ongoing medical needs after primary treatment; these include prevention, surveillance, intervention, and coordination. To operationalize the IOM recommendations related to these domains, the Commission on Cancer (CoC) has established an accreditation standard that requires cancer centers to provide survivorship care plans to survivors treated with curative intent [11]. Further, a number of professional organizations, including the American Society of Clinical Oncology [12], the National Comprehensive Cancer Network [13], and the American Cancer Society offer resources to aid healthcare professionals in summarizing follow-up care. Best practices and considerations to stratify a survivors' risk for recurrence or new primary cancers, late effects, distress screening, rehabilitation, and management of comorbidities can assist providers in delivering appropriate care to each survivor.

The responsibility to deliver survivorship care is a multidisciplinary approach and should not just fall on the shoulders of healthcare professionals. Patients must assume some responsibility for adhering to follow-up guidelines and utilize the survivorship care plan as a road map. As a patient makes the transition from acute survivorship, engagement with, and management of, their own healthcare needs remain vitally important. The coordinating provider must offer education and direction regarding the survivorship plan, and the patient has the autonomy to follow that guidance.

9.8 Incorporating the IOM Domains of Survivorship Care: Prevention, Surveillance, Intervention, Coordination

The IOM defined survivorship as "a distinct phase of care for cancer survivors" that includes four significant components:

- **Prevention** of cancer recurrence, any new cancers, or late effects of treatment
- **Surveillance** for cancer recurrence, spread, or secondary cancers, and assessment of late or long-term effects
- **Intervention** to manage consequences of cancer or late and long-term effects of treatment or consequences of cancer
- **Coordination of care** between specialists and the primary care provider to address all of the patient's healthcare needs

9.8.1 Domains of Follow-Up Care: Prevention and Surveillance

Although cancer survivors have only a 1%–3% risk for getting a secondary cancer (unless a survivor has a germline mutation, then the risk increases to 65%), prevention is an important part of follow-up care. Cancer survivors should be advised to make healthy lifestyle changes, including quit smoking or other tobacco use; achieve and maintain a healthy weight; consume a lower- to moderate-calorie diet, increasing the number of fruits and vegetables; incorporate exercise, including cardiovascular and strength training; follow guidelines for colorectal cancer screening (which includes removal of precancerous polyps); wear sunscreen and undergo regular skin cancer screening; undergo annual mammography; and undergo regular well-person care with a primary care physician. A survivorship care plan can serve as a blueprint for prevention and surveillance based on evidence-based guidelines.

The goal of surveillance is to detect a recurrence at the earliest possible time for better outcomes. Several organizations have established evidence-based cancer screening guidelines specifically for patients with a cancer history. The American Cancer Society (ACS) [3] has created prevention and screening guidelines to direct patients, oncology professionals, and primary care providers. In addition, the ACS published "Nutrition and physical activity guidelines for cancer survivors."

The National Comprehensive Cancer Network (NCCN) [13] has established detection, prevention, and risk reduction guidelines for breast, colorectal, lung, and prostate cancers, as well as guidelines to assess genetic or familial high-risk cancer. NCCN has drafted general survivorship guidelines that should be used in conjunction with the disease-specific guidelines and palliative care guidelines. The survivorship guidelines identify needs that fall into the same four IOM domains of prevention, surveillance, intervention, and coordination of care. Specifically, the guidelines cover:

- Treatment-induced cardiac toxicity
- Anxiety and depression
- Cognitive function
- Fatigue
- Menopause-related symptoms
- Pain
- Sexual function
- Sleep disorders
- Preventive health
- Healthy lifestyle behaviors
- Physical activity
- Nutrition and weight management
- Supplement use
- Immunizations and infections

The American Society of Clinical Oncology (ASCO) [14], the leading professional oncology organization, has created guidelines for surveillance for cancer recurrence for breast and colorectal cancers:

- ASCO Guideline Update: "Breast Cancer Follow-Up and Management after Primary Treatment"
- ASCO Guideline Update: "Colorectal Cancer Surveillance"

9.9 Domain of Follow-Up Care: Intervention

After active treatment is completed, survivors may experience late and long-term effects of the cancer diagnosis and its treatment (Table 9.1). Medical issues may include neuropathy, fatigue, cognitive changes, joint pain, lymphedema, range of motion limitations, early-onset menopause, and sexual dysfunction. Patients may face emotional issues such as anxiety, depression, fear of recurrence, and body image problems. Additionally, a patient may have practical concerns related to the cost of care, insurance, disability, or employment. Effective survivorship care provides interventions to manage any consequences of treatment for each survivor. A transition or survivorship visit where the patient and provider/care team review the survivorship care plan and any subsequent follow-up appointments are opportunities to assess survivors' concerns and to offer appropriate interventions.

ASCO offers guidelines for screening of and interventions for the late and long-term effects of treatment, including fatigue, anxiety and depression, and peripheral neuropathy, as well as recommendations for prostate cancer survivorship [14]. Examples of practice guidelines include:

- "Screening, Assessment and Management of Fatigue in Adult Survivors of Cancer: An American Society of Clinical Oncology Clinical Practice Guideline Adaptation"
- "Screening, Assessment and Care of Anxiety and Depressive Symptoms in Adults with Cancer: An American Society of Clinical Oncology Guideline Adaptation"
- "Prevention and Management of Chemotherapy-Induced Peripheral Neuropathy in Survivors of Adult Cancers: American Society of Clinical Oncology Clinical Practice Guideline"
- "Prostate Cancer Survivorship Care Guideline: American Society of Clinical Oncology Clinical Practice Guideline Endorsement"
- "American Cancer Society/American Society of Clinical Oncology Breast Cancer Survivorship Care Guideline"

9.10 Domain of Follow-Up Care: Coordination

The Institute of Medicine recommended that oncology specialists and primary care providers coordinate with one another to ensure that all of a patient's healthcare needs are met once primary treatment is completed. Survivors' ongoing healthcare needs extend beyond follow-up for cancer and may include screening for other cancers, management of comorbidities, and monitoring of other risk factors. A shared care model allows each provider to focus on their expertise and maintain their relationship with the patient. The survivorship care plan can serve as a useful document shared between the oncology team, the patient, and the primary care provider as a summary of all the pertinent aspects of the cancer and cancer treatment.

Several examples of national standards include:

- American Society of Clinical Oncology Quality Oncology Practice Initiative (QOPI®) [8] includes addressing many aspects of survivorship care and the delivery of a treatment summary.
- The American College of Surgeons/Commission on Cancer "Cancer Program Standards: Ensuring Patient-Centered Care," includes "Standard 3.3 Survivorship Care Plan," including the dissemination of a treatment summary and follow-up plan to survivors who have completed treatment with curative intent [14].

Navigators have been instrumental in addressing these standards and incorporating survivorship care plans into practice. These standards have been challenging to meet due to organizational buy-in, time-consuming construction of the SCP, difficulties with SCP automation within the electronic health record, billing for the development and delivery of the SCP, and tracking outcomes to demonstrate the value of the SCP.

9.11 Summary

Survivorship navigation continues to expand with the growing number of cancer survivors who are thriving with and through their disease. The comprehensive approach to addressing survivorship care requires care coordination and additional competency to address the complex issues affecting cancer survivors. Navigators serve as educators and advocates, facilitate care coordination, and play an active role in the care of cancer survivors. The demands of survivorship care will continue to grow, and navigation will play an invaluable role in meeting the needs of survivors, healthcare systems, and national accreditation standards.

Survivorship Case Study 1

Breast Cancer Survivor

Pamela Goetz

Objectives of the Case Study

- The reader will be able to describe how a survivorship care plan benefits a breast cancer patient after completion of active treatment.
- The reader will learn about the navigator role in survivorship programming.

Intro
The period after cancer treatment ends is a challenging transition for many patients. Cancer programs can ease this transition by providing survivorship care plans and survivorship programming to guide and educate patients.

Background Situation
BR is a 59-year-old woman who was diagnosed with breast cancer, clinical stage IIIB. She received pre-adjuvant AC-T in 2014, then had a left mastectomy with axillary node dissection and no reconstruction, and completed radiation treatment in 2015. BR is single, has no children, and lives alone in a DC suburb. She has friends, neighbors, and family in her support system. BR is not currently working, but was previously employed as a CPA.

At diagnosis, BR expressed concern about insurance issues and stress related to her diagnosis, and the recent death of both of her parents, for whom she was the caretaker. She had not been working for several years due to her parents' illnesses and was hoping to return to work at least on a part-time basis. BR was overdue on many aspects of her health maintenance, and her providers made note to encourage her to get up to date on this after her breast cancer treatment.

Challenges

Upon completion of treatment, BR learned about a survivorship program offered by the cancer center to patients completing active treatment. BR participated in an intake interview with the patient navigator to register for the program series. During the interview, BR articulated her concerns. Regarding medical and physical issues, BR had persistent left axillary cording and hot flashes that affected her sleep. Her radiation oncologist had advised her to start exercising and to lose weight. She also expressed the hope to have delayed reconstruction at some point. In the meantime, she wondered if there are swimsuits for women without breasts. As she put it, her body is a "daily reminder of my condition."

The survivor also admitted that she had been doing some soul-searching on how to move forward now that treatment was completed. Her father had survived melanoma, so this provided her with some perspective on life after cancer. She also had a family history of Alzheimer's, so she felt worried and vulnerable about that. She wondered, "How can I make the experience fade away? How can I be more aware of what I need to know to deal with anxiety?" BR also mentioned that she needs to get back to work.

Solutions

The survivorship navigator recognized a gap in *services* for cancer survivors. With evidence-based guidelines in mind, she designed the survivorship program to support patients to manage the transition after cancer treatment and to develop an individualized health plan. The goals of the program were to educate survivors about the importance of adherence to follow-up guidelines, how a survivorship care plan can provide a road map in managing follow-up care, the importance of achieving a healthy weight through exercise and nutrition, and management of emotional issues related to the diagnosis and recovery. To enable the participants to apply the information learned in the series, health coaching was included to provide expert help in identifying health goals and creating a plan to make lifestyle changes.

During the intake interview for the program, the navigator informed BR that her concerns would be addressed during the survivorship series and/or at a survivorship transition visit. For other issues, the navigator referred the patient to individual resources.

Cording

The navigator confirmed that the patient had been going to physical therapy and in fact had excellent results in dealing with lymphedema earlier in her care. The navigator also assessed if there were any barriers to getting those services. She encouraged the patient to do any at-home exercises that the physical therapist may have prescribed.

Hot Flashes

The patient navigator discussed the benefits of acupuncture for managing hot flashes and provided information on scheduling an appointment with the cancer center's acupuncturist. She also referred the patient to the palliative care nurse practitioner advanced practice provider (APP), who presented at the first sessions of the series on managing late and long-term effects.

Reconstruction and Swimsuits

The navigator provided the patient with recommendations for plastic surgeons and for a swimsuit supplier.

Weight Management

The navigator informed the patient that the survivorship series would include information and guidance on weight management during the nutrition presentation, during the exercise (yoga and Pilates) demonstration, and during the individual sessions with the health coach.

Emotional Challenges

The navigator assured BR that her worries about recurrence, finding a new normal, and general anxiety are common feelings at the transition from active treatment. She let BR know that the series would include a session with the social workers addressing these emotions and making meaning of the cancer experience. The navigator also let BR know that she could meet for individual counseling with one of the social workers to discuss her concerns privately.

Survivorship Care Plan

During the survivorship program, a nurse practitioner informed the attendees about what a survivorship care plan is and how to use it. The patient navigator aided BR in getting an appointment for a survivorship care plan with the nurse practitioner. During the visit, the nurse practitioner reviewed all the treatment BR received, as well as the recommendations for follow-up care and for a healthy lifestyle, including exercise, nutrition, and stress management. Referring back to the earlier health assessment, the nurse practitioner encouraged BR to see her primary care provider to get up to date on all screenings.

Implications

This case study raises some of the commonly faced issues that survivors articulate at the transition after treatment. Navigators are key to supporting patients through the cancer trajectory. Having perspective on a patient's goals at the outset of treatment can guide conversations at the end of treatment as well. At the various points of transition in care, navigators have the opportunity to assess survivors' individual needs and make referrals to services and programs in the cancer center or to services in the community. The survivorship care plan and survivorship programming together can address the medical, emotional, and practical needs of cancer survivors.

Survivorship Case Study 2

Clinical Trial: Chuck, Comanche Nation, Colorectal Cancer Patient

Linda Burhansstipanov
Native American Cancer Research Corp (NACR)
Washington, DC, USA

Objectives of the Case Study

- Identify at least four challenges Chuck experienced that impacted his quality of life and survivorship.
- Describe at least three members of the oncology team and the role(s) they played in helping improve Chuck's quality of life.
- Identify four strategies the oncology team used to address Chuck's quality-of-life issues.

Introduction

Chuck is an enrolled member of the Comanche Nation. He is 55 years old, is of normal weight, has type II diabetes, and is a smoker and a recovered alcoholic (sober for 13 years). He was diagnosed with colorectal cancer. Chuck was treated for 3 months with bevacizumab (Avastin), irinotecan hydrochloride (includes FOLFIRI, folinic acid, and 5-FU), and cetuximab, but his cancer had metastasized. He was successfully enrolled in the National Cancer Institute clinical trial NCT01079780 [15]. This trial was to determine whether giving cetuximab and irinotecan hydrochloride together was more effective with or without ramucirumab (Cyramza).

Background Situation

Chuck joined a cancer support group, but the distance made attending difficult, and the members were not Native. He started meeting with a few local Comanche Nation cancer survivors at one of their homes. Their support group is informal but the three men help one another. They call the community patient navigator on the toll-free number in Denver when they need additional information. The community patient navigator contacts the nurse navigator when the information the three men need or want constitutes medical advice.

Chuck had a lot of fatigue, weakness, dizziness, nausea, vomiting, and severe headaches prior to joining the clinical trial. The headaches and dizziness were of issue because Chuck's work as a ranch hand was conducted on horseback and he fell a few times. Similarly, he had to stop work many times during the day in attempts to calm the nausea and to find a bush where he could vomit. Chuck attempted to remain stoic throughout these symptoms, but the men in his support group insisted he get help. They called the community patient navigator and talked with him via conference call during one of their support group gatherings, and the community patient navigator said he would talk with the nurse navigator to get her involved.

Clinical Challenge

The nurse navigator created a schedule to talk with Chuck's wife to confirm when and how he was taking his medication to keep his blood pressure in normal ranges. She did this the first 3 weeks that Chuck was enrolled in the clinical trial. He complained about the side effects during the trial and had difficulty in recovering from a wound he incurred from the horse fall (he fell on a tree stump and had a deep cut on his shin that would not heal).

Clinical Solution

The nurse navigator talked with the clinical trial nurse, and they worked on a wound management protocol. A volunteer nurse agreed to drive out to the ranch and show Chuck and his wife how to care for the wound, and she traveled once each week to check on the healing of Chuck's wound, because he could not miss any more work at the ranch.

Clinical Challenge

The clinical trial uses ramucirumab; common (10–29% of users) side effects include high blood pressure, diarrhea, and headache. Chuck was enrolled in the trial in spite of his poorly managed high blood pressure. Of note, the dizziness and nausea side effects were lessened once Chuck was in the clinical trial. Chuck continued to have headaches, but less severe than prior to the clinical trials.

Patient Challenge

However, Chuck continued to experience a lot of weakness and fatigue. He had difficulty grooming his horse prior to starting work on the ranch each day. His comments describing the weakness were "I had to sit down two to three times while brushing my horse. Then I had to carry my saddle from the tack room to set on a tie rail. Next, I'd need to move my horse to the tie bar so that I could lift the saddle, rotate around, and heave it onto my horse's back. Luckily, my horse stands real still because I'd have to lean against the tie rail or sit on the ground before I was able to cinch the girth. This whole process took about an hour whereas it used to take 10 min before I was in cancer treatment. This meant I had to get to the ranch a lot earlier. After the saddle was cinched up, I'd have to rest before I got the bridle from the tack room and put it on my horse. I'd rest, lead him over to a mounting block, and get on. Then I'd have to just sit in the saddle and catch my breath…."

Community Solution

"…The Indian guys I work with would get on me about acting like a woman … all of it in fun until I finally told them I was in cancer treatment. Then my buddy, Cal started grooming my horse and saddling him before I even got to the ranch. That was real nice."

Solutions by the Team

Chuck called the community patient navigator early in May and asked him how long the weakness and tiredness were going to last, and if there was anything he could do to feel better. Lance explained that some fatigue could last as long as 2 years, occasionally even longer, but that it would gradually get better. In the meantime, the community patient navigator said he would contact the nurse navigator to get her medical advice and assistance for additional medications that may help. Because Chuck was in the clinical trial, the nurse navigator had to talk with the clinical trial nurse. The clinical trial nurse reached out to the dietitian for help with the fatigue, and also contacted the clinical trial lead physician for a recommendation of medication to alleviate the fatigue symptoms. The nurse navigator talked with Chuck and scheduled a follow-up appointment with her, the dietitian, and the clinical trial nurse to work on strategies to address his issues. During the appointment, the dietitian helped Chuck and his wife understand the importance of high-iron and nutrient-rich foods and supplements. Both were willing to improve his diet but could not afford these foods. The nurse navigator called to find out if the oncology social worker was available and could help with food supplement program. The appointment lasted 4 hours, but by the end, Chuck and his wife drove home with new prescription medication to lessen the fatigue symptoms, dietary supplements free of charge, and food discount coupons to use for shopping at the local market. His wife cooked and Chuck ate the high-iron, nutritious foods.

Community Challenge and Solutions

By July, Chuck was not yet strong enough to dance in the pow wow, but his family and friends danced for him. The community patient navigator also came down to Comanche Nation and danced and prayed for Chuck. Following the pow wow, Chuck took part in three traditional Indian ceremonies with the help of his family and friends throughout the rest of the summer. Because the community patient navigator also was Comanche and involved with Chuck's care, he took part in one of the traditional ceremonies.

By the following year, Chuck was strong enough to dance again (only a few slower dances and widely spaced intervals in between dances). Chuck continues to work on the ranch and gradually returned to performing part-time construction jobs around the community (he could not do this work for 18 months following the completion of his chemotherapy). He is enjoying his family, friends, and community activities, and he talks openly about his cancer experience now, but only when asked. A common concept presented by Chuck when talking with others is the Creator gives us the strength to have this journey and helps us reorganize our priorities to enable us to become more involved in our families and our communities. The cancer and the treatments are very hard, but through our traditions and guidance of the Creator, we become well again.

Implications

Chuck's quality of life was greatly impacted by the side effects of his cancer treatment. Because of the help from the community patient navigator, nurse navigator, clinical trial nurse, the physician (to prescribe fatigue medications), the dietitian (to help Chuck and his wife with a high-iron and nutrient-rich dietary plan), the oncology social worker (for inexpensive and free food supplements), traditional Indian healer (for cleansing and spiritual ceremonies), and his local male support group, Chuck struggled through the side effects to gradually be strong enough to work on the ranch without help from his friends, take part in cultural activities (ceremonies and pow wow dancing and praying), and improve his relationships with his family and friends.

References

1. National Coalition for Cancer Survivorship. Self-advocacy: a cancer survivors handbook. www.canceradvocacy.org/cancer-advocacy/what-is-advocacy. 2009. Accessed 28 Jun 2017.
2. Mullan F. Seasons of survival: reflections of a physician with cancer. N Engl J Med. 1985;313:270–3.
3. American Cancer Society (ACS) Cancer Treatment and Survivorship Facts & Figures 2016–2017. www.cancer.org/content/dam/cancer-org/research/cancer-facts-and-statistics/cancer-treatment-and-survivorship-facts-and-figures/cancer-treatment-and-survivorship-facts-and-figures-2016-2017.pdf. Accessed 25 Jul 2017.
4. Institute of Medicine (IOM). Cancer care for the whole patient: meeting psychosocial health needs. Washington, DC: The National Academies Press; 2007. https://doi.org/10.17226/11993.
5. NCCN Clinical Practice Guidelines in Oncology: Distress management. V.2.2017. www.nccn.org. Accessed 18 Oct 2017.
6. Forsythe LP, Kent EE, Weaver KE, et al. Receipt of psychosocial care among cancer survivors in the United States. J Clin Oncol. 2013;31:1961–9.
7. www.nccn.org/patients/resources/life_with_cancer/pdf/nccn_distress_thermometer.pdf.
8. Howlader N, Noone AM, Krapcho M, Miller D, Bishop K, Kosary CL, Yu M, Ruhl J, Tatalovich Z, Mariotto A, Lewis DR, Chen HS, Feuer EJ, Cronin KA, editors. SEER cancer statistics review, 1975–2014. Bethesda, MD: National Cancer Institute. April 2017. https://seer.cancer.gov/csr/1975_2014.
9. Institute of Medicine and National Research Council. From cancer patient to cancer survivor: lost in transition. Washington, DC: The National Academies Press; 2006. https://doi.org/10.17226/11468.
10. American Society of Clinical Oncology. www.asco.org/practice-guidelines/cancer-care-initiatives/prevention-survivorship/survivorship-compendium. Accessed 25 Jul 2017.
11. American College of Surgeons Commission on Cancer. www.facs.org/quality-programs/cancer/coc/standards. Accessed 25 Jul 2017.
12. American Society of Clinical Oncology Institute for Quality. Quality oncology practice initiative (QOPI®). www.instituteforquality.org/quality-oncology-practice-initiative-qopi. Accessed 25 Jul 2017.
13. National Comprehensive Cancer Network (NCCN). www.nccn.org/. Accessed 25 Jul 2017.
14. American Society for Clinical Oncology (ASCO) Survivorship Guide (for patients). www.cancer.net/survivorship. Accessed 25 Jul 2017.
15. National Institutes of Health, U.S. National Library of Medicine. Irinotecan hydrochloride and cetuximab with or without ramucirumab in treating patients with advanced colorectal cancer with progressive disease after treatment with bevacizumab-containing chemotherapy. https://clinicaltrials.gov/ct2/show/NCT01079780. Accessed 25 Jul 2017.

Patient Resources

American Cancer Society. ACS Guidelines for Nutrition and Physical Activity. www.cancer.org/healthy/eat-healthy-get-active/acs-guidelinesnutrition-physical-activity-cancer-prevention/guidelines.html.

Association of Community Cancer Centers. Survivorship care. www.accc-cancer.org/home/learn/
    Patient-Centered-Care/survivorship-care.
American Society for Clinical Oncology. Survivorship (for patients). www.cancer.net/survivorship.
American Institute of Cancer Research (AICR). www.aicr.org.
Cancer*Care*. www.cancercare.org.
Cancer Support Community. www.cancersupportcommunity.org.
LIVESTRONG at the YMCA. www.livestrong.org/what-we-do/program/livestrong-at-the-ymca.
National Center for Complementary and Integrative Health. https://nccih.nih.gov.
National Coalition for Cancer Survivorship. www.canceradvocacy.org.

Transitioning to End-of-Life Care

10

Lillie D. Shockney

10.1 Defining End of Life

End of life (EoL) can best be defined as the phase entered by a terminally ill patient when further disease-targeted treatments cannot reasonably be expected to provide any benefit and actually are likely to cause a faster death, destroying quality of life along the way. Being able to identify when a patient enters EoL and when continuing with treatment is detrimental are viewed as the most difficult decisions advanced cancer caregivers have to face. Probably there are few if any care decisions that have such a profound impact and implication for patients and their loved ones as those that are made near the EoL [1]. Perhaps the hardest decision is when to stop treatment completely and rely on palliative care. The caregiver may be now the sole person making decisions for their seriously ill loved one and needs to focus on quality of life (QoL) instead of merely extending life. What complicates this further is a rare patient who will respond to a phase I clinical trial, making the issue of continuing treatment versus stopping treatment even more difficult. This is despite the knowledge that phase I clinical trials usually cause serious side effects that can for some destroy what QoL they have that remains. Something that has also been learned from research conducted with family caregivers is that the presence of the patient, no matter what their clinical condition, allows hope and emphasizes the strong sense of responsibility that the caregiver is actually willing to sacrifice everything to keep the patient alive. This basically guarantees that the caregiver continues absorbing all of the patient's attention and becomes the only focus of the caregiver's thoughts, actions, and feelings [2, 3].

There continues to be no consensus, however, of when EoL begins and what is its duration. With hindsight being 20/20, physicians and even family members can reflect backward and see when the patient started to show significant decline and their EoL experience seemed to pick up some speed. Ironically, even

L. D. Shockney, RN, BS, MAS, ONN-CG (✉)
Johns Hopkins University School of Medicine, Baltimore, MD, USA
e-mail: shockli@jhmi.edu

© Springer International Publishing AG, part of Springer Nature 2018
L. D. Shockney (ed.), *Team-Based Oncology Care: The Pivotal Role of Oncology
Navigation*, https://doi.org/10.1007/978-3-319-69038-4_10

otherwise well-designed EoL care guidelines developed by panels of experts do not include a definition of EoL [4–6].

10.2 Understanding the Origin of, Definitions of, and Phases of Hope

Hope has been defined in various ways over time. Research still available online dates back to the 1950s, with work done by Karl Menninger in 1959. He wrote that hope is of critical importance to patients during times of suffering and loss [7, 8].

Understanding the origin of hope actually began with Pandora's box. This is a story from centuries ago that is associated with hope. According to Greek mythology, Pandora was the first woman created. She was very beautiful but also known for being curious and didn't always obey the rules set before her. Zeus, the King of the gods, gave Pandora a gorgeous box with explicit instructions to never open the box. The gift was the box and not what was inside of it. One day her curiosity got the better of her, and she did open it. It was not an act of malice but an act of curiosity. As she cracked the lid just slightly open, out of the box came all of the evil, illnesses, and diseases not previously ever known to mankind. She quickly shut the lid. The only thing that remained trapped inside the box was hope. Hope, however, is what makes human existence in troubled times bearable, according to this myth. This perhaps implies that when all is lost, or seems lost due to feeling totally surrounded by bad and evil, somehow hope survives [9, 10].

10.2.1 Types of Hope

Hope is a complex concept, however. It is one not always understood even by oncology professionals. The reason for the confusion is likely due to there being wide differences as to what an individual, a patient, may be hoping for themselves. It has been studied and published that healthcare professionals prefer to think in terms of therapeutic hope, which is based on therapy and is more related to a cure or remission of the patient's disease [11]. We need to factor into this discussion also the concept of generalized hope, which is, for many, to maintain a high quality of life despite having to deal with a cancer diagnosis. There is also a type of hope known as particularized hope, which is hope for something specific such as being strong enough and able to attend a special family event that is in the near future. There is clearly a necessity for hope to exist. There is also an important dimension between hope and despair [12].

Hope is a universal concept and a necessity to our existence [13]. What happens when life is shortened and ends up being discussed as only lasting for a few months, or perhaps days, or even hours? What then does hope mean to a metastatic cancer patient? To the family and loved ones who cherish the mere existence of this person who is soon to die? Yes, there is still a role for hope at the EoL too. There are different kinds of hope as a patient transitions through the various and to some degree predictable phases of the dying process.

Nurse navigators need to have an ongoing dialogue with our patients and their family caregivers. In doing so, we can better understand what they are singularly or collectively hoping for, and how what we say and do influences their hopes of today and the tomorrows to come. If we don't understand the principles of what fosters hope, as well as what takes it away in the mind's eye, and how to support patients appropriately during their treatment and with palliative care support throughout the continuum of care, then we are failing our patients at a fundamental level. We each must help our patients to live with their cancer instead of dying with their cancer. To do this means we must know what gives them joy, so we can provide care in a way that maintains or restores these joyful moments. It also means understanding their future hopes for themselves and for the family members they leave behind to mourn their loss while celebrating the patient's life, which was hopefully lived well. We must support patients to be optimistic for as long as it is realistic, and have a good understanding of patients' expectations of treatment and ensure they are not being misled or confused about its purpose and likely outcomes. And we need to support patients as their hopes over time go through a transitional process that can only be achieved with our support and use of good communication skills about how to make decisions that are in their best interest [10].

10.2.2 Learning More About the Research Conducted on Hope

A research study on fostering hope in terminally ill patients focused on key questions to ask patients as part of an interview process. They asked five probing questions, listed below [14]:

1. What does hope mean to you?
2. Tell me about your hope. What kinds of things do you hope for?
3. If you could identify a source of hope for yourself, what would it be?
4. What things cause you to lose hope?
5. What helps you to maintain your hope or makes you feel hopeful?

These are not questions that can be asked similarly to inquiring if your patient has any history of heart disease or diabetes. These are thought-provoking questions that require a private environment, a sense of calm when spoken, and adequate time devoted to listening and understanding the answers.

10.2.3 Life Cannot Exist Without Hope

Hope enables people to cope with horrifically difficult and stressful situations and circumstances that otherwise may cause them to simply give up. Some consider it an unused resource, an inner readiness [15]. It is not believed to necessarily be within our conscience. It doesn't come forth into our conscience until we are confronted with a crisis. It is considered by some to be a belief that we can get ourselves to be in a better state by modifying the situation we are in, and in doing so, can figure a way out of the difficulties we are forced to face [16].

Hope is connected to motivation, too. When someone has a strong hope, it usually gives them the strength and fortitude to keep aggressively pushing forward with tackling a difficult situation. This type of motivation is very important in enabling people to reach their goals. Achieving goals cannot happen without hope. The probability of being able to reach it is dependent on how important the goal is to the individual [17].

Although it may be obvious, it is worth stating that hope is about something happening in the future. It is believed to be possible to achieve holding on to hope despite having to cope with metastatic cancer that has many unknowns associated with it. This was eloquently stated by Tone Rustøen, a doctoral student in Norway, two decades ago when she wrote: "Having goals and different choices regarding the future can motivate people to reach them and remind them of the possibilities that are open to them. This will, in turn, increase the possibility for goal attainment. Thus hope is connected to future possibilities" [16].

Why are the questions associated with family relationships important to inquire about when talking with a patient about their diagnosis and treatment? Our interpersonal relationships carry great significance as they relate to hope. A spouse, son, dear friend, or perhaps even ourselves as oncology navigators will provide a patient support and in doing so mention to them something related to their future and how living is important to continue to be able to do. Whether it be witnessing the birth of a grandchild or being present for a family reunion, there are things in their future that they believe will give them joy, and therefore they hope to be able to still be here to experience them. Is it a source of power? Yes, most definitely. It is a fundamental driver of what makes the patient want to achieve specific milestones that for them carry great significance. There are situations too in which the patient feels no particular drive to reach a specific life goal, but someone they love, such as their spouse, asks it of them because that milestone, that hope, carries great significance to the other person and in turn becomes important to the patient—by fulfilling a hope for someone they dearly love.

Hope must be attainable. It must be realistic. Without realism, it is likely to be more of a wish or daydream. Therefore, our charge should be to help our patients refocus their goals and their hopes onto things that can be realistically achieved. Hope is not limited to one specific outcome. It should be looked upon as a process by which we expect something good to happen in the future and develop action plans to achieve that specific goal [18].

Hope, therefore, is perhaps a coping strategy that comes forth when we are in desperate need of it. It is an interpersonal confidant, our power source. No one can exist without having hope about something.

Cancer patients with end-stage disease were asked to provide their definitions of hope. The responses were then categorized, and the following list represents the primary answers given [19].

It is a feeling or expectation that falls into four general categories:

1. Things can go well.
2. Because one thing has gone wrong, it doesn't mean that other things will not go well.
3. You have just as good chances (if not better) as the next person of having the best outcome.
4. You can still enjoy good quality of life, even if life expectancy is uncertain.

In a publication by the National Coalition for Cancer Survivorship entitled *You Have the Right to Be Hopeful*, information from a book authored by Jerome Groopman entitled *The Anatomy of Hope: How People Prevail in the Face of Illness* was provided that serves as a well-constructed summary of the key elements of hope [8, 9]. They are listed below [9]:

Hope constitutes an essential experience of the human condition. It functions as a way of feeling, a way of thinking, a way of behaving and a way of relating to oneself and one's world.

Hope means the desire for personal survival and the ability of the individual to exert a degree of influence on the surrounding world.

Hope is necessary for healthy coping, with its key purposes being the avoidance of despair and the desire to make life under stress bearable.

Hope is a cognitive-affective resource that is a psychological asset. The importance of this asset becomes greater in times of threat.

Hope is mental willpower plus "waypower" for goals. Willpower, in this definition is the driving force to helpful thinking. It is a sense of mental energy that helps move a person toward a goal. Waypower, the second component in the hope equation, is the mental capacity used to find a way to reach goals. It reflects the mental plans or road maps that guide hopeful thoughts.

Hope is a prerequisite for action. It must be flexible and open to possibilities.

10.2.4 Caregivers Desperately Need Hope, Too

Loved ones who have become caregivers, by chance or by choice, also need hope. Hope is defined by some caregivers as the inner strength to achieve future good and to continue caregiving. It is a key psychosocial resource among family members serving as caregivers [20].

Caregivers need respite over time to maintain their hope as well as their own resilience. Dealing with life day in and day out as a constant caregiver is physically and mentally wearing. Guilt occurs, too, when things look grim and the patient is anticipated to die soon only then to rebound from their death bed and resume the chronic EoL care they still need. Caregivers may have surrendered themselves to watching their loved one die and feel a sense of peace as they had hoped they would feel. With the patient not dying at that time, the emotional upheaval it can cause within the caregiver's mind should not be ignored or underestimated. They too need to discuss their hopes and talk through what they are feeling and experiencing. Initially, they may be hoping for quantity of time to be a primary goal so that the patient is alive for as long as possible. As the illness progresses, however, and they witness their loved one's health failing, experiencing physical symptoms such as pain, and losing QoL, their personal hope can change into wanting a good death and for it to occur sooner versus later. So their hopes are twofold—hopes they have for the patient they dearly love and hopes for themselves that they can endure this experience.

10.2.5 All Members of the Multidisciplinary Team Influence Our Patients' and Their Caregivers' Hopes

Each member of the oncology team, including the nurse navigator, influences what our patients hope for and believe is achievable. Great caution and care must be exercised to not overpromise something or only focus on statistics that may be more pessimistic. Patients, however, rely on the words said to them by their treatment team members to give them hope. Sometimes such words are simply to provide a way for patients to feel better about their current situation; however, caution must be exercised in the use of such words and their interpretation. In fact, these words are doing more than just giving hope; these hopes become shared hopes with the treatment team. The bond that is formed with advanced cancer patients and their treatment team, including their navigator, is very significant. This relationship has been formed when patients are at their most vulnerable, easily influenced, and fragile state of mind [10].

10.2.6 It Is Not Possible to Take Away Hope from Our Patients

A primary reason why oncologists sometimes are not honest with patients about their true clinical status, even when it includes deterioration, is the fear they will be taking hope away from their patient. What really happens, however, is not losing hope but instead helping the patient transition through the various phases of hope. Without such a transition over time, the patient may never reach the moment of acceptance and be ready to prepare for a good death experience [10].

10.2.7 There Can Be a Cost to Hope

Although costs vary by tumor type and stage of the disease, the highest costs occur in the last year of a cancer patient's life [21]. Out-of-pocket expenses including copayments, deductibles, lost time from work, and other indirect costs are reaching an all-time high. Patients do not want to leave bad debt for their families to pay associated with their cancer care. Individuals usually are not financially prepared for a diagnosis of advanced cancer, either. As part of the role of a navigator, it is important to discuss with the patient what the expenses will likely be based on the various phases of treatments the patient is potentially going to be receiving. Despite the American Society of Clinical Oncology (ASCO) changing the standard of care many years ago to recommend that the oncology specialist caring for the patient, no matter what the stage of the disease, discuss the risks, benefits, and costs of the treatments with the patient, few physicians have embarked on that portion of the discussion. Navigators, however, are positioned to have such a conversation and help the patient determine if they will need financial assistance through resources that a navigator or financial counselor can provide, whether they want to make their treatment decisions based on expense, as well as make sure that their patient is still the one in the driver's seat, making the decisions about treatments overall. The patient has the right to decline a specific expensive treatment, request a less expensive treatment recognizing that it may not work as well, or even decide to stop treatment altogether. Treatment for treatment's sake is bad care. Patients who receive chemotherapy treatments within a few weeks of their death likely did not receive the appropriate care they needed at that time.

Patients who are guided and choose to discontinue treatment sooner in favor of QoL preservation and more time at home with their families are more satisfied with their care, have fewer expenses, and actually live longer [22].

10.2.8 Helping Your Patient Transition Through Phases of Hope

Transition is a process of changing from one situation or status to the next. Experiencing metastatic cancer requires a series of phases of transition that takes the patient from the point of hearing the diagnosis to reaching EoL. Not all patients successfully complete the psychological transitions to EoL as hoped, however. It requires the patient to adjust to each transitional phase in order to successfully negotiate them. When a transition includes the loss of a previously healthier state of being, that state of prior wellness must be grieved in order to successfully transition to the next phase [23]. There is such a thing as living the experience of hope that our cancer patients experience as they journey through the various phases of their treatment, along with, hopefully, eventual acceptance of their death. Hope is therefore not stagnant. And patients hope for more than just one thing or one outcome to occur.

A hope that someone has that may have been put aside or even lost might rekindle itself based on new information or opportunities. Some of this new information comes from clinicians. The need to listen closely to patients, asking them what they are hoping for at various points in time will provide insight as to where they are across the trajectory of time. It also provides insight as to whether they have rational hopes, whether their hopes differ from those of their loved ones, and how we can best support them through these phases of transformative change.

Just as there are stages our patients go through that define the dying process, there are also phases of hope that a patient experiences.

Due to family dynamics, there can be differences of opinion about what the patient hopes for and what their family members want to happen. There can be a desire to get closure with specific family members and friends so that the patient feels a sense of peace about a previously broken or damaged relationship. Focus sensitivity to where the patient is along the death and dying stages, recognizing that their hopes will evolve as they evolve along the staging process.

Patients undergo multiple transitions during the course of their cancer care. Navigators are positioned in an extraordinary place within their lives to support the patients and their families as they make the transition from one phase to the next. With each transition there is opportunity and need to redefine hope.

10.2.9 Themes of Hope

Research has even been able to define specific themes of hope that cancer patients experience. These themes are [24]:

A hope for a cure
A hope for living as normally as possible
A presence of confirmative relationships
Reconciliation with life and death

This research confirmed that there actually is a structure and process that patients go through as their journey carries them closer to dying. A hope for a cure may be a longshot but still is something they want to keep on the table as a possibility. As long as some type of treatment is being given, then patients feel they still have a chance at experiencing a miracle. And when they acknowledge that cure isn't possible, then they want to live a life that gives them a sense of normalcy, or in essence being able to live in harmony with their disease. There was consistent expression by research subjects that they valued the little things in life with greater appreciation and found simple things to have more meaning and provide them a stronger sense of joy than before [10].

10.2.10 Circles of Hope Domains

J. Donald Schumacher, former president and CEO of the National Hospice and Palliative Care Organization, identified that there are six circles of hope for the terminally ill population, with a very specific focus; patients move through these domains as they approach their life's end. Some of these are incorporated into other research work; however, this focus of identifying the specific things that a patient is hoping for provides more clarity and describes in greater detail the transitional thought processes a metastatic cancer patient experiences as they move from one focus to another until their death. What can be concerning to the oncology specialists as well as family members is that not all patients transition through these specific phases of hope as desired. Our role as clinicians should be to help guide a patient across this continuum of care, focusing on hope and in turn, help reach the next focus of hope until "being remembered well" is their final hope [10].

The six circles of hope are [25]:

1. Hope for a cure
2. Hope for a sudden and long remission of disease
3. Hope for a pain-free existence
4. Hope for the resolution of interpersonal relationships
5. Hope for forgiveness
6. Hope to be remembered well

The final hope, especially as it relates to preparing for EoL, is that the patient has made some kind of contribution to mankind while living their life. The patient needs to feel and believe that they were here for a purpose and that this purpose was in some way fulfilled. This is also why knowing the patients well is so important. Listen to their stories about their lives. These stories will include their successes and their defeats. Sometimes the person best equipped to point out the ways they will be remembered is their navigator and not their family or even themselves. Navigators can objectively listen and learn then feed information back to the patient, recognizing that their life was not in vain. They were here for a purpose and this purpose was fulfilled. There will be situations, however, in which the patient still has unfinished business for which they place all of their hope into believing that this unfinished work—the creation of a foundation, the completion of some community service effort—must be completed before they can die feeling confident of their fulfilled purpose. When time grows short, the patient's navigator needs to work with family members to ensure that they will carry on in their loved ones absence to fulfill this work, thus enabling the patient to die feeling fulfilled.

10.2.11 Having the Desire and Need for Forgiveness

As more and more families are made up of half-siblings, step-parents, and other blending of multiple family groups, the likelihood of hard feelings and the desire to maintain a distance from certain individuals are ever present. When someone is facing their mortality, however, feelings and desires can change. There may be a desire to mend fences among family members and estranged friends. Although this desire is heartfelt on the part of the patient, it may not be met with open arms by the individuals who have been the other half of the longtime feud. Nonetheless, the desire to repair these broken relationships that have built up emotional walls over a lifetime can promote a sense of peace for the patient and the ability to look upon their future with a sense of anticipation. Although there are unique circumstances in which the estranged family member defiantly chooses to not participate, most of the time, perhaps for the sake of peace for themselves too, they will come to the table (or bedside) and welcome closure.

10.2.12 Preparing for One's Death

When it comes to reconciling oneself with life and death, experience has demonstrated that patients express that their hope was to be well prepared for death and experience a good death, having their legal and financial affairs in order, along with arrangements for their funeral and being emotionally ready, as well. With the exception of being emotionally ready, these are all tangible things that can be done. Again, it is a way to feel a sense of control. It also should cause loved ones to realize that the patient is aware of their future timeline and want to still have a say in how things are handled regarding their death and what occurs thereafter, too.

10.2.13 Stages of the Dying Process

It is important to keep in mind what stage of the dying process each of our patients is in at any given moment while under our care. Elisabeth Kubler-Ross delineated five stages of the dying process for an adult human being. This information was learned in nursing school. The first stage is denial caused by the shock of the diagnosis. The patient's hope is that this must be a mistake and the information was misinterpreted or given to the wrong patient. Then comes anger about how unfair it is to be given what appears to be a death sentence and wanting to know why they were picked for this diagnosis by the higher power they believed would always be there for them and help them at all times. What bad or evil thing had they done to cause such a punishment? Next comes the bargaining stage. Secular bargaining happens with us, the patient's clinician, as well as possibly with some family members. For patients who are religious, they are bargaining with God, or another higher power they believe in, requesting some type of reprieve in exchange for their life being saved. When reprieve fails to happen, then patients can slip into depression.

With loss of appetite, loss of energy, and the obvious sense of slipping away slowly, the final stage comes, acceptance of the reality that they are going to die. Hope, however, is not gone. There still are glimmers of it up until the last breath [10].

10.2.14 Family Members Having Different Hopes than the Patient

A patient may have reached a point of acceptance about their impending death and be in the early stages of experiencing a sense of peace when a family member, meaning well, expresses to the patient to "not give up." It is very hard to lose a loved one. It is also straining on a patient mentally to feel emotionally at odds with their family member who has not reached the same stage of the dying process. This can result in patients agreeing to get treatment that they frankly don't want. Who else can be promoting continuation of treatment and the need to "keep trying?" The treating physician, who has been taught to treat the disease. There has to be supportive behaviors exercised to not confuse a patient and establish unrealistic expectations of what is possible (i.e., a cure). Family meetings with the treating clinician are also necessary to ensure that everyone is supporting what the patient needs and wants.

10.3 Unfortunate Consequences of Failing to Plan for the Transition to EoL Care

There are known ramifications if a patient is not smoothly navigated through the various phases of their care, helping them to transition from one phase of hope to another, with the final phase of hope being that of planning to experience a good death. Initially when someone is diagnosed with metastatic disease, they commonly are hopeful and praying for a miracle to occur. Their treating oncologist is usually doing the same, initially. Without continuous communication taking place as treatments over time fail to keep the disease in control, the patient and/or their family members may be still anticipating a cure despite the patient getting progressively much sicker. Nurse navigators have an instrumental role in helping the patient to understand where they are across the trajectory of their disease, promoting improved communication including helping the patient to ask pertinent questions that foster better understanding of their clinical status, and facilitating referrals when appropriate, such as to palliative care. The goals of treatment must shift to goals of care given that the treatments are for curative intent. This can be quite difficult for patients and family members to understand, particularly if the patient had previously been diagnosed with a curative stage of this same disease and had aggressive treatment to prevent distant recurrence. They were accustomed to the goals of treatment being long-term survivorship that is lived cancer-free. This means from the onset when the patient is diagnosed with advanced cancer, the goals of treatment must focus on the patient's goals. Receiving treatment for treatment sake is bad care.

The adverse consequences of failing to plan for the transition to EoL care include [26]:

Increased psychological distress
Medical treatments inconsistent with personal preferences
Utilization of burdensome and expensive healthcare resources of little therapeutic value
A more difficult bereavement

Avoiding or delaying the planning for the EoL until a few days before the patient dies causes mayhem for the patient and the family. It results in the inability for the patient to experience a good death. Approaching such a conversation can be intimidating and awkward without the right tools, resources, and experience. The purpose, however, is to proactively create a plan of care to improve QoL at EoL. This is accomplished by helping the patient to make informed choices about the potential harms of continued aggressive (usually toxic) treatment and compare that choice to the potential benefits of hospice care.

It is critical to focus on the patient's perspective. Researchers have identified five domains of care near the EoL that patients identified as priorities. They are [27]:

Receiving adequate pain and symptom management
Avoiding inappropriate prolongation of dying
Achieving a sense of control
Relieving burden
Strengthening relationships with loved ones

The strongest predictors of QoL were age, good performance status, and a survival time longer than 6 months. Patients in a waiting pattern hoping for a new treatment have worse emotional well-being. The conclusion from such research affirmed that QoL is primarily related to factors such as disease progression and its complications and to the patients' goals relative to any treatment they are receiving [28]. Extensive research has been conducted looking at specific indicators that measure EoL care quality. These are measures that represent a failure in providing quality of care at EoL [29]:

Increasing numbers of patients starting a new chemotherapy treatment within 30 days of their deaths or continuing to receive chemotherapy within 14 days of their death.
Referrals to hospice taking place too close to patients' actual death, making the length of stay in hospice being relatively brief and raising the issue that hospice may be occurring too late [30].
Rates of utilization of ICU stays have been increasing, with patients dying in the ICU setting or being transferred from ICU to a hospice facility.

Rates of do-not-resuscitate (DNR) orders have increased but are completed close to death. (One study analyzing inpatient deaths demonstrated that the median time between signing the DNR and death was 0 days; for outpatient deaths, it was 30 days. This implies that communication about resuscitation preferences is delayed, thus negatively impacting the patients' ability to prepare for EoL) [31]. A key domain of knowledge on which nurse navigators need to be well versed is that of cultural diversity. Patients' race, ethnicity, age, and religious beliefs can directly influence their decision making about EoL, as well as impact even how their clinicians interact with them. The goal of planning such a transition thoughtfully is to increase the probability that a patient in such a serious life-threatening situation will receive high-quality EoL care that matches their informed preferences and choices. There are characteristics that have been identified through research that inform us about what influences the discussion taking place between the treating physician and the patient. They are [29]:

Age: recognizing that cancer remains a disease primarily attributed to older adults—the older the patient is—especially those who are elderly, the less desire the patient has for life-prolonging treatments. Those over the age of 70 are less likely (44%) to want information about survival when making decisions about treatment [32].

Gender: older men are more likely than women to desire prognostic information (56% vs 29% in one study) [32]. Patients who were interviewed in a study before and after a visit with their oncologist to discuss scan results demonstrated that women were more likely to acknowledge the cancer being incurable and to accurately be able to identify the stage of their cancer. Women were also more likely to report after the consultation that discussions took place related to life expectancy [33].

Race: black patients may be more likely to receive intensive treatments near their EoL. These treatments unfortunately may not correlate with the stated preferences by the patient. Even EoL discussions do not decrease the probability of intensive treatments; it is the opposite for white patients [34, 35]. African-American or Asian patients are less likely to enroll in hospice and more likely to receive aggressive treatment, including hospitalizations and ICU admissions, than white patients [36, 37].

Socioeconomic status: patients with Medicaid are less likely to receive hospital care than patients insured through Medicare and are more likely to die in acute-care facilities. Oddly enough, however, in a Medicaid population, black patients are more likely to have had an EoL discussion [38, 39]. Also, Medicare patients who are enrolled in a managed care plan were more likely to enroll in hospice and to enroll for longer periods of time [40].

Religious and spiritual beliefs and values of patients: when a patient's spiritual needs are significantly supported by their clinicians taking care of them, they are more likely to receive hospice care and less likely to receive aggressive care. They also report higher QoL [41].

It is important to respect patients' preferences.

This is an essential component to ensuring the patient is receiving high-quality care. When a patient is given the opportunity to engage in a discussion about their EoL preferences, there is a higher probability that they will receive care that is consistent with these preferences [42]. In a study conducted and published in 2011, it was reported among 128 newly diagnosed advanced-stage lung cancer patients that [43]:

88.2% wanted to be informed about life expectancy (52.7% said they were informed).
63.5% wanted to be informed about palliative care (25% said they were informed).
56.8% wanted to be informed about EoL decisions (31% said they were informed).
None of the patients recalled being asked about their information preferences.

If we don't know how to elicit patients' preferences, however, then we may never be able to effectively and consistently provide them a good EoL experience. There are optimal ways to elicit preferences from patients. Patients have several preferences that carry significance to planning the transition to EoL care [44].

Timing and manner of prognostic information disclosure—patients with life-limiting illnesses desire information about their prognosis and that such information will not take away hope but instead help them transition through the phases of hope [45].
Decision-making role—a passive role is more common among patients who are older and female or had a poorer performance status.
Palliative chemotherapy rather than palliative care without chemotherapy—patients will commonly want to request chemotherapy, even before learning their treatment options. The younger the patients, the greater the probability that they will seek out chemotherapy.
QoL or length of life—patients in studies who were within 6 months of diagnosis rated length of life as being more important to them than QoL. When patients were asked to rate the relative value of QoL or length of life, 55% valued QoL and length of life equally, 27% preferred QoL, and 18% preferred length of life. QoL preferences correlate with older age, male gender, and increased levels of education. Patients with a preference for length of life preferred less pessimistic communication from oncologists [29].

10.4 Focusing on the Patient's Goals of Care

No effective, thoughtful planning for transitioning to EoL care can be accomplished without a discussion about the patient's goals of care. It is a critical component of the process. There must be a clear delineation of the difference between goals of care and goals of treatment, however; otherwise miscommunication can occur. Goals of treatment focus more on shrinking the cancer and preventing further spreading of the disease, while preserving QoL as best can be achieved. A patient's goals of care should be reflective of their interests and needs, once they have accepted that this disease is not curable. Goals of care should be focused on finding meaning in the life they have led, being comfortable, feeling a sense of direction toward a greater understanding of their purpose, and planning to experience a good death, and all the elements that make up such an experience.

Fulfilling hopes and life goals in alternative ways—commonly among younger adult patients, their frustration rests on the issue of no longer being here for their children, not being present to witness them reach specific milestones in their lives and not being here to instill their values in their children, express their love, and provide them words of wisdom. Discussing with the patient their long-term life goals is a very appropriate role for a nurse navigator, social worker, chaplain, or palliative care expert. The key is to not simply note them but work with the patient and their family members to creatively fulfill these future hopes in alternative ways. This can be done through letter writing, having cards for children when they reach specific milestones in their lives, and identifying someone to serve as a surrogate and keep the parent's memories alive for their children. Such alternative methods have proved successful and provide the patient a sense of comfort and control that didn't exist before [46]. It serves as an additional way for the patient to regain some control over the situation. Other examples are of patients who know they will likely die before a grandchild is born. Arrangements can be made for the patient to still "meet" the baby by being present when an ultrasound is done of the fetus. This requires creativity for some hopes and life goals to be achieved in alternative ways. It provides the peace of mind patients need and deserve, however.

10.5   Potential Barriers to Planning the Transition to EoL Care

Although patients' preferences should be a primary driver of the care they receive, we know from experience and research that this is not always or even likely the case. A cause may be that patients lack sufficient opportunity to develop informed preferences. As a result, they can receive care that is not consistent with what their actual values and goals. Barriers that prevent a patient and their doctor from discussing goals of care, prognosis, various options, and patient preferences are [47]:

Patients' interpretations of prognostic information—it is not unusual for patients to not understand that their disease is incurable. One study demonstrated that among solid organ site tumor patients with advanced disease, more than 80% thought when the oncologist said he "was hopeful that the tumor will respond to their next treatment," the word "respond" was misinterpreted as meaning "be cured" [46]. This may be due in part to the methods used commonly by doctors for eliciting feedback from the patient about their understanding of what has been said, relying on a yes or no response. Nurses, however, are trained differently and will ask the patient to repeat what was just said, thus getting a more specific interpretation of how this information was understood or misunderstood. Therefore navigators must be engaged in these types of discussions to ensure the patient does accurately understand what they are being told as a means to prevent confusion, disappointment, or even mistrust happening between the patient and the oncologist [46]. There can be other barriers to ensuring a more accurate interpretation and understanding of prognosis, beyond poor communication by clinicians. Patients can actually interpret information differently for reasons unrelated to how the information was communicated to them. For example, the perspectives of patients with advanced cancer who enroll in phase I clinical trials provide some insights into why these patients might misinterpret their prognosis. Patients can be overly optimistic about the benefit from a phase I clinical trial. The most common reason a patient gives for enrolling in a phase I clinical trial is the belief that this treatment will kill all the cancer cells [48].

Lack of agreement between patients and oncologists—although ideally, numerous conversations between the patient and the oncologist should result in a clear understanding about the patient's prognosis, goals, preferences, options, and decision-making processes, experience shows that frequently they do not reach the same conclusions about these significant issues. Although not well studied at this point, it is reasonable to assume that by not reaching such agreements, the patient's ability to transition to EoL is impacted in a negative way. Patients can be more optimistic than their doctors. Physicians are known to overestimate the length of remaining time a patient has, and the patient have a better estimation of when their death will likely occur [46]. This too may be a reason for the number of days a patient receives hospice care being so short. Optimistic patients have a tendency to want to receive treatments that will lengthen their life, while possibly jeopardizing their quality of life. The amount of information recalled by a patient following a consultation with their doctor is limited due to the use of unfamiliar medical terms, limited time to spend together, stress the patient is feeling during the visit, and lack of retention of accurate information. Goals of treatment and goals of care can be misconstrued as meaning the same thing when they do not. Even a patient's status can be misinterpreted. The doctor may score their performance status higher than the patient does. This can be due in part to a patient camouflaging herself by wearing additional makeup, a well-styled wig, and bright-colored clothing with the hope that she will hear the doctor say how good she looks. What isn't asked is whether the patient feels as good as she looks. This is enabling behavior because the patient wants to hear that she appears to be doing well when in fact she knows that she is feeling worse, which may be a sign that the cancer has spread further [46].

Oncologists' communication behaviors—doctor-patient communication frequently does not fully support informed or shared decision making [29]. The majority of oncologists will disclose that chemotherapy will not cure the patient of their advanced cancer, however, few discuss any alternatives to chemotherapy. If the cancer is incurable but the only treatment discussed is chemotherapy, then the patient will receive chemotherapy. Physicians, as mentioned earlier, are often not skilled in asking the patient about their understanding of the information the doctor has provided. Lack of comprehension is a worrisome problem because it can continue for a lengthy time, with the patient not understanding their options or their approaching EoL. There are also physicians who provide overly optimistic information that is misleading, having the patient believe their condition is better than it actually is or will be. Oncologists frequently do not discuss the anticipated survival benefit of chemotherapy in advanced cancer. Additionally, the doctor doesn't provide the patient information about the potential survival benefit gained by receiving palliative (non-curative) chemotherapy [49]. Those patients whose treating physician discussed prognosis awareness earlier rather than waiting for the patient to be doing poorly had a more accurate understanding of their clinical situation and better communication with their doctor. Doctors, however, prefer in most cases to wait until the patient requests such information rather than volunteer it early on [50].

Oncologists' misconceptions about the harm of EoL discussions—physicians have expressed in interviews and surveys why they are hesitant to have EoL discussions with their advanced cancer patients. They are worried they will be taking away hope and harming them psychologically. Research, however, has demonstrated that this is not the outcome of such thoughtful discussions. Such discussions actually improve psychological adjustment, helping the patient to transition through the various phases of hope [46]. A study showed that explicit disclosure about prognosis and reassurance that the doctor will not abandon the patient were helpful to patients. Being explicit with the information and providing reassurance actually decreased anxiety and feelings of uncertainty [46, 51].

Oncologists' attitudes and preferences—an individual physician's beliefs and attitudes can and do influence how they communicate with their patients. This results in there being wide variance among doctors about how and when they communicate about prognosis and discuss advance directives and how they will approach limiting (or not limiting) treatment near the time of the patient's death. Some physicians do not support shared decision making, taking a paternalistic approach to caring for patients with advanced cancer [52, 53].

Uncertainty about options other than disease-directed treatments—this is another barrier to a patient transitioning to EoL. There can be great confusion regarding some of the language and terminology that are used with a patient. They may have preconceived ideas about what palliative care or hospice care means. They are asked if they have an advance directive without an explanation what this document is. Terms like DNR are foreign to patients and their families. This is important patient education a nurse navigator needs to provide to the patient and family members so that there is less confusion and clearer understanding, and a thoughtful discussion can take place.

10.6   Palliative Care and Hospice for Patients with Advanced Disease

There is a stigma associated with both palliative care and hospice care in the USA. Palliative care has become so misunderstood that some institutions have even changed the terminology to "supportive care." Ironically, the newest definition of palliative care is described as "specialized medical care for people with serious illnesses." The mission is relief from pain and other symptoms, no matter what the serious diagnosis. Patient and family QoL is a primary goal and mission of care. Palliative care can even be provided for those who we anticipate will be cured of their illness [54].

Palliative care is an interdisciplinary model of care that is specifically focused on patients with serious or life-threatening illnesses. It also supports their family members who serve as caregivers at home. The goals of palliative care are to [54]:

Reduce illness burden, relieve suffering, and maintain QoL through interventions that maintain physical, psychological, social, and spiritual well-being.
Improve communication and care coordination.
Ensure that care is consistent with the values and preferences of the patient.
Ensure that dying occurs with minimal suffering and maximum opportunities for closure.

Note the reference above to care coordination. This means that navigation must be a key component of this care delivery model, beginning with making sure the patient has accurate information about what palliative care is and isn't. It is care usually provided by doctors, nurses, social workers, and chaplains. Relief from pain and other uncontrolled symptoms is a priority. The team focuses on the goals of care. Special attention is paid to prevention or relief from distress related to the dying process. Family burden is also a priority. This requires effective communication and understanding on the part of the patient and their family caregivers so that the patient's goals remain the focus. Consider palliative care a philosophy of how to organize and structure patient-centered care. Enhancing QoL, optimizing the patient's functional status, promoting informed and active decision making with the patient, and creating and promoting opportunities for closure and personal growth are all components of this highly specialized field. Palliative care does not have a specific start and end time frame. It can and should be provided simultaneously to the patient receiving life-prolonging care. Helping the patient and family understand these concepts can aid in patients receiving palliative care earlier than they commonly do today.

10.7   Hospice Care

Hospice care also involves a multidisciplinary team that specializes in medical care, pain management, and emotional and spiritual support for patients whose life expectancy is no longer than 6 months. As referenced earlier, oncologists misgauge the length of time a patient may have before their death, which results in patients not getting the full benefit from hospice care.

There are state as well as federal regulations that serve as the criteria for hospice eligibility. It is required that a licensed physician certify that the patient is suffering from a life-limiting illness for which their EoL is projected to be less than 6 months from enrollment. Hospice services are covered by virtually all forms of medical care coverage.

10.7.1 Barriers to Timely Hospice Enrollment: Common Patient and Family Caregiver Barriers

Patients and caregivers assuming that hospice is only for the last few days of life.
Patients still want to receive life-sustaining treatments [55].
Many patients believe hospice means giving up hope [46].
Denial of the patient's own declining health condition.
Patients or family members may have a negative perception of hospice [56].
New cancer treatments, such as those offered in phase I clinical trials, may imply to the patient that they should remain optimistic even though actual clinical benefit is very small or nonexistent [57].

10.7.2 Barriers that Result in Physicians Not Enrolling Their Patients in Hospice

Although physicians are certainly well-meaning individuals, even they can be a barrier for the patient to receive the optimal treatment they need and deserve as their disease progresses. These barriers include:

Oncologists have demonstrated an inability to accurately predict their patients' estimated life expectancy, resulting in patients not learning or being offered hospice care.
Oncologists believe that a referral and transfer of the patient's care to hospice is a reflection of their personal failure to save the patient.
Oncologists believe they are losing control over their medical practice.
Enrolling a patient later than is ideal can result in it being harder for the patient, family, and oncologist to cope with the sudden change, complexities of making such a transfer, and the patient not benefiting much since they only have a few days or fewer in hospice.
Some oncologists still believe that an enrollment in hospice will somehow speed up the patient's death, which is untrue.
Oncologists worry that a hospice referral will be viewed by the patient as their oncologist abandoning them.

10.8   The Role of the Nurse Navigator in Fostering Improvements in Communication and Decision Making

There are some known strategies that can foster improvements in communication and decision making, which can then facilitate the transition to EoL care for patients with advanced cancer. These include:

10.8.1 Promoting Advance Care Planning

One method of doing this is to provide an example of someone who did not have cancer, was in good health, and was in a car accident and on life support for months and finally died. She had no legal written will in place and no legal or financial affairs in order and left behind young children who were shifted from grandparent to grandparent until the court system determined who they would eventually permanently live with and where the young mother's assets would also go. By providing a non-cancer patient example, it makes it easier to discuss and demonstrate that all adults should have advance care plans. This can lead easily then into a discussion about an advance directive, living will, durable power of attorney for healthcare, etc.

10.8.2 Giving Patients Materials to Help Them Prepare for Consultations with Their Oncologist and Other Team Members

List for the patient the following issues that must be discussed with their oncologist:

Their personal goals of care; understanding what all treatment options are including doing no treatment, and comparing risks and benefits of each treatment including the cost of the treatment to the patient; what to expect going forward from the perspective of how decisions are made when treatment needs to be discontinued and a new treatment considered; how side effects will be managed; will the patient still be able to work and for how long; how to cope with uncertainty; and how to be actively engaged in the decision-making steps going forward. The patient usually wants to know about life expectancy too, so ask the patient about this when preparing the list of questions for him/her to take with them for the appointment. Whenever possible, it is ideal if the nurse navigator can accompany the patient, serving as an extra set of ears and eyes, reiterating information that may be confusing or unclear, and serving as an advocate when the patient does not feel comfortable asking questions to which they have expressed they want answers. Also, add to the list of questions about the opportunity to meet and involve palliative care clinicians early in the patient's care.

10.8.3 Using Decision Aids: Some Decision Aids Can Be Provided by Palliative Care Specialists That Can Help a Patient in Making Informed Decisions

Integrating specialized palliative care services into conventional cancer care is ideal but requires buy-in from the oncology team. Having a patient have a good experience with palliative care, however, and sharing that experience with their oncologist opens the door for palliative care specialists to become integral members of the multidisciplinary team from the start rather than be viewed as an add on service later. In 2012, the American Society of Clinical Oncology (ASCO) published a provisional clinical opinion (PCO) advising its membership that "… combined standard oncology care and palliative care should be considered early in the course of illness for any patient with metastatic cancer and/or high symptom burden" [58].

Knowing what the patient's preferences are and sharing that information with all the multidisciplinary team members—this includes having the nurse navigator document this information in the patient's medical record, providing such information if the patient's case is discussed at tumor board, and verbally reiterating it whenever the patient is being seen, receiving treatment, or being discussed for whatever reason. This is one of the best ways to serve as a patient advocate.

Providing clinical predictions of survival based on statistical evidence based information is important. Although physicians have a reputation of over projecting this time line, a private conversation between the oncologist and the nurse navigator could be helpful in comparing a patient's clinical status with that of prior patients for whom they have cared. There can be a shift in the time line by using comparative data. Patients expect and want honesty [46].

10.9 Fulfilling a Final Hope by Orchestrating a Good Death

Terminally ill cancer patients are very concerned about experiencing pain and suffering that is not appropriately relieved, have fears regarding their future, feel frustrated with uncertainty, depressed about their loss of independence, worried about their family, and fear they are being a burden on their loved ones. These are universal concerns for patients with advanced cancers. What do we mean by a good death? Research has been conducted to provide a means of understanding from patients what constitutes a good death. These studies provide insight into the major components of a good death. They are management of pain and suffering, clear decision making, preparation for death, completion, contribution to others, and affirmation of the whole person [59]. There must be a discussion about each of these attributes of a good death with the patient and their loved ones so as to provide them the information they need at specific points in time. No one should die in pain. No one should feel confused or untrusting of how decisions are going to be made with them and potentially for them acknowledging and honoring their final wishes. Patients usually want to know what they might expect during the course of their illness and want to plan for these phases that would eventually lead to their death. Family members also need to learn from their oncology team members what to expect with a special focus on the physical and psychosocial changes that will occur as their loved one transitions into EoL and dies. Patients need to feel a connection spiritually and from that confirm a deep importance in the meaningfulness of their life at EoL; this must include resolutions of conflicts, spending time with family and friends, and even saying goodbye. Contributing to others may seem odd but it is also very important. Giving to others doesn't mean money, although for some it may. It could be a gift of time or gift of information that provides new knowledge. Most will say before their passing that they have learned that family and relationships are important above all else including money and careers. The patient also wants to be acknowledged as a whole person and not defined by their cancer. This too is very important for families to witness.

10.9.1 Elements of a Satisfying EoL Experience

Another study that exposed a clearer understanding of patients' perspective regarding the hope of experiencing a good death was published by Singer et al. This qualitative study resulted in the following domains of quality EoL care being understood as important: receiving adequate pain and symptom management; avoiding inappropriate prolongation of dying; achieving a sense of control and relieving burden; and strengthening relationships with loved ones [27].

Receiving adequate pain control and symptom management, a primary goal of palliative care, has been discussed in some degree here as well as a prior chapter. Avoiding inappropriate prolongation of dying, however, has not been discussed, and deserves to be further understood. Having a DNR order can only happen with the patient if such a discussion takes place between the clinician and the patient. There can be hesitancy to do so, however. There are also family conflicts that can occur from the patient being too ill to speak on their own behalf, leaving it to a family member to make decisions. The family member may want their loved one here "no matter what it takes," forgetting that the patient may be suffering to stay alive. Again, we must go back to what we all agreed to when becoming oncology clinicians—to do no harm. Therefore, decisions about life support, ICU admissions, invasive tests and procedures, as well as treatments should be candidly discussed with the patient, with the family present so that there is a clear understanding about what the patient wants, and why.

Patients also want a sense of control. This applies even when the patient reaches a point at which they are unable to make decisions for themselves. Their proxy is to ensure that the patient's wishes will be carried out.

Spirituality is an element of a good death experience: when approaching EoL, even if a patient says they are not spiritual, they will turn to a higher power of some kind usually for spiritual comfort. During times of uncertainty, human beings are known to feel a stronger sense of spirituality within themselves. It is a natural process associated with uncertainty at the EoL [60]. Spirituality is a broad term and does not necessarily mean the patient or family has now acquired religious feelings or connections. It is considered a part of everyday life and appears in both religious and nonreligious forms including a spiritual meaning of family relationships recognized as the chain of life and seeking meaning, purpose, and transcendence in life. This is, after all, the patient's life and no one else's.

10.10 Case Study: Stage IV Breast Cancer Patient Approaches End of Life

10.10.1 Objectives of the Case Study

Learn the importance of focusing on the patient's goals of care, and that these goals must drive treatment decisions.

Recognize the pivotal role the navigator has in serving as an advocate for their patients.

Identify ways to fulfill the patient's hopes in alternative ways.

10.10.2 Introduction

This case study provides insight into the difficulties patients and their oncology providers face that can be improved or even prevented by having effective communication skills, comfort in discussing death, and a supportive nurse navigator who serves in the pivotal role of the patient's advocate.

10.10.3 Background

10.10.3.1 Clinical

A 31-year-old mother of two preschool children was diagnosed with triple negative stage IV breast cancer 18 months following completion of treatment for stage IIb disease. The location of the metastatic disease was on the lungs, bones, liver, and brain. She had expressed to her doctor that she wanted to "receive treatment up until her last breath" as a way to demonstrate to her children how hard she fought to be with them for as long as possible. Her medical oncologist agreed with this plan, recognizing it as her goal of care.

When the nurse navigator met with the patient and was discussing goals of care and learned the plan that had been put into motion, she discussed with the patient what these two goals of care meant to her. She discussed them individually. The first goal was to live as long as possible because she wanted her children to be able to remember her without looking at a photograph. The second goal was to receive treatment until her last breath so that other family members could tell her children how hard she fought her disease.

10.10.3.2 Challenges
In analyzing these two goals, however, the nurse navigator explained that they were actually in conflict with one another. If she received toxic drugs until her last breath, she would undoubtedly be in the hospital for much of her final weeks, and due to the ages of her toddlers, she would not be able to have them with her at all. So a discussion ensued as to what was the most important goal to the patient.

10.10.3.3 Opportunities
The patient wanted to be remembered by her children, and she wanted as much quality time with them as possible. This totally changed the goals of care, and opened the door to a discussion about palliative care beginning now, along with palliative treatments. A brief discussion about hospice care was also initiated by the nurse navigator to dispel the image and negative stigma it is known to carry. A key element of importance to the patient was her desire to still have her oncologist involved to some degree with her care, even if it was only to touch base with her and her family and see how she was doing while receiving hospice at home when the time came. She didn't want to feel abandoned by her treatment team, especially her oncologist. She felt comforted to hear that commonly patients who transition to hospice sooner live longer and have better QoL. This for her meant more time with her children at home. She also selected from boxes provided by the nurse navigator cards for her children for each milestone they will reach in the future, beginning with birthdays, communion, driver's licenses, graduation, and even wedding and when they each have their own first child. These cards provided her the ability to write to them what she hoped for them at the time of that specific milestone, giving her love and words of wisdom. These were carefully preserved by her husband. If she was still living when the child reached a milestone, then she would hand the child the card; if not, her husband would provide it on her behalf.

The individual who had the most difficulty accepting that the patient would eventually lose her life to this disease was her mother. Her mother wanted to try to control the situation and treated the patient as a child once again. The nurse navigator connected the mother with a national nonprofit organization called Mothers Supporting Daughters with Breast Cancer. This organization provided the mother with written information about what to expect medically with her daughter and matched her to a mother volunteer who several years ago lost her daughter to stage IV breast cancer at approximately the same age and with young children. A primary mission of the organization is support but also to reiterate to the mother that the patient (the daughter) must be the one in charge.

When the cancer spread further, requiring thoracentesis, the patient made the decision to enroll in hospice care at home. She died a good death with the following elements in place:

She knew her purpose for living and that it was valued by others.
She left a legacy, unrelated to leaving money—demonstrating how to live each day with cancer rather than dying each day with cancer.
She gave and received forgiveness.
She was pain-free.
She died with dignity and in the environment of her own choosing—home with family, receiving hospice services.
She left no financial debt for her family to pay associated with her cancer treatment or care.
She was confident she would be spoken of fondly after she was gone.
She felt a spiritual connection to a higher power.

Her funeral was truly a celebration of her life and the impact she had on many people by having lived. Her husband and mother continued to receive hospice support for a year after her death.

The time from the point of diagnosis with stage IV disease to transitioning to hospice care was 13 months. She received hospice at home for 4 months.

Her boys remember their mommy and enjoy listening to her voice recorded in videos and in children's recordable books. Their cards await them in the future.

10.10.4 Implications for Stakeholders

Stakeholders in this scenario include the patient, her immediate family, the oncology team, and the nurse navigator. By providing an opportunity for a thoughtful, candid discussion about goals of care, the focus was off of receiving treatment for treatment's sake and instead focused on the patient's true goals of care. It is imperative that the entire oncology team strive to focus on patient-centered care. The goal should never be extending quantity of life without QoL also being preserved. There must be adequate time for planning EoL care and orchestrating all of the elements the patient needs to experience a good death. This requires proactive planning, time to sit and have thoughtful discussions. If a patient wants to know how many treatment options remain available to her and what the likelihood is that any will work, she deserves to know the answers. During times of such great uncertainty, the patient needs to have provided to her any and all information that can provide her some sense of control, even when the news given is bad.

Future patients are stakeholders, too. The oncology specialists must learn from their experiences with patients and their families so that they can support the patients better who are diagnosed after the ones currently receiving care. Without such lessons, nothing will ever improve.

Conclusion

For decades, patients with advanced cancers were told by their treatment teams how sorry they were that they couldn't be saved or couldn't do more for them. This has fostered behaviors that make it more difficult to be able to prepare a patient and their family for EoL. It is critically important that patients are supported in such a way that they are able to transition effectively to EoL care and experience a good death. To accomplish this outcome, the oncology team taking care of the patient must know the patient well. The goals of care must be based on the patient's goals and no one else's.

Palliative care must be introduced as QoL preservation or QoL restoration so that the stigma associated with the term, palliative care can be undone. It should be a natural part of oncology care, including for patients who will likely survive their disease. Hospice care is designed to last for up to 6 months but commonly continues to only be provided for weeks or even days before the patient's death. Ensuring the patient that they will not be abandoned by their oncologist is an effective way to help engage the patient in considering hospice as a viable option that can preserve QoL for their remaining life.

Nurse navigators are well positioned to be an advocate for the patient and support the patient by recognizing barriers to effective transitioning and create solutions for these barriers. Navigators also need to be mindful of the patient's family caregivers, who also will need support and education. In some instances, family members can have different goals than the patient's goals, believing that the mission is extending the patient's life, forgetting about the importance of QoL to the patient.

In recognition that a patient feels sad that they will miss out on experiencing specific events in the future, it is necessary to be creative and identify alternative ways to still accomplish these hopes and life goals.

Hope is a thread that is ever present. Life cannot be sustained without hope. Navigating a patient through phases of hope is one of the most significant roles a nurse navigator, social worker, and/or chaplain can do for a patient. The final outcome must be a peaceful death for the patient, with family well prepared for loss and ready to celebrate and acknowledge all that their loved one has accomplished while living and what they will continue to accomplish through the various legacies that they have left.

References

1. Faguet GB. Quality end-of-life cancer care: an overdue imperative. Crit Rev Oncol Hematol. 2016;108:69–72.
2. Coelho A, Barbosa A. Family anticipatory grief: an integrative literature review. Am J Hosp Palliat Med. 2017;34(8):774–85.
3. Beng TS, Guan NC, Seang LK, et al. The experiences of suffering of palliative care informal caregivers in Malaysia: a thematic analysis. Am J Hosp Palliat Care. 2013;30(5):473–89.
4. National Institute for Health and Care Excellence. Quality standards for end of life care for adults; October 2013.
5. Emanual LL, von Gunten CF, Ferris FD. The education for physicians on end of life care curriculum. 1999. www.amaassn.org/ethic/epec. Accessed 6 Mar 2017.

6. Institute of Medicine. Dying in America: improving quality and honoring individual preferences near the end of life. Washington, DC: The National Academies Press; 2014. p. 17.
7. Menninger K. The academic lecture: hope. Am J Psychiatr. 1959;116(12):481–91.
8. Clark E. You have the right to be hopeful. 4th ed. National Coalition of Cancer Survivorship; 2008.
9. Groopman J. The anatomy of hope: how people prevail in the face of illness. New York: Random House; 2005.
10. Shockney L. Fulfilling hope: supporting the needs of patients with advanced cancers. New York: Nova Science; 2014.
11. Nuland S. How we die. New York: Random House; 1959.
12. Kylma J, Vehvilainen-Julkunen K. Hope in nursing research: a meta-analysis of the ontological and epistemological foundation of research on hope. J Adv Nurs. 1984;25(2001):364–71.
13. Hinds PS. Inducing a definition of 'hope' through the grounded theory methodology. J Adv Nurs. 1984;9(4):357–62.
14. Herth K. Fostering hope in terminally-ill people. J Adv Nurs. 1990;15:1250–9.
15. Schneider JS. Hopelessness and helplessness. J Psychiatr Nurs Ment Health Serv. 1980;18:12–21.
16. Rustoen T. Hope and quality of life, two central issues for cancer patients: a theoretical analysis. Cancer Nurs. 1995;18(5):355–61.
17. Stotland E. The psychology of hope. San Francisco: Jossey-Bass; 1969.
18. Clyton J, Butow P, Arnold R, et al. Fostering coping and nurturing hope when discussing the future with terminally ill cancer patients and their caregivers. Cancer. 2005;103(9):1965–75.
19. MacCormick T, Simoniam J, Lim J, et al. "Someone who cares": a quantitative investigation of cancer patients' experience of psychotherapy. Psycho-Oncology. 2001;10:52–6.
20. Duggleby W, Williams A. Living with hope: developing psycho-social supportive program for rural women caregivers of persons with advanced cancer. BMC Palliat Care. 2010;9:3.
21. Mariotto AB, Yabroff KR, Shao Y, et al. Projections of the cost of cancer care in the United States, 2010–2020. J Natl Cancer Inst. 2011;103:117–28.
22. Smith TJ, Hillner BE. Concrete options and ideas for increasing value in oncology care: the view from one trench. Oncologist. 2010;15:65–72.
23. Evans WG, Tulsky JA, Back AL, et al. Communication at times of transitions: how to help patients cope with loss and re-define hope. Cancer J. 2006;12:417–24.
24. Benzein E, Norberg A, Saveman BI. The meaning of the lived experience of hope in patients with cancer in palliative home care. Palliat Med. 2001;15:117–26.
25. Taylor C. Rethinking hopelessness and the role of spiritual care when cure is no longer an option. J Pain Symptom Manag. 2012;44(4):626–30.
26. National Library of Medicine, National Institutes of Health. Planning the transition to end-of-life care in advanced cancer. NCBI Bookshelf. Health professional version. https://www.ncbi.nlm.nih.gov/books/NBK223164. Accessed 21 Jan 2016.
27. Singer PA, Martin DK, Kelner M. Quality end of life care: patients' perspective. JAMA. 1999;281(2):163–8.
28. Jones JM, McPherson CJ, Zimmerman C, et al. Assessing agreement between terminally ill cancer patients' reports of their quality of life and family caregiver and palliative care physician proxy ratings. J Pain Symptom Manag. 2011;42(3):354–65.
29. www.ncbi.nlm.nih.gov/books/NBK223164
30. Bergman J, Saigal CS, Lorenz KA, et al. Hospice use and high intensity care in men dying of prostate cancer. Arch Intern Med. 2011;171(3):204–10.
31. Levin TT, Li Y, Weiner JS, et al. How do-not-resuscitate orders are utilized in cancer patients: timing relative to death and communication-training implications. Palliat Support Care. 2008;6(4):341–8.
32. Elkin EB, Kim SH, Casper ES, et al. Desire for information and involvement in treatment decisions: elderly cancer patients' preferences and their physicians' perceptions. J Clin Oncol. 2007;25(33):5275–80.

33. Fletcher K, Prigerson HG, Paulk E, et al. Gender differences in the evolution of illness understanding among patients with advanced cancer. J Support Oncol. 2013;11(3):126–32.
34. Loggers ET, Maciejewski PK, Paulk E, et al. Racial differences in predictors of intensive end-of-life care in patients with advanced cancer. J Clin Oncol. 2009;27(33):5559–64.
35. Mack JW, Paulk ME, Viswanath K, Prigerson HG. Racial disparities in the outcomes of communication on medical care received near death. Arch Intern Med. 2010;170(17):1533–40.
36. Smith AK, Earle CC, McCarthy EP. Racial and ethnic differences in end-of-life care in fee-for-service Medicare beneficiaries with advanced cancer. J Am Geriatr Soc. 2009;57(1):153–8.
37. Haas JS, Earle CC, Orav JE, et al. Lower use of hospice by cancer patients who live in minority versus white areas. J Gen Intern Med. 2007;22(3):396–9.
38. Mack JW, Chen K, Boscoe FP, et al. Underuse of hospice care by Medicaid-insured patients with stage IV lung cancer in New York and California. J Clin Oncol. 2013;31(20):2560–79.
39. Sharma RK, Dy SM. Documentation of information and care planning for patients with advanced cancer: associations with patient characteristics and utilization of hospice care. Am J Hosp Palliat Care. 2011;28(8):543–9.
40. McCarthy EP, Burns RB, Ngo-Metzger Q, et al. Hospice use among Medicare managed care and fee-for-service patients dying of cancer. JAMA. 2003;289(17):2238–45.
41. Paragament KI, Smoth BW, Koenig HG, Perez L. Patterns of positive and negative religious coping with major life stressors. J Sci Study Relig. 1998;37(4):710–24.
42. Mack JW, Weeks JC, Wright AA, et al. End of life discussions, goal attainment, and distress at the end of life: predictors and outcomes of receipt of care consistent with preferences. J Clin Oncol. 2010;28(7):1203–8.
43. Pardon K, Deschepper R, Vander Stichele R, et al. Are patients' preferences for information and participation in medical decision making being met? Interview study with lung cancer patients. Palliat Med. 2011;25(1):62–90.
44. Na H, Ditto PH, Danks JH, et al. Micromanaging death: process preferences, values, and goals in end of life medical decision making. Gerontologist. 2005;45(1):107–17.
45. Fried TR, Bradley EH, O'Leary J. Prognosis communication in serious illness: perceptions of older patients, caregivers, and clinicians. J Am Geriatr Soc. 2005;51(10):1398–403.
46. Shockney L. Fulfilling hope—supporting the needs of patients with advanced cancers. New York: Nova Science Publishing; 2014.
47. Quill TE, Holloway RG. Evidence, preferences, recommendation—finding the right balance in patient care. N Engl J Med. 2012;366(18):1643–5.
48. Agrawal M, Grady C, Fairclough DL, et al. Patients' decision making process regarding participating in phase I oncology research. J Clin Oncol. 2006;24(7):4479–84.
49. Audrey S, Abel J, Blazeby JM, et al. What oncologists tell patients about survival benefits of palliative chemotherapy and implementations for informed consent: qualitative study. BMJ. 2008;337:a752.
50. Daughtery CK, Hlubocky FJ. What are terminally ill cancer patients told about their expected deaths? A study of cancer physicians' self- reports of prognosis disclosure. J Clin Oncol. 2008;26(36):5988–93.
51. van Vliet LM, van der Wall E, Plum NM, et al. Explicit prognostic information and reassurance about nonabandonment when entering palliative breast cancer care: findings from a scripted video-vignette study. J Clin Oncol. 2013;31(26):3242–9.
52. Koedoot CG, De Haes JC, Heisterkamp SH, et al. Palliative chemotherapy or watchful waiting? A vignetes study among oncologists. J Clin Oncol. 2002;20(17):3658–64.
53. Kozminski MA, Neumann PJ, Nadler ES. How long and how well: oncologists' attitudes toward the relative value of life-prolonging v quality of life-enhancing treatments. Med Decis Making. 2011;31(3):380–5.
54. Center to Advance Palliative Care. Public opinion research on palliative care: a report based on research by public opinion strategies. New York: The Center to Advance Palliative Care; 2011.
55. Casarett D, Van Ness PH, O'Leary JR, et al. Are patients preferences for life sustaining treatment really a barrier to hospice enrollment for older adults with serious illness? J Am Geriatr Soc. 2006;54(3):472–8.

56. McCarth EP, Burns RB, Davis RB, Phillips RS. Barriers to hospice care among older patients dying with lung and colorectal cancer. J Clin Oncol. 2003;21(4):728–35.
57. Mintzer DM, Zagrabbe K. On how increasing numbers of newer cancer therapies further delay referral to hospice: the increasing palliative care imperative. Am J Hosp Palliat Care. 2007;24(2):126–30.
58. Smith TJ, Temin S, Alesi ER, et al. American Society of Clinical Oncology provisional clinical opinion: the integration of palliative care into standard oncology care. J Clin Oncol. 2012;30(8):880–7.
59. Steinhauser KE, Clipp EC, McNeilly M, Christakis NA, et al. In search of a good death: observations of patients, families and providers. Ann Intern Med. 2000;132(10):825–32.
60. Flaherty D. Between living well and dying well: existential ambivalence and keeping promises alive. Death Stud. 2017:1–8. https://doi.org/10.1080/07481187.2017.1396643.

The Role of Navigation Around Tumor Board Participation

11

Sharon Gentry

11.1 Multidisciplinary Oncology Care

The complex world of oncology care with different types of tumor-specific disease, diverse stages, genetic variants, and cellular molecular peculiarities along with the individual patient's physical, psychosocial, and comorbidity distinctions requires multiple cancer specialties to assess and evaluate the unique patient in order to offer the best evidence-based care. The National Cancer Institute defines multidisciplinary care as a treatment planning approach or team in cancer treatment that includes the primary disciplines of medical, surgical, and radiation who are experts in their different specialties (National Cancer Institute Dictionaries) [1]. Other extended members of this team or ancillary support include the primary care physician; nurse practitioner; physician assistant; pathologist; radiologist; nurse navigator; clinic nurse; clinical trial staff; social worker; psychologist; genetic counselor; clergy; speech, occupational, or physical therapist; as well as others such as administrative assistants. Horvath and colleagues summed up the importance of this concept in oncology care as "many people working together may reach more intelligent solutions than an individual working alone" [2].

11.1.1 Multidisciplinary Clinic versus Individual Specialty Consultation

This type of oncology care is often given in multidisciplinary clinics where the patient is seen by all physicians in one visit and access ancillary support as needed or in a traditional setting where individual patient visits to each specialty are made over different days with referrals made to ancillary support. Multidisciplinary team

S. Gentry, RN, MSN, ONN-CG, AOCN, CBCN
Novant Health Derrick L. Davis Cancer Center, Winston-Salem, NC, USA
e-mail: ssgentry@novanthealth.org

© Springer International Publishing AG, part of Springer Nature 2018   227
L. D. Shockney (ed.), *Team-Based Oncology Care: The Pivotal Role of Oncology Navigation*, https://doi.org/10.1007/978-3-319-69038-4_11

care has resulted in better clinical and process outcomes for patients and consistent communication among the team and patients [3]. The nurse navigator role has been recognized in multidisciplinary clinic care as they often refer patients to the multi-disciplinary clinic and see that the necessary staging studies are completed prior to the consultative visit [4, 5]. Wilcox and Bruce emphasize the role of a nurse naviga-tor as a coordinator for the multidisciplinary clinic with primary roles of educating the patient on their disease as well as the chosen treatment after the clinic visit, assisting the patient in scheduling necessary appointments prior to the clinic consul-tation and being a conduit for communication on behalf of patients to the nurses and physicians who provide their care [5]. Seek and Hogle describe a nurse practitioner navigation model for thoracic patients that coordinates the necessary care for the clinic, refers to ancillary staff as needed, and is a consistent contact for questions and education [6].

11.2 Cancer Conference (Tumor Board)

Common to each delivery of care setting is the cancer conference or tumor board review in which the multidisciplinary care team, along with the extended members, reviews in real time and discusses the individual cancer diagnosis and treatment options of the patient without the patient present. The final treatment decisions are dictated by the patient's own treating physician, who presents the case for this consultative purpose. As each case is analyzed from the point of view from each multidisciplinary team member, the opportunity for the interjection of the latest knowledge from medical meetings, updates in ASCO standards, changes in NCCN standards, medical journals, or webinars, is increased. Tumor boards have positive effects on cancer care. They serve to educate all providers involved in the patient's care [7], increase appreciation of the different team members' perspectives on the treatment approach [7, 8], alter and assist in evidence-based treatment manage-ment decisions [7, 9–11], increase adherence to National Comprehensive Cancer Network guidelines [10, 12], and enhance clinical trial enrollment [13, 14]. With the advancement of technology, virtual tumor boards are allowing smaller, rural institutions to access tumor boards that specialize in a particular type of cancer, and a real-time discussion of cases and treatment is conducted regardless of the physi-cal location of the patient and care team [15]. This was seen in the survey of nurse navigators—"To ensure any and all members of the multidisciplinary team are able to attend, we have AV feed between the cancer center and the main hospital to ensure rounding physicians as well as surgeons preparing for early cases are given the opportunity to participate." "'Skype'-type tumor boards are used for specific disease type from our clinic that is located in one state to a clinic in another state." Continuing medical education (CME) credit is granted for tumor board attendance, and this can be used for members of the multidisciplinary team in retaining certification.

11.2.1 Who Requires Tumor Board Participation?

In the American College of Surgeons Commission on Cancer (CoC) Program accreditation, there are five eligibility requirements that are the foundation for the basic structure of an accredited program and one is a cancer conference policy [16]. The policy requires all accredited cancer programs to have a general multidisciplinary cancer conference that meets as determined by their cancer committee and subspecialty conferences are optional. It allows the institution to set the composition of their multidisciplinary team as well as attendance rates. CoC does mandate that organizations present at least 15% of new cancer cases seen at their institution and that 80% of the cases must be presented prospectively, so this requirement can influence frequency and subtype of conferences. Treatment planning must use national, evidence-based guidelines, and options for clinical trials must be proposed.

The National Accreditation Program for Breast Centers accredits established breast centers with the goal to improve the quality of evaluation and management of patients in diverse settings in the United States, and an interdisciplinary Breast Cancer Conference is one of the three critical standards that an organization must be in compliance in order to receive accreditation [17]. Standard 1.2 states that the Breast Program Leadership establishes, monitors, and evaluates the interdisciplinary breast cancer conference frequency, multidisciplinary, and individual participant attendance, prospective, and total case presentation annually, including American Joint Committee on Cancer (AJCC) staging and discussion of nationally accepted guidelines [17]. It requires the discussion to include history and findings, imaging studies, pathology, as well as pre- and posttreatment interdisciplinary discussion. Conference frequency is dependent upon annual caseload as depicted in Table 11.1. Multidisciplinary attendance is mandated for physician representatives from diagnostic radiology, pathology, surgery, medical, and radiation oncology with nurses, fellows, cancer registrars, genetic counselors, social workers, clinical trial nurses, and/or other research leaders suggested for participation. The discussion elements of clinical trials, genetic risk, and reconstructive options are suggested. During an accreditation visit, the surveyors attend a breast conference.

Table 11.1 Interdisciplinary breast cancer conference frequency

Analytic case load	Required conference frequency
100 cases or less	Every other week or twice monthly or included in a weekly cancer conference at a designated time to allow for maximum attendance and present 85% of these cases prospectively
100–250 cases	Every other week or twice monthly or more frequently at the discretion of the BPL
250+ cases	Weekly

NAPBC Standards Manual 2014 Edition https://www.facs.org/~/media/files/quality%20programs/napbc/2014%20napbc%20standards%20manual.ashx

11.3 Navigation and Tumor Boards

The National Cancer Institute Community Cancer Center Program (NCCCP) networked with oncology programs across the country to develop a Navigation Assessment Tool for cancer programs to understand how to develop a navigation program [18]. This tool identifies 16 core measures as a framework for a program to set goals, benchmarks, and grow navigation services. One measure is navigator responsibilities, and it evolves from the navigator being responsible for patient support to the expectation of the navigator being an active member of a disease-specific tumor or multidisciplinary conference. Often, a core responsibility of a nurse navigator's job description calls for nurse navigator role advocacy in tumor conference participation, assisting with conference material preparation and providing patient follow-up after the discussion [19, 20]. The Academy of Oncology Nurse and Patient Navigators (AONN+) domain titled Coordination of Care in-Patient/Care Transitions recognizes the nurse's role to be competent in tumor board participation [21]. The Oncology Nursing Society Oncology Nurse Navigator Core Competencies for a novice nurse navigator calls for participation in the coordination of the plan of care with the multidisciplinary team and cites tumor board as a method for this activity [22].

Despite the nurse navigator scope of practice including attending multidisciplinary team meetings, there is no standardized expectations of the patient or clinical navigator in this role. In 2010, the Advisory Board Company completed a survey on navigator responsibilities and the role to coordinate a multidisciplinary conference or clinic was in the top seven activities, but there were no specific tasks explained for this function [23]. Although many specialists attend tumor boards and contribute to the decision-making process, only a few, such as the nurse navigator, remain involved in a patient's care after the team meeting. PubMed and CINAHL were searched for articles between 2000 and 2017 with the word strip navigators, cancer conference, tumor board, and multidisciplinary cancer conference to explore exactly what a navigator contributed to a cancer conference or tumor board. The results revealed no entire publication devoted to the topic and sparse comments in publications on the subject.

11.3.1 Role of a Navigator Around Tumor Board Activities

AONN+ has conducted sessions on this topic at its annual conferences [24, 25], has published highlight articles on the subject [24, 26], and has website videos on why navigators should attend tumor boards [27–29]. To further explore the role of a navigator around tumor board activities, AONN+ asked its members to reply to a survey titled Multidisciplinary Tumor Board Questionnaire in the spring of 2017.

Three hundred eighty-three navigators responded with 87% being clinical (nurse/social worker) and 13% working as a patient navigator in the community or healthcare institution. Sixty percent were from a community teaching institution or hospital and 25% were from an academic setting with the remaining from an independent practice, government hospital, or community foundation. Breast, lung, and colorectal were the largest disease-specific responders, but there was representation for all tumor types including hematologic as well as general tumor board. Seventy-one percent met once a week and others met every 2 weeks (18%) or monthly (11%). Eighty-three percent met for an hour, 14% for 1.5 hours, and 3% for 2 hours.

11.4 CME Accredited

Eighty-four percent said their tumor board was CME accredited. Tumor boards are an example of activities that are planned and presented as a regularly scheduled series, planned by and presented to the accredited organization's professional staff as defined by the Accreditation Council for Continuing Medical Education [30]. The ACCME identifies, develops, and promotes standards for quality continuing medical education utilized by physicians in their maintenance of competence and incorporation of new knowledge to improve quality medical care for patients and their communities. Nurses can also use CME for their certification application and renewal. This is a reflection of how a tumor board is an opportunity for all providers involved in the patient's care to educate others on the team about their specialty contributions as well as receive understanding of the different team members' perspectives on individual treatment. Tumor boards provide postgraduate trainees a meaningful educational opportunity [31].

> "The board is very informal and collegial. The atmosphere is one of openness and learning about best options for the particular patient from those at the table."
> "We are lucky to have staff dedicated to ensuring a well run conference and physicians from all disciplines dedicated to discussion as well. Several departments have also required staff attendance at conferences, which boosts attendance in general."

Sarff and colleagues report that offering CME credit is not a major factor in tumor board attendance, but when they reviewed the CME evaluations of a gastrointestinal tumor board, the average response on the participant question satisfaction survey was excellent and nearly half implied that the tumor board information would change their practice [32]. Our survey revealed that some navigators have a role in the CME process.

> "I do the CME application and put the names in for the credits."
> "It is my job to communicate with CME office for all completed CME documents, checklists, sign in sheets, agendas and evaluations. Since it is more frequent than a guest speaker, our evaluations are done quarterly with a yearly overview for CME documentation purposes."
> "I monitor attendance to ensure everyone has signed in to earn their CMEs and arrange for faculty speakers on specific topics of interest to the interdisciplinary team."

Navigators did identify the value of learning from tumor boards for themselves as well as the medical oncology fellows. Several described it as a great place to learn with excellent experience gained from open discussions that expanded their understanding of diagnostics, disease site–specific knowledge, and best options of care for the particular patients and on how to interact with other departments that also work with the patients.

"The value gained helps to expand my knowledge so I can help the patients more."

"Coming to Tumor Board is always a learning opportunity. There is always room for learning, especially with unique cases and patients with other health issues that come into play with cancer care. Interdisciplinary team members also keep each other updated in their field of specialty and keeps patient care and recommendations up to date."

"Aside from benefitting the patients, it is the only time our entire team is together and it is sort of a team building time as well."

"Wonderful way to network and get to know the other members of the team, very informative and educational."

"It has definitely helped with communication within our team."

The survey looked at the navigator role in three phases of tumor board participation—case preparation, activities during the actual tumor board, and follow-up after the discussion.

11.5   Prior to Tumor Board Discussion

In case preparation, the literature mentions identification of cases by the navigators, from the primary care physician or sent by the referring provider [4, 27, 33]. Navigators frequently coordinate the cases by collecting, preparing, or expediting materials such as records and tests from pathology, radiology, and other ancillary departments as well as identify clinical trials [4, 24, 25, 27, 28, 34, 35]. Other tasks are identifying specific questions a physician wants answered or listing patient concerns [24, 27]. And some navigators coordinate attendance by notifying each patient's physicians that their patient's case is being presented [24, 36].

Twenty-four percent of the survey responders did not assist in this phase. Table 11.2 summarizes the survey responses in tumor board case preparation. For the navigators who helped prepare for tumor board, the top three navigation tasks were identifying cases to present, gathering materials for case presentation, and scheduling patient diagnostics. Several other activities reflect the coordination of care domain or competency as patient's were assessed for barriers to care, psychosocial needs, social history, financial status, genetic risk, as well as distress, and then navigators prepared to identify community resources to benefit patients' needs. Others survey responders mentioned using National Comprehensive Cancer Network (NCCN) guidelines in preparation for group discussion plus arranging to discuss survivorship issues. The care coordination activities promote a patient-centered aspect and highlight the unique contribution of navigation in the multidisciplinary team. One survey responder

Table 11.2 What is your role in case preparation? (Select all that apply)

Answer choices	Number of total responses/percentage
Identify cases to present	156/46%
Schedule patient diagnostics	86/25%
Prepare materials for case presentation	146/43%
Others	159/47%

Others—53% reported no role in tumor board participation. Manage room setup and availability and preparation to discuss patient were frequent comments in this answer.

commented, "it is essential that navigators are familiar with patients' medical, family, surgical history as well as the social and economic status prior to the discussion."

Administrative or clerical tasks such as sending email, meeting invitations, and reminders, acquiring the meeting location and food, as well as developing a PowerPoint on the cases were noted.

"ONN arranges breakfast, prepares the NCCN guidelines, uploads all the information on flash drive and then brings it for presentation."

"I work with the registrar to facilitate tumor board. We get materials together for radiologist, pathologist and all physicians who have taken care of the patient. We set up and clean up the room."

"I set up tumor board, establish the call in conference line, bring all of the paperwork, fill out all of the forms for tumor registry (for CoC), and moderate and advocate."

"If film or pathology are outside we help get those CDs and slides."

11.6 During Tumor Board

Table 11.3 reflects the answers on the survey question—What do you do during the tumor board? The number one response of listening and/or note-taking to understand the plan to educate the patient on his or her treatment regimen was not indicated in the previous published navigation material. This immersion is a reflection of the positive attributes of the tumor board discussion that serves to educate providers involved in the patient's care and promote evidence-based treatment management decisions.

"We enjoy attending and listening to discussions so we know what's going on with our patients."

"For me it's very helpful to know and understand exactly what's going on with the patient and how they determine the recommendations from the various input from all the physicians attending."

Table 11.3 What do you do during the tumor board? (Select all that apply) (328 total responses)

Answer choices	Number of total responses/percentage
Actively lead or run the tumor board	44/13.41%
Present cases	49/14.94%
Present unique information on patients as advocates	186/56.71%
Discuss individual barriers to care	187/57.01%
Promote NCCN guidelines	75/22.87%
Suggest local resources	115/35.06%
Document discussion	134/40.85%
Listening/note-taking to understand the plan to educate the patient on his or her treatment regimen	262/79.08%
Identifying and adding potential clinical trial options that are appropriate, etc.	65/19.82%
Others	23/7.01%

Actively presenting unique information on patients, acting as their advocate, and discussing individual barriers to care with suggested resources are a common theme in the limited publications on this subject as well as normal tasks among the navigators in this survey [24, 27–29, 37]. Comments such as advocating for the patients since they are more than pathology [27], seeing the patient not just as a disease [28], and championing the unique needs of each patient by bringing the whole story to the table [25] visually indicate navigation's resilient role in representation of the patient. The survey also reflected this theme.

> "Physicians are open to the knowledge and resources provided from the Nurse Navigator; often unknown case information is brought to the attention of the presenting physician."
> "I am available to share any pertinent information I can add since I have already met the patient."
> "We bring an element beyond the images on the screen. We bring the patient and the family to the table (not literally)."
> "I am able to lend a firsthand account as to his day to day life—what limitations he has disclosed, his goals of care, who he lives with, who he is responsible for, what his activity level is when all is going well for him, etc. We, as NN, need to be the voice of the patient."

Others discuss presenting the patient's beliefs, values, and preferences; life goals with a balance for work if employment is essential; and also the perspective of the family and caregiver needs [27, 29, 38].

> "I am able to share info about the patients the doctors usually aren't aware of—like social issues, financial, etc."
> "Psychosocial and barriers to care are the biggest role in our TB for the NN."
> "Nurse Navigators are a vital part of coordinating patient care across the continuum. Tumor Board Physicians often want to focus on medical issues but the RNs input related to the psychosocial, financial, and socioeconomic challenges related to each individual case is vital."
> "My primary role is a patient advocate and to bring to the board psychosocial needs, patient goals/life events, and patient strengths and barriers. I also bring the overall multidisciplinary care plan and actual timeline of patient care received or scheduled that is often referenced by team members for coordination of needed and anticipated care."
> "I can also help anticipate barriers and problems and be proactive with the patients."
> "The navigator is in a unique situation to advocate for patients' needs and to ensure that barriers are overcome."

Clinical trial discussion in tumor board has been a way institutions have increased their clinical trial enrollment especially among the minority and underserved populations [39]. Other surveyed navigators described bringing in support services such as genetics, nutrition, physical therapy, and survivorship care plans in the tumor board discussion and using electronic orders for referrals during the tumor board.

> "This is the venue for discussing appropriate clinical trials and referrals for genetic testing."
> "You are often the only voice for the patient with information that is often vital to the treatment plan. Examples include genetic information, barriers to treatment such as fear, religious, financial, etc...."

Some answers reflected activities such as signing professionals in for CME credit, collecting the CME forms, setting up the room, distributing materials, and arranging guest speakers.

11.6.1 Legal Implication

A comment by a navigator raised a point that navigators need to be aware of the privacy of prospective planning conferences such as a tumor board. "Concerns about liability for participating physicians were addressed by contacting the hospital legal department and developing a policy that protected the discussion as a quality assurance educational activity. The discussion was documented by the registry but was not discoverable in the event of litigation." Burton and Mathis addressed this to navigators in their presentation at the Academy of Oncology Nurse Navigators 4th Annual Navigation and Survivorship Conference and described it as peer-review privilege protection designated by the individual's healthcare institution [25].

Gross explains that the concern is that a defendant of a patient could subpoena the records of a tumor board in a malpractice case, but the confidentiality of the proceedings is protected because of the tumor board's peer-review function [40]. He stresses that the protection of tumor board participants depend on being granted committee status and cites the Illinois Supreme Court case of Darling v Charleston Memorial Hospital in 1965 and a 1985 Texas Health Code statute, which stated that the records of any hospital committee defined in the hospital's bylaws should be confidential and not considered part of the public record [40]. The CoC policy requires all accredited cancer programs to have a general multidisciplinary cancer conference as part of the foundation for the basic structure of an accredited program, and so each healthcare institution should have peer-review protected status per their legal department [16].

The Advisory Board Company provided insights about the protection of tumor board discussions from malpractice suits and noted it was a rare occasion that this information was sought by an attorney [23]. They stressed the confidentiality of the discussions among the team members and not to widely disseminate confidential documents. During tumor board discussions, the patient's initials or case number is referred to instead of name identification.

11.6.2 Who Documents?

Documentation of the discussion was a role noted by several navigators, but the cancer registry staff was the main group that recorded the outcome of each case. For the navigators who performed this role, the electronic health record (EHR) was the most frequent documentation avenue noted, and then they or an administrative assistant relayed the information to the patient's care team.

"I enter a Tumor Board note into the EHR with a statement that identifies me as the note taker and not a decision maker."

"I have recently begun completing the necessary registry documents which has seen an increased compliance. Additionally, I ensure staging is discussed for all cases presented."

In some institutions, the physician will dictate in the EHR after the discussion or update and then sign off on recommendations entered by the navigator. One navigator remarked, "The name of the patient, why presented, physician lead, and treatment considerations are recorded and kept on a password protected drive that the team can get to for prospective review if necessary." A few navigators mentioned the recommendations being recorded as minutes of a meeting.

The CoC and NAPBC guidelines, as well as an Excel spreadsheet, were referenced as a template for the documentation. The CoC mandates the following be reviewed [16]:

- Discussion of stage, including prognostic indicators, and treatment planning using national, evidence-based treatment guidelines
- Options for clinical trial participation
- Cases may be discussed more than once and counted each time as a prospective presentation as long as management issues are discussed

NAPBC states that open discussion by for all conference participants should include [17]:

- Consideration of nationally recognized guidelines at the conference and that these guidelines are available for reference during the conference
- Visual display of pathology slides and radiology imaging and a discussion regarding radiology-pathology correlation
- Discussion regarding clinical trials, genetic risk, and reconstructive options
- A presentation of relevant H and P elements, including family history
- A discussion of stage, risk profile, and surgical options/presurgical options

A few navigators commented that there was no formal documentation, but they took notes and could answer questions about the discussion if a physician should call after the conference. They did remark that they felt the physician should be routinely present to understand the entire discussion leading up to recommendations.

11.7   Follow-Up

Table 11.4 reflects the two main roles that navigators report performing after the tumor board session is communicating recommendations to the team as noted above via EHR, as well as making sure the suggested plan is carried out. Messier described communicating discussion outcomes with primary care physician and team physicians via a post-clinic summary letter [24], and Burton and Mathis disseminated

Table 11.4 What do you do to follow up after the tumor board? (Select all that apply)

Answer choices	Number of total responses/percentage
Communicate board recommendations to team or patient	188/58.20%
Arrange further diagnostics/screenings	136/42.11%
Make sure plan is carried out	193/59.75%
Others	68/21.05%

Other answers had common themes of no follow-up tasks, documentation of tumor board, and navigate patient according to discussion.

recommendations to each physician but did not specify the route [25]. The survey showed that navigators commonly completed summaries and sent them to referring physicians with primary care physicians and surgeons noted specifically. Navigators also communicated with physicians who were not present.

To promote initiation and compliance of treatment, Messier confirms treatment plans with support staff and monitors patient progress on the plan [24]. Burton and Mathis follow to implement recommendations and assess any barriers, and this method was reflected in the survey answers [25]. The surveyed navigators described meeting with the referring physician to verify if he or she is going to implement the suggested recommendations and then making sure the plan is coordinated and carried out. Specific ways to promote patient treatment were to correlate patients to education and needed resources to keep them on track with care, coordinate care with survivorship or palliative care clinics, meet with the patient to talk about financial needs, and reinforce what the physician communicates to the patient.

The third most common role after tumor board was to arrange further diagnostic testing or screenings. Forty-two percent of the respondents schedule patients for appointments that were recommended by the tumor board, or they ensured the patient had appropriate follow-up appointments. Some navigators delegated this to other team members to do the scheduling and arranging unless it was a "complicated" patient. One navigator explained this was done by the specific physician office such as medical oncology or radiation. "I assist as needed with follow-up recommendations if the case was difficult or complicated." Interestingly, it was noted that "there is more participating among physicians now with navigation follow-up and facilitating communication among the team."

Other tasks navigators noted after tumor board were to log statistics for the CoC, remind physician to sign off on documentation, log recommendations into a spreadsheet, share plan with the nursing staff, and type summary for CMEs.

11.7.1 Who Tells Patient?

The navigators were asked who was responsible for telling the patient the results of their case after the tumor board presentation. The medical oncologist was the primary healthcare team member noted, but surgeons and radiation oncologists were also responsible. Over 50% of those answers commented that this duty fell to the physician who presented the case or whoever saw the patient next. Navigators were included in the group that may see the patient first after the tumor board presentation. "Whoever is presenting the case is usually responsible, although many times the navigator is asked to communicate to the patient." Eleven percent of the navigators had this responsibility, and Schafer and Swisher was the only published reference that expressed appropriately communicating recommendations to the patient [36].

A common theme in this question was the physician discussing tumor board recommendations with the patient, and then navigators followed up with appointments to address the next steps of care. Also, the navigator talked with the patient after the physician had explained the plan of care to reinforce and answer questions. "When there is a change in treatment plan recommended it is up to the medical oncologist primarily to discuss it with the patient. The nurse navigator plays a very important role in supporting the patient by assisting in coordinating appointments and advocating for him/her throughout the whole process." This was described as supporting the patient to make sure they were aware of tumor board outcome, discuss upcoming therapy, conduct any necessary teaching, and assess for other psychosocial needs. This support was reflected as a two-way communication with navigators contacting the patient to answer any questions as well as patients having access to the navigator for treatment clarification. The navigators in a multidisciplinary clinic after the tumor board session were responsible for writing a patient summary or minutes of the meeting to present to the patient before leaving the clinic.

11.8 Administrative Help

The last question on the survey inquired about any administrative help the navigator had with the tumor board. This inquiry raised comments that reflect an ongoing issue in the navigator role—expectation of the navigator to perform non-nursing tasks. The survey showed this in the tasks prior to tumor board discussion with clerical tasks such as sending email, meeting invitations, and reminders, setting up the room and arranging food, developing a PowerPoint on the cases, as well as getting materials such as outside records, pathology, and scans. During the case presentation, navigators were filling out forms for CME, signing professionals in for CME credit, collecting the CME forms, and distributing materials. Follow-up nonclinical tasks included logging statistics for the CoC, reminding physicians to sign documentation, log recommendations into a spreadsheet, and typing summaries for CMEs. Navigators summed up this concern with their comments.

> "I understand the practice of using the NN to prep cases, gather films, take notes and run A/V equipment. But when you assign the NN tasks that are primarily clerical, it takes away from her ability to practice as a nurse. It also has a negative impact on the way the tumor board members view the NN. As an NN my role should be helping educate and communicate the plan to the patient—not driving around town gathering radiology films and slides. Administrative assistants and secretaries are in a perfect position to take notes, gather slides, etc. The nurse should be empowered to share information with the team about the patient and aid in patient education etc…"

"Although tumor board is VERY important, I feel more like a secretary than a nurse navigator. I put together a paper packet on each patient reviewing all testing, labs, path. I present 12 cancer patients a week. I spend 80% of my time preparing for the conference. I'd rather spend that time with patients."

"It can take a couple of hours a week depending on the caseload. It can be time intensive with no clerical assistance."

There is no one correct way to run a tumor board, and each cancer center will determine the presentation based on the accreditation needs of the institution. Programs are aware of this conflict in tasks around the tumor board and navigation.

"We have tried to lessen the clerical duties as we spend an inordinate amount of time preparing for tumor boards."

"It takes me 24 hours to prepare for a conference; no time to navigate. We recently hired clerical support to allow me to navigate patients more and clerical less."

"The NN strictly is nursing—our tumor conference coordinator, who is an MA by background, orders food, sends the patient list to the team, and does all clerical work, the nurse strictly does nursing work."

Forty percent of the responders to this question described administrative help in the form of administrative assistants, tumor board coordinators, and cancer registry staff. Cancer registrars are critical in helping support the role of nurse navigation in tumor boards since they provide oversight to make sure CoC standards are met and monitor patient outcomes and treatments to make sure patients are treated according to national treatment guidelines. The survey comments did show the team of cancer registrars, administrative assistants, and nurse navigators working together. "Our cancer registry coordinates all roles with getting information for the presentation—medical records, pathology assistant, navigation, genetics, social work, and clinical trials for preparation."

A synopsis of the comments demonstrating this team approach appears to have the navigator identify cases for review or receive the requests for patient case presentation from a physician. Then the navigator completes a template for each patient that was designed by the institution for the tumor board (Figs. 11.1, 11.2, and 11.3).

"The template we have designed includes information listed: name date of birth, age, doctors, imaging, path, question, clinical history, path and stage, recommendations, national guidelines, applicable clinical trials, plastic surgery."

"Our basic template: Patient name, Diagnosis, Work-up: Labs, tumor markers; Diagnostics: CT, MRI, PET, EUS, Colonoscopy, etc…; Surgical intervention: Medical oncology, Radiation oncology; Patient history; Family history; Comments and Recommendations."

The template is then used by an administrative assistant to inform team members of the cases presented, and each healthcare discipline prepares their part, such as radiology and pathology formulating their slides, and brings their voice to the table. The cancer registry and administrative staff set up the room, sign people in for CME, and complete all required CoC paperwork. One navigator summed it up as "My team consists of an AV staff for projecting imaging/path; staff to set up the room (i.e., tables/chairs, microscope, coffee/tea/water); medical assistants in the

Breast Tumor Board   Date_____

Initials DOB Age Gender				
Health Menopause HRT BMI Smoking				
PCP Surgeon Med Onc Rad Onc Plastic Navigator				
Fam Hx				
Mammo US MRI Other				
Biopsy Surgery				
Histology Grade ER/PR Her2 LVI Margins LN OncoType				
Genetics				
Clinical Trials				
Social Rehab				
Stage NCCN				
Issues to Discuss				
Plan				

Permission to share granted by HSHS St. Vincent Hospital Cancer Centers

Fig. 11.1 Breast tumor board

different physicians' offices, usually surgeons, who request outside path slides and imaging. I do my best to support everyone working at the top of their license, and luckily have great team and administrative support."

11.9   Metrics Around Tumor Board

In 2016, 35 baseline metrics that any navigation program could evaluate and monitor despite the individuality of the patient navigation program were developed using the AONN+ domains for certification [41]. The metrics focus on three outcomes

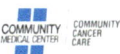

Multidisciplinary Cancer Conference

	Cancer Conference Date:
Patient Name:	
DOB: Age:	

MCC Attendees:

CONFIDENTIAL
Summary of Cancer Conference Findings and Recommendations
Report prepared by _____

Diagnosis:
AJCC stage: Clinical/Provisional: Pathological/Surgical:
Providers: PCP:

Evaluation and Treatment Guideline Discussion

Medical Oncologist: New patient appointment on

Radiation Oncologist: New patient appointment on

Surgeon: New patient appointment on

Reconstructive Surgeon: New patient appointment on

Pathologist: Pathology slides reviewed:

Radiologist:

Social Work:

PT/OT/ST: Oncology PT on

Oncology Nurse Navigator:

Genetics:

Treatment Plan:

1.

2.

3.

Medical Oncology Signature: _____ Date:
Radiation Oncology Signature: _____ Date:

2837 Fort Missoula Rd.
Missoula, MT 59804

Authors Roni Nelson, RN, Terri Paxinos, RN & Kimberly Hardwick, RN

Permission to publish granted from Community Medical Center

Fig. 11.2 Multidisciplinary cancer conference

that patient navigation can influence—clinical outcomes, patient experience, and return on investment. To address the validation of the role of navigation around the tumor board, several standardized metrics can be utilized from the domains of navigation.

Lancaster General Health **CHEST TUMOR BOARD EVALUATION**
DATE:

CASE MRN#/DIAGNOSIS	PROSPECTIVE TREATMENT DISCUSSED Y/N	CASE IS NOT ELIGIBLE FOR STAGING (CHECK BOX)	STAGING DISCUSSED	NCCN GUIDELINES DISCUSSED Y/N	CANDIDATE FOR CLINICAL TRIALS Y/N	CASE NOTES/RECOMMENDATIONS	Letter to be sent
			T N M Stage		Trial #		
			T N M Stage		Trial #		
			T N M Stage		Trial #		
			T N M Stage		Trial #		
			T N M Stage		Trial #		

Completed by:

Nurse Navigator: _____

Facilitator: _____

Permission to share from Lancaster General Health

Fig. 11.3 Thoracic template

From the domain of Coordination of Care in-Patient/Care Transitions, the number of navigated patients per month referred to clinical trial department can be monitored at the tumor board. The goal would be to see an increase in this number as the navigator works with the research staff to assess clinical trial eligibility of presented patients. Another Coordination of Care in-Patient/Care Transitions metric would be treatment compliance defined as the percentage of navigated patients who adhere to tumor board recommendations as monitored and supported by navigation. This same metric could also look at the percentage of treatment plans that follow the NCCN guidelines [42]. Again, the goal would be to see an increase with the support of navigation in the follow-up phase after the tumor board.

If no-show rates are an issue for the institution after tumor board treatment plan recommendations are developed for the patient, the operations management domain metric to monitor the number of navigated patients who do not complete a scheduled appointment per month can be applied. The outcome goal would be that the implementation of a navigation follow-up would reduce the number of no-shows or cancellations.

11.10 Conclusion

The navigator participates in the tumor board within their professional role boundaries as designated by their healthcare institution needs and job description. Being an active multidisciplinary team member early in the care of the patient allows the navigator to proactively recognize the need for a tumor board consult. Understanding the patient's unique circumstances prior to the presentation allows the navigator to champion the unique needs of each patient. Attentively participating and listening during the case presentation promotes adherence to planned treatment by implementing appropriate patient education and reinforcement as well as anticipating future patient needs. Follow-up allows the navigator to support patients during transitions of care and be proactive regarding future issues related to treatment goals. The following comments best sum up the information gained by asking navigators what is their personal experience around tumor boards.

> "When I mention to the patient that their case will be reviewed in a tumor board by other physicians, they feel good knowing that it is a multidisciplinary approach and there is agreement amongst other MDs."
>
> "In my institution, the nurse navigators are the key players before, during and after all of the tumor boards. The NNs are crucial in the documentation and dissemination of thoughts and recommendations to external providers as well as making sure that recommended tests/consults/treatments/etc…are carried out/implemented."
>
> "Ultimately, the patients are receiving much better and more appropriately being treated since the initiation of our tumor board."
>
> "Since we started the nurse navigation program at our organization, we have assisted in developing and implementing three new tumor conferences."
>
> "Tumor Board is a very educational experience. The multidisciplinary team works together to achieve the best treatment plan."
>
> "We work with the multidisciplinary team to have everything ready for discussion. We run the equipment, maintain the patients' charts, add any pertinent info to the conversation, offer resources, schedule appointments as appropriate, and complete summaries after discussion to disseminate to various providers."

11.11 Case Study

The cancer conference or tumor board review allows a real-time discussion of a patient's diagnosis and treatment options in a multidisciplinary care team setting where the individual team members provide their latest specialty knowledge to meet the unique needs of individualized patients care. The navigator is an extended member of this team and acts as an advocate to present unique information on patients as well as discuss individual barriers to care with suggested resources. The navigator brings the whole story to the table that is not limited to the disease diagnosis or pathology staging. After the story is presented, the navigator continues to remain involved in the patient's care supporting the suggested plan with needed education and resources.

CS is a 53-year-old African-American female who had a focal asymmetry within the superior lateral left breast on routine annual bilateral screening mammogram. Diagnostic mammogram and ultrasound on the left breast demonstrated a hypoechoic solid margin with ill-defined margins measuring 8 × 7 mm. Biopsy of the radiographic abnormality revealed invasive ductal carcinoma of the right breast. The breast nurse navigator (BNN) met with CS 3 days after her biopsy as she came back to the regional community breast clinic for her results. After the radiologist explained the cancer diagnosis and recommended a preoperative breast MRI due to breast tissue density and patchy areas of dense tissue, the BNN spent time with CS and her husband to provide education on breast cancer type, prognostics, and description of next steps based on an individual assessment of family history and patient needs. To schedule the next appointments, the BNN has an oncology nurse breast cancer pathway developed by the breast oncology team to dictate how referrals are made based on individual patient pathology and needs. Her family history revealed a maternal grandmother with ovarian cancer at the age of 60, a paternal aunt with ovarian cancer at the age of 55, and a maternal uncle with pancreatic cancer at the age of 61. There is no family history of breast cancer. Because the patient was estrogen negative, progesterone negative, and HER2 negative on the prognostic panel, a genetic referral was indicated for triple-negative breast cancer in a woman under the age of 60. The BNN explained how genetic results can influence an informed decision for surgical care, and an appointment was arranged for a genetic consult 2 days later. CS was motivated for the additional testing to help make surgical decisions as well as the information it could provide to her family since she has a 16-year-old daughter and two sisters. The BNN acknowledged the radiologist recommendation for a breast MRI but explained the need for genetic results prior to making that appointment.

Since CS works full time as an administrative assistant and is the primary breadwinner with her husband on a disability for cardiac issues, a surgeon consult was scheduled for the same afternoon as genetics, so she could limit time missed at work. CS expressed appreciation of the BNN being a "financial steward" for her with the MRI explanation and scheduling of appointments. The BNN picked up on her financial concern and offered the resource specialist to reach out to her to explore additional financial help as her care plan developed. Also, CS voiced concerns about how her daughter would handle the breast cancer news since a classmate had lost her mother with breast cancer last semester. The BNN discussed ways to explain the diagnosis to her daughter and offered additional counseling for the patient, husband, and daughter as needed. Otherwise, CS reports good social support with family, friends, and church members.

Clinical trials were not mentioned at this point since no neoadjuvant trials for sub-centimeter triple-negative breast cancer were available. Treatment trials would be discussed later due to the amount of information that was covered in the first visit.

CS reports menarche at age 13. She is G2 P1 and denies the use of any oral contraceptive pills or hormone replacement therapy. She had a bilateral tubal ligation after the birth of her daughter. Her last menstrual period was 7 months ago and is perimenopausal. She denies the use of any hormone replacement therapy. Overall, she has been feeling well and denies any other complaints. The Women's Midlife Health Clinic specializing in postmenopausal care and symptoms was briefly discussed in case of a future need, and clinic information was added to her breast cancer care educational packet.

CS' past medical history includes hypertension that is under control by diet and exercise, seasonal allergies, asthma that is allergy induced but under control at this time, and bilateral cataracts. Exercise and diet are important to CS since her father died of cardiac arrest at the age of 50.

The other team members' roles of medical oncology and radiation oncology were introduced, and referrals to these specialties were deferred to the surgeon due to genetics and the sub-centimeter size of the tumor. Since CS had a Ki-67 of 70%–80%, the BNN introduced the idea that chemotherapy would be a future discussion. After all questions were answered to the patient's satisfaction, it was stressed to CS and her husband to call the BNN team as needed and contact numbers were provided.

A second BNN was able to see CS and her husband prior to the genetic consult to follow up on any new questions or concerns. Her daughter was having difficulty with the news of her mother's diagnosis, and the BNN offered counseling services for the patient and daughter. The counselor contact was given to CS so she could arrange a convenient time for herself and daughter. The BNN contacted the counselor to make her aware of the incoming call. The BNN also explained the different genetic panels for breast cancer patients and that the genetic counselor would discuss the best option for her. This proactive education was insightful by the BNN since CS called the day after and confirmed a larger panel was ordered that would take 3 weeks for results. CS questioned whether she should wait or just go ahead and get surgery scheduled. The BNN allowed CS to ventilate her fears and supported her decision on getting the best answer regarding her personal diagnosis and family history through genetic results. The BNN also confirmed that a counseling visit had been scheduled.

Later the BNN was notified CS had been informed of her genetic panel results, and the results showed variant of uncertain significance. It was stressed by the genetic counselor to CS that this variation should not be used to make any medical management decisions. The BNN reiterated this information in a follow-up call. The BNN confirmed that the surgeon's office did order a breast MRI as previously recommended by the radiologist and also scheduled the medical oncology and radiation oncology visits. CS shared that she and her daughter did see the counselor and the session helped her daughter's anxiety around CS' breast cancer diagnosis.

A breast MRI was performed and revealed post-biopsy changes in the left upper outer part of the breast with no evidence of multifocal or contralateral disease. After seeing the radiation oncologist, CS elected to have a left breast lumpectomy. After seeing the medical oncologist preoperatively to start the discussion on chemotherapy, a follow-up phone call by the BNN addressed a common myth that patients verbalize during this phase of care. "If I have a bilateral mastectomy, I will not need chemotherapy." The reasoning behind her need for possible chemotherapy was discussed as the medical oncologist had explained, and the myth was debunked for her understanding. The electronic medical record has been a positive to team communication in this instance where the BNN can see what was discussed at the oncologist visit around chemotherapy and the surgeon visit for options of care.

The BNN was present the day of surgery for last-minute questions, support during the sentinel lymph node injection, and reiterated post-op activities and arm exercise program. Pathologic findings at surgery revealed a poorly differentiated invasive ductal carcinoma. The invasive ductal carcinoma measured 1.2 cm in greatest dimension with all margins free of tumor, and three lymph nodes were examined; none contained metastases. Based on evidence showing an earlier start date for chemotherapy for appropriate patients, this system adopted the practice of scheduling a medical oncology visit within 2 weeks after surgery [43]. The BNN also puts cases on the breast tumor board template based on pathology and individual patient needs; an administrative assistant then takes the template and notifies each multidisciplinary member so they can come prepared to discuss the individual case. CS was scheduled for a multidisciplinary discussion prior to the post-op medical oncology visit.

In the tumor board preparation phase, the BNN recognized CS as appropriate to present based on criteria set by the cancer conference policy criteria. In preparing the patient information on the template, the BNN was knowledgeable on breast presentation history, family history, genetics, medical history, psychosocial needs and resources, and prehabilitation requirements. The administrative assistant notified physician representatives from diagnostic radiology, pathology, surgery, medical and radiation oncology, as well as supporting services of genetic and clinical trials.

During the tumor board, the BNN added the psychosocial history with emphasis on CS' role as primary insurance carrier for the family, her employer's support to help her continue work during treatment, connection to the resource specialist for financial help, her caregiver's role for a disabled husband, and current counseling for patient and daughter. A discussion around the dosing of treatment to decrease side effects was part of the tumor board looking at her best avenue to continue to support CS to work as much as possible. The BNN takes notes on the template during the tumor board and sends them via email to active team members in CS' care the same day. The physician who first sees CS after the tumor board is the person to discuss the team's recommendations.

After the tumor board, the BNN continues to navigate the patient through recommended treatment with resource support as needed. At the medical oncology visit after the tumor board, CS had recovered quite well and resumed many of her activities of daily living as well as full-time clerical work. A physical therapy consult to address lymphedema had been arranged by the BNN based on pathology results after the tumor board discussion. CS was prepared to hear a discussion on chemotherapy due to the BNN proactively describing how the Adjuvant Online was used to assist with treatment decisions. She was reminded that a clinical trial may be presented as an option of care or as a supportive route for this early stage of disease. After a medical oncology discussion with CS, her husband, and her daughter, CS elected treatment with Adriamycin/Cytoxan followed by weekly Taxol. Her goal to continue to work was supported given that much of her job does not directly deal with the public and is an office-type employment. She also chose to have a right chest port placement prior to chemotherapy. A follow-up call after this visit revealed that CS had a good understanding of her treatment plan and that the inclusion of her daughter in planning visits was decreasing the teen's anxiety.

The BNN met with the patient and her husband at her first chemotherapy infusion to support the chemotherapy teaching with an emphasis on steroid drop feelings and hair loss. Options for nausea care and a dietary consult were discussed since premedication could exacerbate her diet and exercise controlled diabetes. Also, the breast navigation pathway uses an evidence-based practice of referring all triple-negative breast cancer patients to a dietician for a discussion on a low-fat diet to improve survival [44].

Another evidence-based practice in the pathway is calls to each chemotherapy patient after their first treatment or change in chemotherapy agents to decrease emergency room use by using telephone triage [45]. Actually, CS called the evening of her first treatment with nausea unrelieved by her current prescription. She was directed to the on-call service for a different nausea medication. A follow-up call the next morning by the navigator revealed she did get a different medication that was more effective. She was able to eat and drink, and understood to call the on-call clinic if needed again. She was called 2 days later when most patients experience a drop from the premedication steroids or nausea medication effect so the BNN could verify that the patient's nausea plan of care is adequate. Again, if all planned options are not effective, the patient is put in contact with the medical oncology staff and not sent to the emergency room.

CS did complete her chemotherapy as well as radiation therapy and worked full time during treatment. She was able to continue to exercise, and this continuation of her normal lifestyle patterns allowed her daughter to realize that breast cancer did not always have a fatal outcome. CS received her survivorship care (SCP) plan on her follow-up visit to medical oncology after radiation completion. The BNN contributed to the plan with financial resources, counseling, genetic, dietician, and physical therapy consultations. The BNN did acknowledge on the call after the SCP was in place that consistent contact would not be continued by the BNN team. The patient can always call them for any education and support needs concerning future breast care.

Acknowledgments   The author would like to acknowledge the work of AONN+ staff on creating, dispatching, and collecting the responses of the survey titled Multidisciplinary Tumor Board Questionnaire in the spring of 2017.

References

1. National Cancer Institute Dictionaries. Multidisciplinary. 2017. www.cancer.gov/publications/dictionaries/cancer-terms?cdrid=335079.
2. Horvath L, Yordan E, Malhotra D, Leyva I, Bortel K, Schalk D, et al. Multidisciplinary care in the oncology setting: historical perspective and data from lung and gynecology multidisciplinary clinics. J Oncol Pract. 2010;6(6):e21–6. https://doi.org/10.1200/JOP.2010.000073.
3. Pradesa J, Remueb E, van Hoofc E, Borrasa J. Is it worth reorganising cancer services on the basis of multidisciplinary teams (MDTs)? A systematic review of the objectives and organisation of MDTs and their impact on patient outcomes. Health Policy. 2015;119(4):464–74. https://doi.org/10.1016/j.healthpol.2014.09.006.
4. Hunnibell L, Rose M, Connery D, Grens C, Hampel J, Rosa M, Vogel D. Using nurse navigation to improve timeliness of lung cancer care at a veterans hospital. Clin J Oncol Nurs. 2012;16(1):29–36. https://doi.org/10.1188/12.CJON.29-36.
5. Wilcox B, Bruce S. Patient navigation: a "win-win" for all involved. Oncol Nurs Forum. 2010;37(1):21–5. https://doi.org/10.1188/10.ONF.21-25.
6. Seek A, Hogle W. Modeling a better way: navigating the healthcare system for patients with lung cancer. Clin J Oncol Nurs. 2007;11(1):81–5. https://doi.org/10.1188/07.CJON.81-85.
7. Keating N, Landrum M, Lamont E, Bozeman S, Shulman L, McNeil B. Tumor boards and the quality of cancer care. J Natl Cancer Inst. 2013;105(2):113–21. https://doi.org/10.1093/jnci/djs502.
8. Lamb B, Green J, Benn J, Brown K, Vincent C, Sevdalis N. Improving decision making in multidisciplinary tumor boards: prospective longitudinal evaluation of a multicomponent intervention for 1,421 patients. J Am Coll Surg. 2013;217(3):412–20. https://doi.org/10.1016/j.jamcollsurg.2013.04.035.
9. Pillay B, Wootten A, Crowe H, Corcoran N, Tran B, Bowden P, Crowe J, Costello A. The impact of multidisciplinary team meetings on patient assessment, management and outcomes in oncology settings: a systematic review of the literature. Cancer Treat Rev. 2015;42:56–72. https://doi.org/10.1016/j.ctrv.2015.11.007.
10. Saghir N, Charara R, Kreidieh F, Eaton V, Litvin K, Farhat R, Khoury K, Breidy J, Tamim H, Eid T. Global practice and efficiency of multidisciplinary tumor boards: results of an American Society of Clinical Oncology International survey. J Global Oncol. 2015;1(2):57–64.
11. Charara R, Kreidieh F, Farhat R, Al-Feghali K, Khoury K, Haydar A, Nassar L, Berjawi G, Shamseddine A, Saghir N. Practice and impact of multidisciplinary tumor boards on patient management: A prospective study. J Global Oncol. 2016;3(3):242–9. https://doi.org/10.1200/JGO.2016.004960.
12. Brauer D, Strand M, Sanford D, Kushnir V, Lim K, Mullady D, Tan B, Wang-Gillam A, Morton A, Ruzinova M, Parikh P, Narra V, Fowler K, Doyle M, Chapman W, Strasberg S, Hawkins W, Fields R. Utility of a multidisciplinary tumor board in the management of pancreatic and upper gastrointestinal diseases: an observational study. HPB (Oxford). 2017;19(2):133–9. https://doi.org/10.1016/j.hpb.2016.11.002.
13. Kuroki L, Stuckey A, Hirway P, Raker C, Bandera C, DiSilvestro P, Granai C, Lagare R, Sakr B, Dizon D. Addressing clinical trials: can the multidisciplinary tumor board improve participation? A study from an academic women's cancer program. Gynecol Oncol. 2010;116:295–300. https://doi.org/10.1016/j.ygyno.2009.12.005.
14. Kehl K, Landrum M, Kahn K, Gray S, Chen A, Keating N. Tumor board participation among physicians caring for patients with lung or colorectal cancer. J Oncol Pract. 2015;11(3):e267–78. https://doi.org/10.1200/JOP.2015.003673.
15. Shea C, Teal R, Haynes-Maslow L, McIntyre M, Weiner BJ, Wheeler SB, et al. Assessing the feasibility of a virtual tumor board program: a case study. J Healthc Manag. 2014;59(3):177–93.
16. American College of Surgeons Commission on Cancer. Cancer conference policy. 2016. www.facs.org/quality-programs/cancer/coc/standards
17. National Accreditation Program for Breast Centers. Interdisciplinary breast cancer conference. 2014. www.facs.org/~/media/files/quality%20programs/napbc/2014%20napbc%20standards%20manual.ashx

18. Swanson J, Strusowski P, Mack N, Degroot J. Growing a navigation program using the NCCCP Navigation Assessment Tool. 2012. http://www.accc-cancer.org/oncology_issues/.../JA12-Growing-a-Navigation-Program.pdf. Accessed 28 May 2017.

19. Newcomer B. A national system approach to oncology patient population management across the continuum of care: how we standardized navigation. Nurs Admin Quart. 2014;38(2):138–46.

20. Malone P, Bruno L, Hayden B, Carlson J. Development and evolution of an oncology nurse navigation program: from formation to fruitation. J Oncol Navig Surviv. 2014;5(5):19–24.

21. Academy of Oncology Nurse & Patient Navigators. Core competencies for oncology nurse navigator–certified generalists. 2017. www.aonnonline.org/certification/nurse-navigator-certification

22. Oncology Nursing Society. 2017 Oncology nurse navigator core competencies. 2017. www.ons.org/sites/default/files/2017ONNcompetencies.pdf

23. Advisory Board Company. Six opportunities to get the most out of your patient navigation program. 2016. www.advisory.com/research/oncology-roundtable/resources/2016/patient-navigation.

24. Messier N. The navigator's role in coordinating multidisciplinary clinics and tumor boards. J Oncol Navig Surviv. 2010;1(6):21.

25. Burton E, Mathis L. The nurse navigator's participation in tumor boards: a valuable communication vehicle presentation at the Academy of Oncology Nurse Navigators 4th Annual Navigation & Survivorship Conference November 14–17, 2013 in Memphis, TN; 2013.

26. Fala L. Highlights form the fourth annual navigation and survivorship conference. J Oncol Navig Surviv. 2014;5(2):4–15.

27. Shockney L. Why navigators should attend tumor boards. 2017. www.aonnonline.org/education/video-library/178-why-navigators-should-attend-tumor-boards.

28. Delarama F. Role of the oncology nurse navigator in tumor boards and multidisciplinary settings. 2014. www.aonnonline.org/education/video-library/512-role-of-the-oncology-nurse-navigator-in-tumor-boards-and-multidisciplinary-settings.

29. Skinner N. Role of the oncology nurse navigator in tumor boards and multidisciplinary settings. 2014. www.aonnonline.org/education/video-library/518-nancy-skinner-role-of-the-oncology-nurse-navigator-in-tumor-boards-and-multidisciplinary-settings.

30. Accreditation Council for Continuing Medical Education. Resources for planning and monitoring regularly scheduled series (RSS). 2017. www.accme.org/education-and-support/video/tutorials/resources-planning-and-monitoring-regularly-scheduled-series.

31. Gatcliffe T, Coleman R. Tumor board: more than treatment planning—a 1-year prospective survey. J Cancer Educ. 2008;23(4):235–7.

32. Sarff M, Rogers W, Blanke C, Vetto J. Evaluation of the tumor board as a Continuing Medical Education (CME) activity: is it useful? J Cancer Educ. 2008;23(1):51–6.

33. Gentry S, Sellers J. Navigation considerations when working with patients. In: Blaseg K, Daugherty P, Gamblin K, editors. Oncolgy nurse navigation delivering patient-centered care across the continuum. Pittsburgh, PA: Oncology Nursing Society; 2014. p. 71–120.

34. McMullen L. Oncology nurse navigators and the continuum of cancer care. Semin Oncol Nurs. 2013;29(2):105–17.

35. Johnson F. The process of oncology nurse practitioner patient navigation: a pilot study. Clin J Oncol Nurs. 2016;20(2):207–10. https://doi.org/10.1188/16CJON.207-210.

36. Schafer J, Swisher J. Cancer care coordination with nurse navigators. 2006. www.sg2.com/wp.../05/Cancer-Care-Coordination-with-Nurse-Navigators.pdf.

37. Plante A, Joannette S. Monteregie Comprehensive Care Centre: integrating nurse navigators in Monteregie's oncology teams: the process—part 2. Can Oncol Nurs J. 2009;19:72–7. PMID: 19757765.

38. Bellomo C. Nurse navigation certification learning guide—care coordination. J Oncol Navig Surviv. 2016;7(5):30–2.

39. Germain D, Dimond E, Olesen K, Ellison C, Nacpil N, Gansauer L, Carrigan A, Igo K, Gonzalez M. The NCCCP Patient Navigation Project using patient navigators to enhance clinical trial education and promote accrual. Oncol Issues. 2014;May–June:44–53.

40. Gross G. The role of tumor board in a community hospital. CA Cancer J Clin. 1987;37(2):88–92.

41. Academy of Oncology Nurse Navigators. Standardized metrics source document. 2017. https://www.aonnonline.org/metrics-source-document. Accessed 17 Jun 2017.
42. Strusowski P, Stapp J. Patient navigation metrics. Oncol Issues. January–February:62–9.
43. Shockney L. The evolution of patient navigation and survivorship care. Breast J. 2014;21(1):104–10. https://doi.org/10.1111/tbj.12353.
44. Xing M, Xu S, Shen P. Effect of low-fat diet on breast cancer survival: a meta-analysis. Asian Pacific J Cancer Prev. 2014;15(3):1141–4. PMID: 24606431.
45. Sprandio J. Oncology patient-centered medical home and accountable cancer care. Commun Oncol. 7(12):565–72. https://doi.org/10.1016/S1548-5315(11)70537-X.

Navigation and Clinical Trials

Sharon Gentry and Linda Burhansstipanov

12.1 What Are Clinical Trials and How Do They Relate to Patient Navigation?

A "clinical trial" is a study designed to answer a specific scientific question. It is conducted with people and designed to find better ways to diagnose, prevent, and treat cancer. Clinical trials are one stage of a thorough research process (i.e., basic research to preclinical studies with computer, molecular, or animal models to clinical trials conducted with people). Trials are categorized into different "phases" of the research process. Taken collectively, phases I through IV illustrate "translational" research (i.e., from the bench to the bedside). Participants of clinical trials are told to not expect personal improvement but that they are helping others diagnosed with cancer in the future. Ideally, they *DO* benefit, but because clinical trials are "research," there are no guarantees, and it is important to not be misleading in any way when recruiting a patient to a clinical trial. Not all research studies are categorized as "clinical trials" even if they use a control or comparison group. Clinical trials follow a very regimented protocol that documents all steps and processes.

- Phase I trials address "safety" to determine the best and safest way to give a new treatment and to determine the maximum tolerated dose for one or more schedules of medication. Patients enrolled in phase I typically have advanced disease (i.e., metastasized), and they have not been helped by other known treatments. Basically, there are no better treatments to offer the patient.

S. Gentry, RN, MSN, ONN-CG, AOCN, CBCN (✉)
Novant Health Derrick L. Davis Cancer Center, Winston-Salem, NC, USA
e-mail: ssgentry@novanthealth.org

L. Burhansstipanov, MSPH, DrPH
Native American Cancer Research Corporation, Pine, CO, USA
e-mail: lindab@natamcancer.net

© Springer International Publishing AG, part of Springer Nature 2018
L. D. Shockney (ed.), *Team-Based Oncology Care: The Pivotal Role of Oncology Navigation*, https://doi.org/10.1007/978-3-319-69038-4_12

- Phase II trials address "efficacy" to determine how well a new medication or treatment works in a specific tumor type. These trials typically include a few participants (e.g., 25). These patients have been (1) untreated or (2) have shown little to no response to previous treatment or (3) have relapsed after standard treatment. The goal is to have the tumor become smaller and/or people to "feel" better after the treatment protocol is completed.
- Phase III trials compare "new" treatments of care with "standard" treatment of care. They are conducted on the same stage and type of cancer. These trials are conducted with large numbers of participants (hundreds to thousands of individuals), and the participants are followed for long-term effects for several years. These include regularly scheduled medical check-ups while undergoing the new treatment of care regimen. In this phase, the researchers are looking at the patient's response to the treatment, changes/improvements in survival, toxicity, and impact on quality of life. Patients are randomly assigned to the standard treatment or new treatment. Of note, there are NO "sugar pills" or placebos in NCI treatment trials, and they are rarely used in pharmaceutically supported trials. "Cure" is the goal for those receiving adjuvant care (e.g., hormonal and some targeted therapies), and for those with metastatic disease, the goal of phase III is to extend their lives and still preserve quality of life.
- Phase IV trials are post Food and Drug Administration (FDA) approval of the medication or device. These trials are designed to answer additional questions since receiving the original FDA approvals. For example, a chemotherapy drug may have been approved for breast cancer and then is used for prostate or colorectal cancer.

Patient navigators (both community and nurse navigators) can play essential roles in clinical trials. Because they typically have a trusted role with the patient, they can make certain patients be included in discussions about their possible participation in a clinical trial, particularly minorities and populations that are underrepresented (i.e., LGBTQ, elders, poor, African-American) in clinical trials. What does that last phrase mean? More than 90% of clinical trial participants are white, are well-educated, belong to middle to upper socioeconomic class, and have private health insurance; and until the mid-1990s, almost all were heterosexual males. Medically underserved populations are often excluded from clinical trials because of the belief held by some healthcare providers that the medically underserved are less likely to comply with study protocols and treatment guidelines. Additionally, many barriers exist that make medically underserved populations less likely to consider enrollment. One of the most important is the lack of information about clinical trial participation and access [1]. The community and nurse navigator can collaborate with the clinical trial recruiter to help the patient understand eligibility criteria and what the clinical trial is able to provide or offer. For example, several clinical trials require medications that a patient's insurance will not cover, but such issues can be negotiated with the pharmaceutical company for patients who are from underrepresented populations. A Native Sister (patient navigator who works with American Indians) did this in the mid-1990s with an American Indian breast cancer patient who could not afford tamoxifen. The Native Sister contacted the pharmaceutical company and discussed the lack of inclusion of American Indian patients in the Tamoxifen Prevention Trial, and thus, little to nothing was known about indigenous peoples' side effects to the medication. The pharmaceutical company agreed to provide tamoxifen for 3 years to the patient who wanted to take part in a local breast cancer clinical trial.

The community and nurse navigator help the patient, recruiter, and healthcare providers collaborate to allow for inclusion (i.e., recruitment), which is essential for retention in the clinical trial. For example, people who live in poverty are likely to have transportation issues to and from the clinical facility conducting the trial. The navigator helps address such structural barriers to retention. Similarly, a trial that requires a patient to take medication immediately upon awakening may encounter issues with a culture that mandates the first thing the individual does each morning is pray, not take a pill. The navigator can help explain that praying prior to taking the medication is an acceptable modification that allows for inclusion in the study.

Also the timing of when to discuss clinical trial participation may be best determined by a navigator. A newly diagnosed patient who is very upset throughout her initial consultation with the oncologist may not be emotionally ready to hear about clinical trials. The navigator can still screen the patient to be a candidate but arrange for the discussion to happen a few days later, once the patient is calmer and more able to listen to such treatment options.

12.2 Where Is the United States with Clinical Trial Participation?

Clinical trials support evidence-based practice for oncology patients, but only 3% of adult cancer patients participate in clinical trials [2]. Patients on clinical trials receive closer follow-up and more prompt interventions of side effects, leading to decreased morbidity and mortality, increased survival, and an overall increase in quality of life. The lack of enrollment was reflected when the National Cancer Institute performed an analysis on the Cancer Therapy Evaluation Program (CTEP) trials and discovered that 40% of trials, as well as three out of five phase III trials, failed to achieve minimum patient enrollment [3]. Yet, even when there is enrollment in a clinical trial, the underrepresented populations may be in the observation group rather than the treatment interventions. For example, the Women's Health Initiative study was designed to examine the major causes of death and disability in older women (cardiovascular disease, cancer, and osteoporosis). The study had two study arms: clinical trial and observation study. The clinical trial arm included interventions such as dietary modification and/or hormone replacement therapy. The goal was to include 20% from minority populations, but they only reached 17.5%, and of those, most were in the observation arm of the study only [4]. This is a concern because the lack of inclusion demonstrates the protocol was based on urban, middle class women and required rigor that was not practical for real-life environments (e.g., the nutrition component required several visits to the clinical setting to collect survey data and/or lab specimens that were not feasible to women who experienced travel issues or had the time to participate in so many surveys or clinic visits). Another concern is that it is not known if minority elder women have higher prevalence of side effects to medications such as hormonal replacement therapy in comparison to non-Hispanic women. Another concern with clinical trial participation is that despite federal policies along with educational initiatives on the local and national levels to assure diversity participation, enrollment remains low in racial/ethnic minorities, underserved populations, and rural communities [5]. A contributing factor is not all cancer patients are informed about the treatment option of participating in a clinical trial and patients from minority groups that are eligible are less probable to be approached to enroll [6–9]. Similarly, patients of all races and underrepresented populations cite issues with not understanding what the recruiters are talking about (i.e., too much jargon, literacy level is too high, rate of speech too fast) [10, 11]. Yet, 60% of children with cancer get treatment by means of a clinical trial, and physicians theorize that the higher survival rate for children is due to the enrollment of this group in cancer clinical trials over many years [12]. Patient navigation is emerging as a means to bridge this gap in enrollment. Thus, the community or nurse navigator helps explain the clinical trial using easy-to-understand language, integrates more questions and answer processes to the discussion, and asks the patient about how their family may or may not be able to support taking part in the clinical trial. When issues arise that interfere with compliance, the navigator works with the patient, clinical trial recruiter, and healthcare providers to find strategies to address the issue(s) and allow the patient to continue to participate in the trial.

Traditionally, clinical research trials started in academic medical centers and moved out into the community setting in 1983 with the development of the National Cancer Institute (NCI) Community Clinical Oncology Program (CCOP) and the minority-based CCOP [13]. This allowed access to cancer research in the community where the majority of patients received their care. The inclusion of women and minorities was promoted in 1993 with the National Institutes of Health guidelines for all sponsored research requiring their presence in clinical and government-sponsored human subject research, including phase III trials [7]. In 2007, the NCI launched a Community Cancer Center Program (NCCCP) to promote the conduction of research at community cancer centers and to address healthcare disparities such as racial or ethnic minorities, rural participants, and the elderly in trials [13]. Community and nurse navigation were introduced along with a minority matrix, a tool to appraise issues related to accruing a community's underserved population, to improve accrual to clinical trials in the NCCCP setting [14]. Many sites expanded outreach patient navigators and nurse navigators when a key to overcome the accrual issues was the trusting relationship between the navigator and the patient that developed as other aspects of care were addressed. The relationship development and not just focusing on clinical trial enrollment allowed the navigator to introduce a clinical trial at an earlier stage of care (e.g., prevention and/or early detection trials). The exposure of clinical trial education allowed the patient to be more receptive to participation. Similarly, it addressed one of the most frequently repeated comments from underrepresented populations, "If I take part in a clinical trial, I am being a guinea pig?" These individuals frequently also cite that they will not be given a real treatment or given a placebo only. Navigators share that all cancer clinical trials include treatments and there are NO placebos and that guinea pigs are not given a choice. All clinical trial participants have the right to choose to withdraw from any study. In turn, the preparation of the patient for a clinical trial had a positive influence on physicians referring to clinical trials. Accrual to clinical trials was enhanced by the navigator's ability to educate on clinical trials, advocate for trial inclusion in treatment, and serve as a bridge between the research team and the patient [15].

The NCI sponsors and conducts thousands of cancer clinical trials across the United States as well as other government agencies such as the Department of Defense and the Department of Veterans Affairs [16]. Clinical trials involve ways to detect, diagnose, or stage cancer and study forms of treatment such as surgery, radiation therapy, and complementary and even alternative medicines. Oncology clinical trials also include prevention, quality of life, and supportive care. Other main sponsors of trials are pharmaceutical and biotechnology companies, which must demonstrate that medicines or devices are safe and effective before they can be released to the public [12]. Doctors, medical foundations, volunteer groups or advocates, and other nonprofit organizations can sponsor clinical trials too. Community and nurse navigators play roles with any clinical trial regardless of the sponsor. They are the common bond and communication for trusted information with the patient.

12.3 National Mandates

Clinical trial participation is encouraged and mandated by national oncology organizations. The National Comprehensive Cancer Network (NCCN), which provides comprehensive standards for clinical policy in oncology that are continually updated by a review of clinical trials along with expert medical judgment emphasizes on the page of every standard "that the best management of any cancer patient is in a clinical trial" [17]. The Patient Navigation Research Program (PNRP), a collaboration of multiple sites across the United States that evaluated patient navigation through randomized groups in populations of racial/ethnic minority and low socioeconomic status with a focus on four cancers (breast, colorectal, cervical, and prostate), developed a set of "common" data points using the NCCN guidelines as the major focus of clinical outcomes [18].

The Commission on Cancer (CoC) accreditation recognizes oncology programs that have established data-driven performance measures that provide high-quality, multidisciplinary, and patient-centered cancer care [19]. Standard 1.9 Clinical Research Accrual from the CoC requires a certain percentage of patients from the cancer program to be accrued to cancer-related clinical research studies each year [19]. Policies and procedures have to be established to provide cancer-related clinical research information to patients, and there must be a screening process to identify participant eligibility. This screening process has been an avenue for navigation involvement.

The American Society of Clinical Oncology (ASCO) and the National Cancer Institute recommended patient navigation as a strategy to evaluate in order to improve patient enrollment in clinical trials [20]. The consensus was that navigation is a personalized approach to help patients overcome barriers of education, communication, and logistics, which are issues identified that decrease clinical trial participation.

The NCI and the radiation research program within the NCI initiated the Cancer Disparities Research Partnership (CDRP) in 2002 to address and increase access of underserved and health disparate communities to clinical trials [21]. Funding was provided to develop the infrastructure for a clinical research program, including the establishment of community outreach/education and navigation programs, in order for patients to access NCI-sponsored radiation oncology-based trials. In 2006, the access was expanded to other NCI-sponsored trials beyond radiation, such as surgical and medical oncology, since there were limited trials to address locally advanced disease in the health disparate population. Underserved and health disparate communities are willing to participate in trials when offered at their local cancer center. Patient navigation was a critical component to inform this population about clinical trials and yearly trial accrual increased by 60% [21]. Navigators also reduced the number of missed appointments and addressed other barriers for participation.

The NCCCP recognized the need for cancer programs to understand how to develop a navigation program and networked with member oncology programs across the country to develop a Navigation Assessment Tool [22]. This tool identifies 16 core measures as a framework for a program to set goals and benchmarks and grow navigation services. One measure is engagement with clinical trials, and it starts with the basic step of the navigator understanding clinical trials and evolves to the highest level where a navigator engages with a research team to assist patients with trial participation, especially the underserved population. As programs develop, facilitating screening and access to clinical trials is a core responsibility for a nurse and is reflected in the job description [23].

12.4   Navigation Organizations

Navigation and oncology nursing organizations propose the involvement of navigators in the recruitment and education of patients to clinical trials. The Academy of Oncology Nurse & Patient Navigators (AONN+) outline in the framework for navigation role delineation and core competencies for oncology patient navigators states the expectation of navigation in clinical trials [24]. The functional domain of education, prevention, and health promotion delineates the difference between a patient navigator and a nurse/social work navigator (Fig. 12.1). In the educational function area of the Oncology Nursing Society Oncology Nurse Navigator Core Competencies, nurse navigators are to be competent to promote awareness of clinical trials to patients, families, and caregivers [25].

The fundamental goal of the patient navigation concept was to assist oncology patients by eliminating barriers to timely care in underserved and health disparate

Patient Navigation Framework	Navigation Functions Across Domains		
Domain	Community Community Health Worker	Community/Healthcare Institution (Patient Navigator)	Healthcare Institution Nurse Navigator/Social Work Navigator
Education, Prevention, and Health Promotion: *Promoting healthy behaviors and lifestyle, including integrative and wellness approaches.*	Provide general health promotion at the individu al and community level, including physical activity, healthy eating habits, stress reduction, sunscreen use, tobacco cessation, and reduction of other risky behaviors to reduce risk of cancer and chronic disease	Educate patients on practical concerns and next steps in treatment with regard to what to expect. Identify the educational needs of patients to advocate on their behalf with the care team. **Inform patients of the importance and benefit of clinical trials and connect them with additional resources.**	Assess educational needs of patients. Identify the educational needs of patients to advocate on their behalf with the care team. **Inform patients of the importance and benefit of clinical trials and connect them with additional resources.** **Provide clinical education** about diagnosis, treatment, side effects, and posttreatment care (specific to nurse navigators). Educate patients and caregivers on biopsychosocial concerns regarding their diagnosis and treatment (specific to social work navigators).

Fig. 12.1 Patient navigation framework [24]

communities by circumnavigating the hospital and human services bureaucracies [26]. Underserved and health disparate communities are underrepresented in clinical trials due to multiple barriers from the patient, physician, and healthcare system [5]. As navigation programs are being planned and developed to enhance clinical trial enrollment, administrators of navigation programs, as well as team members, need to be aware of learned barriers to clinical trial participation associated with underrepresented populations (Table 12.1). Developing strategies to overcome barriers to clinical trial participation is essential for trial recruitment and retention.

Almost all community-based organizations that work within the cancer field are also supportive of participants taking part in clinical trials. Many times the issues are very basic. For example, American Indians generally have many struggles accessing standard care, primarily due to lack of insurance and insufficient funding via the Indian Health Service. By taking part in a phase III treatment trial, at a minimum the patient receives standard care.

Table 12.1 Barriers to participation in clinical trials

Patient	Fear of clinical trials
	Lack of trust with clinical trials
	Lack of trust with research
	Lack of awareness of trials
	Lack of access to healthcare
	Lack of transportation
	Concerns about receiving a placebo
	Interference with work/family duties
	Out-of-pocket expenses
	Lack of access to trial opportunities
	Lack of insurance or insurance coverage
	Fears of additional cost
	Age
	Culturally specific health beliefs
	Low socioeconomic status
	Fear of negative results or side effects
	Dislike of randomization
	Complexity of clinical trial process (paperwork involved)
	Historical factors
Physician	Nonsupportive attitude toward clinical trials
	Viewing clinical trials as a last resort treatment option
	Ineligibility of patient due to time lapse from diagnosis to treatment
	Lack of clinical trial knowledge/availability
	Time involvement—finding trial, educating patient, informed consent
	Not having research staff on location in community
	Not referring patients to clinical trials
	Not following up on clinical trial referral
	Poor doctor–patient communication
	Lack of cultural training to address patient
Systemic bureaucracies	Limited community involvement in study design
	Lack of community marketing/outreach
	Lack of resources to promote trials—CME programs, educational material
	Lack of staff to screen all new oncology patients
	Lack of research staff infrastructure
	Lack of available suitable trials
	Real and perceived costs of conducting clinical trials (research personnel)
	Lack of stipends to compensate physician practices for time and space
	Clinical trial staff not representative of population sought for participation
	Not addressing patient barriers to clinical trials

Heller C, Balls-Berry JE, Nery JD, Erwin PJ, Littleton D, Kim M, Kuo WP. Strategies addressing barriers to clinical trial enrollment of underrepresented populations: a systematic review. Contemporary Clinical Trials. 39(2):169–82. http://doi.org/10.1016/j.cct.2014.08.004.
Baquet CR, Henderson K, Commiskey P, Morrow JN. Clinical Trials—The Art of Enrollment. Seminars in Oncology Nursing. 2008;24(4):262–269. http://doi.org/10.1016/j.soncn.2008.08.006.
Wujcik D, Wolff SN. Recruitment of African Americans to National Oncology Clinical Trials through a Clinical Trial Shared Resource. Journal of Health Care for the Poor and Underserved. 2010;21(1 Suppl):38–50. http://doi.org/10.1353/hpu.0.0251.

12.5   Strategies to Address Barriers

Patient navigation is a key to address the barriers between the community and the cancer center. Engaging navigators as a community member for input on study design and recruitment for underserved minorities they serve can be a proactive approach to promote clinical trial awareness and increase enrollment [27, 28]. Placing a culturally competent navigator as a member of the clinical trial team can promote patient participation [7]. A navigator can increase patient clinical trial access, awareness, and knowledge as well as appropriately match trials for patients [29]. As an example, the protocol may be to recruit children diagnosed with leukemia only from children's hospitals, but based on unpublished data collected from the "Native American Cancer Education for Survivors," fewer than half of American Indian children received care from children's hospitals. By having members of communities who are un- or underserved by clinical trials on the study teams, recruitment settings can be expanded to allow for inclusion.

As well as being aware of barriers, programs can learn from the different applications of navigation models to promote clinical trial participation. Some strategies involve patient navigators who are often used in communities to address barriers to care and health disparities. They can introduce the concept of a clinical trial to community members, provide basic education on the clinical trial process, and address logistics of barriers to clinical trial participation. Clinically licensed navigators such as nurses can further assess education needs and strategically screen patients for trials based on pathological presentation. They can provide detailed education and be a link to the research teams. A blended model using patient and clinical strategies can cover outreach in the community with patient navigation and clinical support in the healthcare institution.

12.5.1 Patient Navigation Strategies

One of the earliest reported models for patient navigation and clinical trials came from the NCI CDRP program in South Los Angeles at the Centinela Freeman Regional Medical Center (CFRMC) where the minority, low-income population of patients came from a service area with 20 different spoken languages [30]. Initially the Urban Latino African American Cancer (ULAAC) program planners acknowledged the case managers and clinical social workers already working in the system but felt they did not have the availability for the priority of the program, which was for each navigator to have as much time as needed for patient support. Taking the time to explain a trial in clear and logical terms has been a recommendation to overcome barriers to participation in ethnic, minority patients [31]. The nurse navigators' cost would exceed available funding from the CFRMC budget, and since patient navigators would receive a small hourly stipend, cost was a decisive factor in choosing patient navigators over nurses [30]. Diverse patient navigators were selected, especially cancer survivors from the surrounding community, who could relate to other patients in the community and barriers to care they would face. Key transition players were a medical social worker and oncology nurse as liaisons between the patient navigators and the case management staff as well as a clinical research coordinator that was a resource for all staff in the program.

ULAAC creatively used a community advisory board of nonmedical volunteers who provided perspectives on clinical trial acceptance and a community medical advisory board of local practicing physicians who advised on clinical trial applicability and need in the area [30]. The patient navigators interacted with the community boards for effective use of community resources and the professional staff for coordination of care. The patient navigators were trained to identify individual as well as systemic concerns that impeded patient flow of care and to address clinical trial participation when appropriate. The navigators consistently supported patients whether they opted to enroll in a study or declined to join. The navigators, as well as the advisory board, echoed the community's suspicion of clinical trials and reluctance to promote enrollment at the start of the program. This misgiving was addressed in the navigator training with additional educational sessions, role-playing, and testimonies from survivors who were in clinical trials.

Overall, the early inclusion of a navigator in discussions with patients about clinical trials is associated with an increased rate of participation [30]. Patients had the option to accept navigation services or not at the initial intake visit at CFRMC, and 80% of eligible patients for a clinical trial that had a navigator present at initial discussion accepted the proposal. The majority of patients declining a clinical trial also chose no navigation support. The inclusion of lay navigation was a viable model to increase clinical trial participation in this minority community.

Another program from the NCI CDRP program was titled Walking Forward and served the American Indians (AIs) in western South Dakota via Rapid City Regional Hospital where the cancer mortality rate for this population is 30% higher than the overall rate in the US population [32]. A community-based participatory research methodology was used to collaborate with patients, physicians, and community members to primarily encourage enrollment of American Indians in clinical trials. A step-by-step approach starting with a community and patient survey in the AI population to understand barriers to cancer care, as well as cancer-related behavior, was the foundation of the navigation program. The top barrier in this rural area was transportation due to distance and cost and second was mistrust and dissatisfaction with medical providers. With the barriers in mind, the patient navigation program was designed to overcome them and build trust within the community of healthcare. A key feature was having culturally competent navigators with local representation in the community and the hospital who could communicate in the native language. Another key approach was the radiation oncologist changed the recruitment protocol. His initial visit was with the patient who had just been diagnosed with cancer. He spent an average of 90 minutes with the patient making certain the patient understood their diagnosis, treatment options, and clinical trial opportunity. He would not enroll the patient until they had gone home, discussed everything with the family, and then returned for a second visit. This second visit also averaged 90 minutes and included talking through the entire clinical trial process with the family. Barriers raised by family members were addressed by both the community and nurse navigator. Almost all patients enrolled in the clinical trials and almost none withdrew (i.e., 100% retention). This team approach allows the community navigator to stress cancer screening and education, promote the concept of clinical trials, and address external barriers (transportation, cultural issues), while the hospital-based navigators can assist in overcoming in-clinic barriers, facilitate care, and bestow follow-up support [33]. With the navigation engagement efforts by visibility and accessibility in the community, trust increased in the AI population, and thus clinical trial enrollment was increased to 70% for AI cancer patients [32]. Navigation also supported program efficacy measured in reduction of treatment delays and completion of radiation, as navigated patients compared to non-navigated patients had fewer delay days or incomplete radiation regimens. The ultimate goal of decreasing AI mortality by enhancing participation in clinical trials will allow this population to "walk forward" in good health with the support of patient navigation [32].

In 2010, Stanford University observed that only 12% of Asian patients enrolled in gynecologic (GYN) clinical trials despite this population making up 18% of the referral population, and no one from this population participated in cervical trials [34]. They adapted the ULAAC program concept to create a navigation program for the Asian population since one did not exist. Using community contacts, six volunteer, bilingual Chinese cancer survivors were recruited and then trained by the Stanford clinical trial staff. All Chinese GYN patients, and then breast Chinese ethnicity due to low GYN enrollment, were given the option of a navigator. Sixty-seven percent chose to have a personal navigator for 2 months as well as receive a clinical trial booklet in Chinese. The telephonic as well as personal contact by the navigator improved knowledge and attitudes about clinical trials and demonstrated an increase in trial participation from 3 to 5% [34]. Patient navigation demonstrated high patient satisfaction levels as educational barriers and support to resources allowed patients to be more active in treatment decisions, specifically clinical trials.

Three NCI-affiliated cancer centers located in South Carolina and Georgia that were supported by the Medical University of South Carolina conducted a nonrandomized, prospective study to evaluate the effect of a patient navigation intervention on clinical trial education and enrollment on lung and esophageal cancer patients [35]. A patient navigation model was selected over a nurse navigator model due to cost as well as time needed to focus on nonclinical sociocultural, economic, and individual barriers that impede clinical trial recruitment. A clinical trial nurse was their supervisor. For the patients who opted for clinical trial navigator support, the intervention started at the clinical team appointment where treatment options, including a clinical trial, were discussed. At this visit, the patient navigator watched the clinical trial video with the patient, as well as screened for barriers that could interfere with trial participation. Henceforth, the navigator helped the patient overcome barriers to care, communicated reminders to enhance clinical trial compliance, was a liaison between the patient and clinical team, and provided psychosocial support through referrals or personal contact. Using this approach, patient clinical trial knowledge improved, 95% of patients enrolled in a clinical trial, and all were satisfied with the navigation services. Interestingly, all patients agreed they would recommend a clinical trial to a friend [35].

Fouad and colleagues hired and trained lay individuals in the role of patient navigators to enhance the recruitment of African-Americans (AAs) for retention in cancer clinical trials at a NCI-designated comprehensive cancer center [36]. The Increasing Minority Participation in Clinical Trials (IMPaCT) project trained lay individuals who matched the patient demographics in the area to reflect the social network theory that informal leaders in the community are recognized by their neighbors as reliable sources for advice and support. The patient navigators offered their services to patients that had been identified by the program manager as eligible for a clinical trial. The two main roles were education on clinical trials and support to address system and patient barriers to trial participation. In 5 years, 80.4% of AAs who were eligible for a trial enrolled, and 72% agreed to receive patient navigation support. The navigated population had a 74.5% trial completion rate compared to 37.5% of those who did not receive navigation support, and the participation of African-Americans in cancer clinical trials increased from 9% to 16% [36].

Patient navigators identify educational needs of patients and advocate on their behalf with the research care team. They can inform patients of the importance and benefit of clinical trials, as well as connect them to resources needed to enhance their participation in this option of care. Nurse navigators can also identify, educate, and connect as patient navigators, but their clinical expertise allows them to assess the educational needs for clinical trials in relation to diagnosis, treatment, side effects, and posttreatment care.

12.5.2 Nurse Navigation Strategies

Nashville General Hospital reflects 55% of their hospital admissions as African-Americans (AAs) and is a NCI CDRP program with a primary goal to attract more African-Americans (AAs) to clinical trials in a community [7]. It progressed through phases of identifying barriers to clinical trial participation, screening each newly diagnosed patient for eligibility, and a biannual review to ensure studies were open, as well as available, to the current screened disease site and stages of patients. The review was a proactive approach to identify the population of patients who did not have an available study and adjust the institution's future research selection. Navigation was added in 2009 after the initial model used the research nurse to review the clinical trial after the physician had spoken to the patient about treatment options [7]. Prior to nurse navigation support, the research staff was responsible for resources such as transportation, prescriptions, and caregiver support.

With the assistance of navigation, this program has seen an accrual rate to clinical trials of 50% minority-based population [37]. The nurse navigator assists in overcoming barriers of psychosocial issues such as fears of the randomization process and blinding concept by using clinic-based education to answer questions about clinical trials [38]. They address health system issues by coordinating community resources to meet housing and transportation needs. Also, their value was noted in communication issues with patients during the recruitment and enrollment process, as well as treatment adherence, since the needs of each newly diagnosed patient are assessed and shared weekly with the research staff [37].

Holmes and colleagues united the roles of an oncology research nurse with a patient navigator to address the low clinical trial participation of blacks in the South Central Los Angeles area with support through the University of Southern California Norris Comprehensive Cancer Center and Charles R Drew Medical Society [28]. The previous strategies of enhancing clinical trial participation by providing child care at the campus, assisting with transportation, and conducting outreach presentations to community churches and advocacy groups were not successful. A breast cancer surgeon coordinated the navigation with a private breast surgeon, surgical oncologist and medical oncologist, local health department, and ambulatory care center in the targeted community. A monthly stipend was given to the physician to offset navigator's use of office space and supplies. The oncology nurse navigator had a twofold purpose—educating patients about cancer including possible clinical trial treatment options and logistics of care and assisting the community physicians' knowledge about available clinical trials and completing trial documentation. Within 2 years, 86% of the black eligible patients were enrolled in at least one protocol, and the accrual of this population increased from 3% to 7% by the nurse navigator going out weekly to individual community practices. Also, the nurse navigator enrolled 34 nonblack patients to clinical trials showing the application was feasible to other minority groups [28]. The success of the program was contributed to the development of a noncompetitive relationship with community providers, a trusting rapport between the nurse navigator and the patients, patient choice among trials, the cancer center's financial commitment for navigation resources, and collaborating with community organizations. The relationship building between the nurse navigator and patient created a positive encounter with clinical trials, and those patients were more likely to enroll in an additional clinical trial. The nurse navigator assessment revealed that education of trials was not the main limiting factor, but there were no appropriate clinical trials for the patients' case.

12.5.3 NCCCP Project

In 2010, the NCCCP initiated a demonstration project called the NCCCP Patient Navigation Project to add value to the core indicator of engagement with clinical trials [29]. Fifteen sites across the United States volunteered to participate in assessing the engagement of patient navigators to increase underserved and minority populations in clinical trials. The sites could select trials for cancer types that were more prominent in their community or service area. The focus was on engagement with the navigators as the key link to interact with clinical research teams in order to increase patient awareness and education on trials prior to meeting the healthcare

NCCCP PATIENT NAVIGATION INFORMATION

	Pt ID	Race	Ethnicity	Age	Did you discuss	clinical trials ?	If clinical trials were not discussed, please indicate reason
					yes	no	
1							
2							
3							

	Did you provide clinical trial education?		Did you refer the patient to the clinical trials research team?		Barriers and challenges encountered	Strategies to overcome these barriers and challenges	Partnerships and resources used for outreach and clinical trial recruitment
	yes	no	yes	no			
1							
2							
3							

Fig. 12.2 NCCCP Patient Navigation Project Data Collection Tool

provider who would then discuss treatment that would include a trial option. Also, navigators would identify potential trial participants early in their patient relationship and refer patients to the research team with the idea to increase trial enrollment. A spreadsheet to capture population demographics, barriers, and challenges related to a clinical trial discussion with strategies to eradicate them, as well as resources encountered to promote clinical trials, was utilized to document key data points (Fig. 12.2).

Sanford Medical Center (SMC) at the University of South Dakota in Sioux Falls serves a predominantly rural Caucasian population within a 250-mile radius [29]. The NCCCP Patient Navigation Project allowed SMC to establish a nurse navigation department with six disease-specific nurse navigators. The nurses were supported by two lay navigators—one worked with the refugee and immigrant population and the other assisted with logistics of getting care and support group resources. Initially, the nurse navigators had limited clinical trial advocacy skills, but after 3 years, they were engaging with the research team, especially at the tumor board conference, and assisting with specific trial referrals for the underserved population. For each tumor site, an underserved target population was identified, barriers to trial enrollment were identified, and strategies to overcome the barrier were developed. For example, in a head and neck trial that targeted Native Americans, the

Indian Health Service physicians did not support research due to the side effect risks their patients may encounter. The team provided education on benefits of research and followed up with those that did enroll patients and shared trial outcomes. The project was a driving force for strong partnerships among the navigators and research team as well as healthcare team members in the SMC area.

St. Joseph Hospital of Orange, Orange County, California, is a nonprofit Catholic hospital that serves an area of Hispanic, white, and Asian communities [39]. They used the NCCCP Patient Navigation Project to build their disease-specific navigator's clinical trial awareness and education base in order for the navigators to empower patients to ask physicians about clinical trials as a treatment option [40]. A focal point of interaction for the clinical trial engagement was with the patient at time of diagnosis as well as with the research nurses during the cancer conferences of each disease site. The community outreach nurse navigator was credited with serving patients who are normally underserved in trial enrollment. To address their limited referrals to clinical trials in the colorectal area, they collaborated with the research personnel to educate physicians and the community, as well as encouraged the navigator to support screenings.

In South Carolina, Spartanburg Regional Healthcare consists of three hospitals in a rural area that serves mainly whites and African-Americans [41]. This system had nurse navigators and clinical research nurses, but they did not interface with each other. Their focus with the NCCCP Patient Navigation Project was for each patient to be screened for clinical trial eligibility at the disease-specific multidisciplinary conference. Over time with monthly meeting interaction and leadership commitment between two separate departments, the nurse navigators and disease-site research nurses developed a synergistic relationship to educate patients on clinical trials as a treatment option. The navigators address specific barriers to care, prescreen patients for eligibility, and, with strong coordination skills, often reach out to primary care physicians to manage comorbid conditions that may impact eligibility. To increase the African-American participation in a prostrate trial, they worked together to educate about the trial and provided culturally relevant information on the risks and benefits while discussing multiple treatment options with this targeted population.

A common foundation for each avenue to increase clinical trial participation is built on the trusting relationship that the navigator establishes with each patient. Historically, navigators have used their gifts of interpersonal skills and knowledge of community resources to assist patients in making better sense of the medical world around them [42, 43]. Fillion and colleagues describe this as relational continuity in navigation, where a therapeutic relationship between patients develops as the navigator accumulates knowledge of the patient as a person and is easily accessible and trusted to bridge the cancer care process [44]. The timing of the clinical trial introduction in the navigation strategy was early in the formation of the patient and navigator relationship so it was a symbiotic appearance of clinical trial and navigation. The clinical trial programs that used navigation as an opportunity for success set the infrastructure to address barriers stemming from mistrust and system complexity first, and this allowed the discussion of clinical trials to be conducted when the patient was not distressed on other issues of care.

Each of the patient and nurse navigation strategies or models to facilitate clinical trial participation shares common characteristics of community engagement within their service area, acknowledgment of barriers to trial enrollment with strategies to address them prior to program development and integration of the process within the oncology care team by raising healthcare provider awareness. Because there is no standardization or development of training with navigation and clinical trials, various ways to introduce clinical trial education to navigators were employed.

12.6   Oncology Clinical Trial Navigation Training

The patient navigation training to enhance skills for clinical trial enrollment and participation was based on navigation training and curriculum from the Patient Navigation Research Program and enhanced by the supporting healthcare system institutions [45]. Walking Forward was an exception as this program used the Native American Cancer Research (NACR) to support patient navigator training [1, 32]. NACR has a culturally specific and effective "Clinical Trials Education for Native Americans" curriculum [1]. IMPaCT training was designed as three modules by the University of Alabama at Birmingham that focused on patient navigation, clinical trial training using the NCI Cancer Clinical Trial publications, and case management, as well as data management explanations [36].

Bryant and colleagues, who worked with the Medical University of South Carolina program, published a project on how to deliver and evaluate an evidence-based navigation training using strategies from the Patient Navigation Research Program with the addition of knowledge and understanding of clinical trials [46]. The majority of common adult learning principle structures reflected among the programs were didactic sessions addressing the roles, responsibilities, and boundaries of navigation, basic cancer information, documentation, Health Insurance Portability and Accountability Act (HIPAA), resources to address barriers, communication skills, clinical trial overview, and a strong emphasis on cultural competencies [30, 34, 46]. The training also included role-playing, shadowing, vignettes, patient encounters, and biweekly conference meetings. Steinberg and colleagues used an interactive training model where they asked navigators to list barriers to care they encountered as a patient, and then discussion was held to show ways the obstacles could be addressed [30]. McClung and colleagues developed a question-and-answer booklet for patients in Chinese and English, and over half the patients reported not reading the entire booklet [34]. Personal navigation contact was preferred.

ENACCT Training Course was a part of the Medical University of South Carolina program training to enhance recruitment and retention in clinical trials with the medically underserved [34]. This program is a free web-based training to help healthcare providers increase clinical trial participation with the focus on strategies, efforts, and resources for increasing minority accrual [47]. ENACCT training is from the EMPACT consortium that was formed by members from the University of Minnesota, the University of Alabama at Birmingham, the Johns Hopkins University, the University of California Davis, and the MD Anderson Cancer Center of The University of Texas in 2009 [47]. The ultimate goal of this group is to reduce health disparities by increasing recruitment and retention of racial and ethnic minorities into clinical trials. It is a resource for any navigation program working with clinical trial metrics.

The nurse navigation training was institution-specific with common strategies of matching disease-specific nurse navigators with disease-specific research nurses, attending shared meetings or conferences, and using multidisciplinary or tumor board interaction. Sanford Medical Center recognized the nurse navigators' discomfort with discussing clinical trials and developed a script to guide discussions between nurse navigators and patients [48]. In each program, as the separate departments of navigation and research evolved with their interactions, navigators gained the confidence and skills to assist with specific trial referrals for underserved populations.

12.7 Metrics

Navigation, patient or nurse, does have a positive influence on patient clinical trial education and participation in assorted communities with an emphasis on the minority populations and medically underserved. The navigation and clinical trial studies reflect that each program is developed to meet the needs of the patients of the communities and institutions where the program is created and measures to evaluate the success of programs are tailored to the program goal [28, 49]. The projects reviewed discuss various measures that were employed to increase recruitment and retention of oncology patients in clinical trials—infrastructure development with patient navigators to address barriers to clinical trial participation [28, 32], increasing clinical trial knowledge to favorably change attitudes toward trial participation [32, 35], positive patient satisfaction with patient navigation involvement in clinical trial awareness [34], increasing community physicians' knowledge about clinical trial availability and completing trial documentation [28], and navigator interaction with clinical research teams to increase patient participation in trials [50]. Other measures with navigation can include the number of patients educated on clinical trials with documented barriers and interventions [51], the percentage or number of patients who complete a clinical trial eligibility screening per specified population, reasons eligible patients refuse enrollment, the number that completes the entire trial, and reasons why a trial was not completed.

In 2015, the Academy of Oncology Nurse & Patient Navigators (AONN+) recognized the broad range of measures that validate that the role of navigation in all areas of oncology patient care were not standardized due to the individuality of navigation program to meet the needs of their patients and institution goals [52]. A team was formed under the direction of Tricia Strusowski, RN, MS; Elaine Sein, RN, BSN, CBCN; and Danelle Johnston, MSN, RN, ONN-CG, OCN, and after a comprehensive literature search on the topic of navigation metrics, three main categories of metrics were recognized to standardize national metrics to measure programmatic success—business performance/return on investment clinical outcomes, and patient experience. Two standards that can apply to any navigation program were recognized under the coordination of care domain [53] (Table 12.2). The long-term goal would be to see the impact of patient navigation in promotion and completion of clinical trials to have an influence on survival of patients [49].

12.8   Case Study

Introduction. *Chuck is an enrolled member of the Comanche Nation. He is 55 years old, is of normal weight, has type II diabetes, and is a smoker and a recovered alcoholic (sober for 13 years). He was diagnosed with colorectal cancer and was treated for 3 months with bevacizumab, irinotecan hydrochloride, and cetuximab, but his colon cancer metastasized. It was early November, and he has been listed as 25 on the Indian Health Service's Purchased Referred Care (formerly called Contract Health Services) referral list since June and was unlikely to receive care prior to next March.*

Background Situation. While the Native Brother and community patient navigator who understands the very complex Indian Health Service clinical structure and referral procedures following tribal protocols was in the hospital with Chuck for follow-up, he talked with the nurse navigator about ongoing clinical trials. She and the community patient navigator discussed Clinical Trial NCT01079780—National Cancer Institute [54].

Challenges. During this discussion, nurse navigator and community patient navigator recognized that Chuck's high blood pressure was not well controlled and could be a barrier to trial participation. Chuck was inconsistent in taking his medication, and according to his wife, his systolic blood pressure was over 160 and diastolic blood pressure was over 90 mmHg 2–3 times each week.

Solutions (Clinical). The nurse navigator and community patient navigator talked with the clinical trial recruiter about exceptions to the protocol. After some negotiation and after receiving permission from the NCI to accept Chuck into the clinical trial in spite of his high blood pressure [55], the community patient navigator initiated discussions with Chuck and his wife about clinical trials. To keep the patient's best interests and trust in care options, the community patient navigator first determined the clinical trial was available to Chuck before discussing it with him and his caretaker.

Solutions (Community and Clinical). Chuck and his wife were relieved that he might be able to get into high-quality cancer care. They raised a concern but were concerned that if he was in a clinical trial, he would be a guinea pig and be given a sugar pill rather than the real treatment. The community patient navigator clarified to Chuck and his wife that all cancer clinical trials had actual treatments and did not use sugar

Table 12.2 Domain: Coordination of Care/Care Transitions

Metric #4: Clinical Trial Education	Definition: Number of patients educated on clinical trials by the navigator per month

Patient Experience (PE), Clinical Outcome (CO), Return on Investment (ROI): PE, CO
Other Domains with Same Metric: Patient Empowerment
Rating of Metric 1–10 (1 = Low, 10 = High): 10
Source documentation, including key points that support metric selection.
Source:
AONN+ and ONS Core Competencies
Commission on Cancer: www.facs.org/quality%20programs/cancer/coc
St. Germain D, Dimond E, Olesen K, et al. The NCCCP Patient Navigation Project: using patient navigators to enhance clinical trial education and promote accrual. Oncol Issues. 2014;May–June:44–53.
• Benchmark source: Clinical trial accrual
• Educating patient navigators and engaging them with research staff result in navigators who are better prepared to discuss clinical trials with patients. In turn, this education led to increased navigator awareness of treatment options and helped navigators decrease patient anxiety during treatment discussions with their providers
Ghebre R, Jones L, Wenzel J, et al. State-of science of patient navigation as a strategy for enhancing minority clinical trial accrual. Cancer. 2014;120(Suppl 7):1122–1130.
• Benchmark source: Accrual
• The project was a catalyst to developing a strong partnership between nurse navigators and the clinical research team. For the first time, all the nurse navigators became more informed about how research processes are carried out in the clinical setting, and they became advocates for research. The three programs described in this article have demonstrated that—despite some challenges—educating patient navigators and engaging them with research staff result in navigators who are better prepared to discuss clinical trials with patients. In turn, this led to increased navigator awareness of treatment options and helped navigators decrease patient anxiety during treatment discussions with their providers, realizing one of the project's aims: to empower patients to discuss relevant clinical trials with their physicians. These metrics help measure the impact of the navigators' efforts, potentially justifying their use in this area and supporting the navigation program's return on investment

Metric #5: Clinical Trial Referrals	Definition: Number of navigated patients per month referred to clinical trial department

Patient Experience (PE), Clinical Outcome (CO), Return on Investment (ROI): PE, CO
Other Domains with Same Metric: Coordination of Care
Rating of Metric 1–10 (1 = Low, 10 = High):
Source documentation, including key points that support metric selection.
Holmes D, Major J, Lyonga D, et al. Increasing minority patient participation in cancer clinical trials using oncology nurse navigation. Am J Surg. 2012;203(4):415–422. doi: 10.1016/j.amjsurg. 2011.02.005.
• Oncology nurse navigation is an effective outreach strategy for increasing clinical trial participation among black patients with cancer encountered in a community setting. The oncology nurse navigator is able to inform patients about and enroll eligible patients in clinical trials. Oncology nurse navigation is able to provide personalized patient support and ensure that patients move efficiently through the complex healthcare system while ensuring that patient concerns are anticipated, addressed, and resolved. The oncology nurse navigates the minority patient through the entire clinical trial screening, treatment, and follow-up process, thereby increasing the odds that a patient will participate in cancer research

(continued)

Table 12.2 (continued)

Paskett E, Harrop JP, Wells K. Patient navigation: update on the state of the science. CA Cancer J Clin. 2011;61:237–249.
• Comparable to the 2008 review by Wells et al., 9 recent studies in cancer patient navigation have focused on improving care across the breadth of the cancer care continuum. In the present review, articles were centered on cancer screening rates,59–61,73,77,81,82,85,9, 68,69,84,92,93 cancer treatment outcomes,58,65,66,74,86,94,98,99 and clinical trial enrollment
Reprinted with permission from AONN+

pills or placebos. The nurse navigator invited the clinical trial recruiter to discuss and illustrate the clinical trial arms of the three standard chemotherapy medications versus using the same three standard medications plus one additional drug. This additional medication (ramucirumab) was believed to increase the effectiveness of one (cetuximab) of the three standard drugs. The community patient navigator expanded on this idea by telling Chuck that at a minimum, he would be receiving the current "standard of care" for his type of colon cancer. The clinical trial recruiter gave greater details on when, where, and how the clinical trial visits needed to take place.

Challenges. At this point, the navigation team of the community patient navigator and nurse navigator interacted with the clinical trial recruiter to address the barriers Chuck and his wife cited surrounding the clinical trial option. Barriers raised were transportation since visits were 90 minutes from home, scheduling conflicts with Chuck's erratic work schedule, how to reschedule yet remain on the study protocol, and how to recognize and report side effects.

Solutions. The community patient navigator and the family planned out how to realistically comply with the clinical trial study protocols, as well as have monies for food for family members during chemotherapy treatments and cover gasoline costs. Because Chuck did not have health insurance, the community patient navigator and nurse navigator contacted the social worker at the cancer center for help. Chuck mistakenly believed that Indian Health Service was insurance, which it is not and never has been. The social worker contacted the pharmaceutical company which had an "Access to Care" program that provided co-pays to eligible patients who are taking specific chemotherapy medications. The eligibility criteria were that the patient had no insurance and had an annual income less than $100,000. Chuck easily qualified.

Challenge. The community patient navigator also raised the issue of combining traditional Indian ceremonies and healing medicines while taking part in the clinical trial. The clinical trial recruiter did not know anything about traditional Indian medicine, and the only ceremony she knew about was sweat lodge.

Solution (Community). The community patient navigator explained how Comanche ceremonies were much more extensive than taking part in a sweat and that he and Chuck needed to visit with the traditional Indian healer about the medicines before they could provide information to the clinicians to confirm there would not be any contraindications between the clinical trial medications and traditional medicines. On the community patient navigator's next visit to Comanche Nation, he scheduled a visit with Chuck, his family, and the traditional Indian healer. After a very lengthy and productive visit, the community patient navigator returned to the healer's home with him and was given samples of the plants, herbs, and teas that would be included in poultices and drinks that would be part of Chuck's "cure." The community patient navigator brought these back to the clinical trial recruiter.

Solution (Clinical). To ascertain that there were no contraindications between the clinical trial medications and traditional Indian medicine, the oncology team was expanded to include the hospital nutritionist. She was consulted to examine the plants, herbs, and teas to identify what they were so that they could determine any medical conflict with the clinical trial medications. She subsequently had to reach out to labs outside the clinical setting, to analyze the plants, herbs, and teas the healer was recommending to Chuck. These lab tests came back with no contraindications, and Chuck was able to participate in daily traditional Indian medicine and Western medicine with a clinical trial.

The navigation team that kept Chuck and his family as the center of their care was able to champion the unique needs of the patient within the systemic and community care systems. As more team members were needed, such as the clinical trial recruiter, social worker, and dietitian, the layers of support increased around the patient. Key strategies were team discussions around patient eligibility prior to offering a clinical trial option and addressing patient-identified barriers to care. The inclusion of tribal healing and teas allowed the patient to retain his individual identity to self and community.

Conclusion

Clinical trials involve more than new cancer drugs, but a major barrier to new drug availability is the 8 years from the time a cancer drug enters clinical trials until it is approved with only certain people meeting the eligibility to take part in different clinical trials [56]. Since clinical trial participation calls for a trusting relationship between the patient and the healthcare system, navigation is an inside track for the patient to use on this journey. Navigation can be applied from the outreach through survivorship continuum of care to positively promote the culture of research for the patient. Misconceptions that start in the community can be addressed with correct information, logistics of getting to a cancer center with trials or taking the trials out into the community can be disentangled, clinical trials introduced at an earlier stage of care can increase patient receptivity to participation with a culturally competent navigator, and creation of a synergistic relationship between research staff and nurse navigators can raise healthcare provider awareness.

References

1. Burhansstipanov L, Krebs LU, Bradley A, Gamito E, Osborne K, Kaur JS. Lessons learned while developing "clinical trials education for native Americans" curriculum. Cancer Control. 2003;10(5):29–36. PMID: 14581902.
2. Institute of Medicine (US) Forum on Drug Discovery, Development, and Translation. Transforming clinical research in the United States: challenges and opportunities: workshop summary. Washington, DC: National Academies Press, US; 2010. p. 6. Clinical Trials in Cancer. https://www.ncbi.nlm.nih.gov/books/NBK50895/

3. Cheng S, Dietrich M, Dilts D. A sense of urgency: evaluating the link between clinical trial development time and the accrual performance of Cancer Therapy Evaluation Program (NCI-CTEP) sponsored studies. Clin Cancer Res. 2010;16(22):5557–63. https://doi.org/10.1158/1078-0432.CCR-10-0133.
4. Fouada MN, Corbie-Smith G, Curb D, Howard BV, Mauton C, Simon M, Talavera G, Thompson J, Wang CY, White C, Young R. Special populations recruitment for the Women's Health Initiative: successes and limitations. J Control Clin Trials. 2004;25:335–52.
5. Baquet CR, Henderson K, Commiskey P, Morrow JN. Clinical trials—the art of enrollment. Semin Oncol Nurs. 2008;24(4):262–9. https://doi.org/10.1016/j.soncn.2008.08.006.
6. Ulrich CM, James JL, Walker EM, Stine SH, Gore E, Prestidge B, Michalski J, Gwede CK, Chamberlain R, Bruner DW. RTOG physician and research associate attitudes, beliefs and practices regarding clinical trials: implications for improving patient recruitment. Contemp Clin Trials. 2010;31(3):221–8.
7. Wujcik D, Wolff SN. Recruitment of African Americans to National Oncology Clinical Trials through a clinical trial shared resource. J Health Care Poor Underserved. 2010;21(1 Suppl):38–50. https://doi.org/10.1353/hpu.0.0251.
8. Ford JG, Howerton MW, Lai GY, Gary TL, Bolen S, Gibbons MC, Tilburt J, Baffi C, Tanpitukpongse TP, Wilson RF, Powe NR, Bass EB. Barriers to recruiting underrepresented populations to cancer clinical trials: a systematic review. Cancer. 2008;112:228–42. https://doi.org/10.1002/cncr.23157.
9. Joseph G, Dohan D. Diversity of participants in clinical trials in an academic medical center: the role of the 'Good Study Patient?'. Cancer. 2009;115:608–15.
10. Brawley O. Recruitment of minorities into clinical trials. In: National Cancer Advisory Board, editors. Conference summary: recruitment and retention of minority participants in clinical cancer research. U.S. Department of Health and Human Services, National Cancer Institute, National Institutes of Health (NIH Pub. No. 96-4182); 1996.
11. Burhansstipanov L. Overcoming psycho-social barriers to Native American cancer screening research. In: National Cancer Advisory Board, editor. Conference summary: recruitment and retention of minority participants in clinical cancer research. U.S. Department of Health and Human Services, National Cancer Institute, National Institutes of Health (NIH Pub. No. 96-4182), November 1996. p. 40–2.
12. Cancer.Net. About clinical trials. 2007. www.cancer.net/navigating-cancer-care/how-cancer-treated/clinical-trials/about-clinical-trials. Accessed 8 Mar 2017.
13. Dimond EP, St. Germain D, Nacpil LM, Zaren HA, Swanson SM, Minnick C, et al. Creating a "culture of research" in a community hospital: strategies and tools from the National Cancer Institute Community Cancer Centers Program. Clinical Trials (London, England). 2015;12(3):246–56. https://doi.org/10.1177/1740774515571141.
14. Gonzalez M, Berger M, Bryant D, Ellison C, Harness J, Krasna M, et al. Using a minority matrix and patient navigation to improve accrual to clinical trials. Oncol Issues. 2011;March/April:59–60.
15. Gonzalez M, Berger M, Bryant D, Ellison C, Harness J, Krasna M, et al. Using a minority matrix and patient navigation to improve accrual to clinical trials. March/April: Oncology Issues; 2011. p. 59–60.
16. National Cancer Institute. Cancer clinical trials factsheet. 2017. www.hahv.org/wp-content/uploads/2016/01/clinical-trial-fact-sheet.pdf
17. National Comprehensive Cancer Network. About NCCN. 2017. https://www.nccn.org/about/default.aspx
18. Freund K, Battaglia T, Calhoun E, Dudley D, Fiscella K, Paskett E, et al. National Cancer Institute Patient Navigation Research Program: methods, protocol, and measures. Cancer. 2008;113(12):3391–9. https://doi.org/10.1002/cncr.23960.
19. Commission on Cancer. Cancer program standards: ensuring patient centered care. 2016. https://www.facs.org/quality-programs/cancer/coc/standards
20. Denicoff A, McCaskill-Stevens W, Grubbs S, Bruinooge S, Comis R, Devine P, et al. The National Cancer Institute-American Society of Clinical Oncology cancer trial accrual

symposium: summary and recommendations. J Oncol Pract. 2013;9(6):267–76. https://doi.org/10.1200/JOP.2013.001119.

21. Wong RSL, Vikram B, Govern FS, Petereit DG, Maguire PD, Clarkson MR, et al. National Cancer Institute's Cancer Disparities Research Partnership Program: experience and lessons learned. Front Oncol. 2014;4:303. https://doi.org/10.3389/fonc.2014.00303.

22. Swanson J, Strusowski P, Mack N, Degroot J. Growing a navigation program using the NCCCP Navigation Assessment Tool. 2012. www.accc-cancer.org/oncology_issues/.../JA12-Growing-a-Navigation-Program.pdf. Accessed 5 Feb 2017.

23. Newcomer B. A national system approach to oncology patient population management across the continuum of care: how we standardized navigation. Nurs Adm Q. 2014;38(2):138–46.

24. Willis A, Reed E, Pratt-Chapman M, Kapp H, Hatcher E, Vaitones V. Development of a framework for patient navigation: delineating roles across navigator types. J Oncol Navig Surviv. 2013;4(6):20–6.

25. Oncology Nursing Society. Oncology nurse navigator core competencies. 2017. www.ons.org/sites/default/files/ONNCompetencies_rev.pdf. Accessed 5 Mar 2017.

26. Freeman H. Patient navigation: a community centered approach to reducing cancer mortality. J Cancer Educ. 2006;21(1):S11–4. https://doi.org/10.1207/s15430154jce2101s_4.

27. Moffitt K, Brogan F, Brown C, Kasper M, Rosenblatt J, Smallridge R, et al. Statewide cancer clinical trial navigation service. J Oncol Pract. 2010;6(3):127–32. https://doi.org/10.1200/JOP.200006.

28. Holmes D, Majo J, Lyonga D, Alleyne R, Clayton S. Increasing minority patient participation in cancer clinical trials using oncology nurse navigation. Am J Surg. 2012;203(4):415–22. https://doi.org/10.1016/j.amjsurg.2011.02.005.

29. Germain D, Dimond E, Olesen K, Ellison C, Nacpil N, Gansauer L, Carrigan A, Igo K, Gonzalez M. The NCCCP Patient Navigation Project using patient navigators to enhance clinical trial education and promote accrual. Oncology Issues. 2014;May–June:44–53.

30. Steinberg ML, Fremont A, Khan DC, Huang D, Knapp H, Karaman D, Forge N, Andre K, Chaiken LM, Streeter OE. Lay patient navigator program implementation for equal access to cancer care and clinical trials. Cancer. 2006;107:2669–77. https://doi.org/10.1002/cncr.22319.

31. Gorelick P, Harris Y, Burnett B, Bonecutter F. The recruitment triangle: reasons why African Americans enroll, refuse to enroll, or voluntarily withdraw from a clinical trial. J Natl Med Assoc. 1998;90:141–5.

32. Kanekar S, Petereit D. Walking forward: a program designed to lower cancer mortality rates among American Indians in Western South Dakota. South Dakota Med. 2009;62(4):151–9.

33. Guadagnolo BA, Petereit DG, Helbig P, Koop D, Kussman P, Dunn EF, Patnaik A. Involving American Indians and medically underserved rural populations in cancer clinical trials. Clinical Trials (London, England). 2009;6(6):610–7. https://doi.org/10.1177/1740774509348526.

34. McClung EC, Davis SW, Jeffrey SS, Kuo M-C, Lee MM, Teng NNH. Impact of navigation on knowledge and attitudes about clinical trials among Chinese Patients undergoing treatment for breast and gynecologic cancers. J Immigr Minor Health. 2013;17(3):976–9.

35. Cartmell KB, Bonilha HS, Matson T, Bryant DC, Zapka JG, Bentz TA, et al. Patient participation in cancer clinical trials: a pilot test of lay navigation. Contemp Clin Trials Commun. 2016;15(3):86–93. https://doi.org/10.1016/j.conctc.2016.04.005.

36. Fouad M, Acemgil A, Bae S, Forero A, Lisovicz N, Martin M, et al. Patient navigation as a model to increase participation of African Americans in cancer clinical trials. J Oncol Pract. 2016;12(6):556–63. https://doi.org/10.1200/JOP.2015.008946.

37. Cancer Partnership. Clinical Trials Program at Metropolitan Nashville General Hospital. 2017. www.cancer-alliance.org/research/clinical-trials-program-at-metropolitan-nashville-general-hospital. Accessed 26 Mar 2017.

38. EMPACT. General approaches to minority recruitment for cancer clinical trials: a presentation by the EMPACT consortium. 2012. http://tuh7143yoi527qz2743fa3x7.wpengine.netdna-cdn.com/wp-content/uploads/2012/05/General_Approaches_e508.pdf.

39. St Joseph Hospital. St Joseph Hospital community health needs assessment report. 2014. /www.sjo.org/For-Community/Community-Benefits-Plan.aspx.

40. Germain D, Dimond E, Olesen K, Ellison C, Nacpil N, Gansauer L, et al. The NCCCP Patient Navigation Project using patient navigators to enhance clinical trial education and promote accrual. Oncology Issues. 2014;May–June:44–53.
41. Gibbs Cancer Center & Research Institute. 2016 Annual report. 2016. https://gibbscancer-center.org/news-media/annual-reports/#1457639866050-77e7953e-4cd2.
42. Natale-Pereira A, Enard KR, Nevarez L, Jones LA. The role of patient navigators in eliminating health disparities. Cancer. 2011;117:3543–52. https://doi.org/10.1002/cncr.26264.
43. Gunn CM, Clark JA, Battaglia TA, Freund KM, Parker VA. An assessment of patient navigator activities in breast cancer patient navigation programs using a nine-principle framework. Health Serv Res. 2014;49:1555–77. https://doi.org/10.1111/1475-6773.12184.
44. Fillion L, Cook S, Veillette A, Aubin M, de Serres M, Rainville F, et al. Professional navigation framework: elaboration and validation in a Canadian context. Oncol Nurs Forum. 2012;39(1):E58–69. https://doi.org/10.1188/12.ONF.E58-E69.
45. Calhoun EA, Whitley EM, Esparza A, Ness E, Greene A, Garcia R, et al. A national patient navigator training program. Health Promot Pract. 2010;11(2):205–15. https://doi.org/10.1177/1524839908323521.
46. Bryant D, Williamson D, Cartmell K, Jefferson M. A lay patient navigation training curriculum targeting disparities in cancer clinical trials. J Black Nurses Assoc. 2011;22(2):68–75.
47. EMPACT. ENACCT's free E-learning series primary care provider training program. 2017. http://empactconsortium.com/resource/enaccts-free-e-learning-series-primary-care-provider-training-program.
48. Germain D, Dimond E, Olesen K, Ellison C, Nacpil N, Gansauer L, et al. The NCCCP Patient Navigation Project using patient navigators to enhance clinical trial education and promote accrual. Oncol Issues. 2014;May–June:44–53.
49. Ghebre RG, Jones LA, Wenzel J, Martin MY, Durant R, Ford JG. State-of-the-science of patient navigation as a strategy for enhancing minority clinical trial accrual. Cancer. 2014;120(7):1122–30. https://doi.org/10.1002/cncr.28570.
50. Germain D, Dimond E, Olesen K, Ellison C, Nacpil N, Gansauer L, Carrigan A, Igo K, Gonzalez M. The NCCCP Patient Navigation Project using patient navigators to enhance clinical trial education and promote accrual. Oncol Issues. 2014;May–June:44–53.
51. Bellomo C, Christensen D, Strusowski T. Seasoned navigator: a case study on care transitions in genomic testing and timely treatment decision-making. J Navig Surviv. 2016;7(4):33–4.
52. Academy of Oncology Nurse Navigators. Standardized metrics source document. 2017. www.aonnonline.org/metrics-source-document. Accessed 5 Mar 2017.
53. Strusowski T, Sein E, Johnston D, Gentry S, Bellomo C, Brown E, et al. Standardized evidence-based oncology navigation metrics for all models: a powerful tool in assessing the value and impact of navigation programs. J Navig Surviv. 2017;8(5):220–43.
54. Irinotecan Hydrochloride and Cetuximab with or without Ramucirumab in treating patients with advanced colorectal cancer with progressive disease after treatment with Bevacizumab-Containing Chemotherapy.
55. NCI had no American Indians enrolled in the study and were willing to allow Chuck to take part to determine if the medications reacted differently among this underserved population.
56. Innovation Cancer. Clinical trials. 2015. www.innovationcancer.com/For-Patients/Clinical-Trials.aspx.

Understanding Role Delineation of the Multidisciplinary Team Members

13

Elizabeth F. Franklin, Linda House, and Elizabeth Glidden

13.1 Multidisciplinary Cancer Care Team

There are various terms to describe the professionals who make up the cancer care team. "Multidisciplinary" has been used to describe different professionals working individually with a patient. "Interdisciplinary" has been used to refer to multiple professionals working as a team with a common goal in support of the patient. "Transdisciplinary" has been used to describe the team of professionals working together under a shared model with common language [1].

In this chapter, we use the term multidisciplinary, not to make a meaningful statement regarding the various descriptors but because we will be outlining the specific roles of each individual professional. These individuals do work together as a team, but our goal is to describe the roles of the professionals and respect the boundaries required for each person on the cancer care team to ethically and competently adhere to their job duties [2]. However, there must be cooperation and communication to cut across these boundaries in order to best serve the patient [1]. At the end of this chapter, a case study will illustrate the importance of true transdisciplinary professionalism and collaboration.

13.1.1 Members of the Multidisciplinary Cancer Care Team

Depending on patient goals and needs, different members of the cancer care team can serve as the "expert" at different times [3]. Some members will be present

E. F. Franklin, LGSW, ACSW (✉) · L. House, RN, BSN, MSM
Cancer Support Community, Washington, DC, USA
e-mail: efranklin@cancersupportcommunity.org; linda@cancersupportcommunity.org

E. Glidden, MPH
American Cancer Society, Washington, DC, USA
e-mail: elizabeth.glidden@cancer.org

© Springer International Publishing AG, part of Springer Nature 2018
L. D. Shockney (ed.), *Team-Based Oncology Care: The Pivotal Role of Oncology Navigation*, https://doi.org/10.1007/978-3-319-69038-4_13

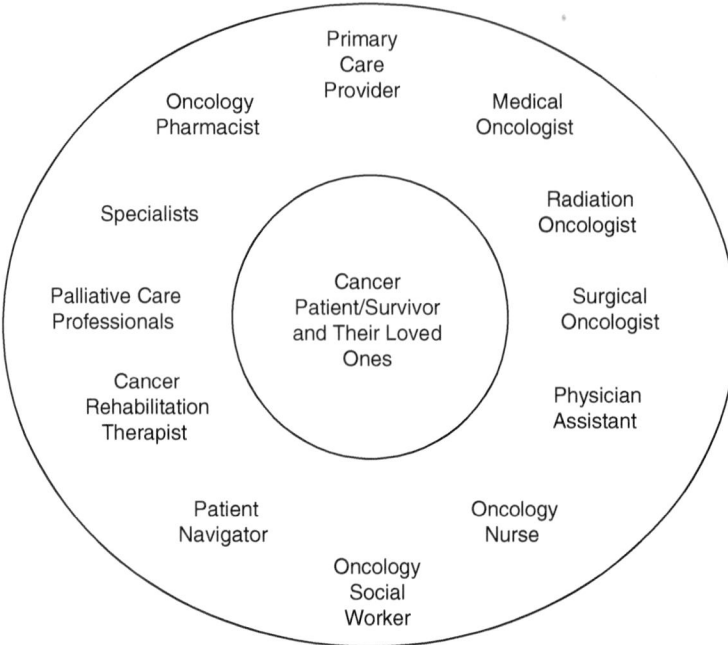

Fig. 13.1 Members of the patient-centered multidisciplinary cancer care team

throughout the patient's journey, while others will be present only at specific points [3]. While it is important for team members to have shared goals, it is equally as important for them to have clear roles, responsibilities, and accountabilities [4].

Figure 13.1 illustrates members of the multidisciplinary cancer care team which include, but are not limited to, the following individuals and professionals.

13.2 Cancer Patient

A cancer patient is a person who has been diagnosed with any type of cancer. The patient is at the center of the multidisciplinary care team and drives the treatment decision-making process. According to the IOM [5], patient-centered care can be defined as care that is respectful of and responsive to individual patient preferences, needs, and values, and ensures that patient values "guide all clinical decisions." Patient-centered care involves good communication between the patient and care team, evidence-based information to educate the care team (including the patient) about treatment options, and a shared decision-making process [4].

This shared decision-making process centers around the relationship of the patient and the care team. Together, they make decisions and select treatment plans that both incorporate clinical evidence and consider patient preferences and values [6]. Shared decision-making includes medical treatment as well as psychosocial and palliative care [4]. The benefits of shared decision-making include more knowledgeable and prepared patients, more trusting relationships between patients and providers, and greater satisfaction for all parties involved [6]. However, true shared decision-making can be difficult due to emotional, financial, or logistical challenges facing the patient along with potential health literacy barriers and a lack of experience with the healthcare system [4].

When the cancer care team is functioning well together, they can provide truly patient- and family-centered care. Patient- and family-centered care is "an innovative approach to the planning, delivery, and evaluation of health care that is grounded in mutually beneficial partnerships among health care providers, patients, and families" [7] (p. 596). Patient- and family-centered care is beneficial to not only the patient and family but also the providers and the institution.

According to the IOM [4], the multidisciplinary cancer care team should "provide patients and their families with understandable information on cancer prognosis, treatment benefits and harms, palliative care, psychosocial support, and estimates of the total and out of pocket costs of cancer care" (p. 116). This information should be personalized and provided at key decision-making points along the cancer continuum [4].

13.2.1 Primary Care Physicians

Primary care physicians (PCPs) are generalists who provide comprehensive care to patients on a regular basis [4]. PCPs specialize in general internal medicine or family medicine and are often the first point of contact for patients diagnosed with cancer. In fact, a typical family physician will have three to four patients who receive a new diagnosis of cancer each year [8]. Klabunde et al. [9] found that 90% of PCPs fulfilled general medical roles for cancer patients such as managing comorbid conditions. Of those surveyed, 19% reported heavy involvement in cancer care roles [9]. PCPs can be a mainstay of information, support, and advice through cancer diagnosis and treatment [8]. When patients are followed by both an oncologist and a PCP, they are more likely to receive preventive care and care for non-cancer chronic illness that is consistent with guidelines [8]. PCPs will be caring for more and more cancer survivors, going forward, with oncology specialists also following the patients long-term. Therefore, more ongoing education for PCPs will be taking place nationally in medical school training, continued education at professional conferences, and continued education programs locally, regionally, and nationally.

13.2.2 Medical Oncologists

Medical oncologists diagnose and treat cancer using chemotherapy, hormonal therapy, biological therapy, immunotherapy, and targeted therapy [10]. The medical oncologist may be the main provider for a cancer patient or may offer supportive care or coordinate treatment with other specialists [10]. Medical oncologists are also responsible for helping patients manage the side effects of chemotherapy [11].

Medical oncologists utilize chemotherapy to treat cancer, to slow tumor growth, or to ease cancer symptoms such as pain [11]. Chemotherapy can be administered in a variety of ways, including intravenously, orally, topically, or by injection [11]. It can also be administered at home, during a hospital stay, in a doctor's office, or in a clinic [11]. Neoadjuvant chemotherapy can be used before other types of therapy such as surgery or radiation. Adjuvant chemotherapy is utilized after other types of therapy to destroy cancer cells that may remain in the body [11].

13.2.3 Surgical Oncologists

Surgery is the oldest form of cancer treatment and can be part of a curative treatment plan for many patients [12]. A surgical oncologist focuses on the surgical treatment of tumors [12]. This may be the complete removal of a tumor, the partial removal of a tumor otherwise known as "debulking," or easing of cancer symptoms by the removal of tumors that are causing pain or pressure [13].

Surgeons are "responsible for the preoperative diagnosis of the patient, for performing the operation, and for providing the patient with postoperative surgical care and treatment [14]. Surgeons can work in private practice, academic medicine, institutional practice, hospitals, ambulatory surgery settings, government service programs, and the uniformed services [14].

In addition to their primary role, surgeons may also work with colleagues to provide expertise on "biopsy techniques, optimal image guidance, the likelihood of achieving clear margins…and what role there is, if any, for surgical management of more advanced disease" [12]. Surgery can take place before or after chemotherapy and/or radiation as a comprehensive approach to addressing the disease [12].

13.2.4 Radiation Oncologists

Radiation oncologists treat cancer using radiation or high-energy x-rays or other particles [15, 16]. Radiation therapy is used to destroy cancer cells and slow tumor growth, and can be used alone or in combination with other types of treatment [15]. Over half of all cancer patients receive radiation therapy [15]. The therapy can be delivered through external beam, whereby radiation comes from a machine outside the body, or through internal radiation therapy or brachytherapy, whereby radioactive material is placed inside or on the body to treat the cancer [16]. A patient may receive radiation therapy before (neoadjuvant), during, or after (adjuvant) surgery [16]. Radiation can also be given with chemotherapy, sometimes called chemoradiation or radiochemotherapy [16].

The radiation oncologist conducts the therapy, monitors safety, evaluates progress throughout therapy and adjusts as needed, and addresses side effects with the patient [15]. Physicists and dosimetrists work with the radiation oncologist to determine the exact radiation plan [16].

13.2.5 Specialists

In addition to oncologists, there are other physicians who may diagnose and treat cancer patients. Hematologists diagnose and treat blood disorders, including cancer [4]. Urologists may treat prostate cancer, pulmonologists treat early-stage lung cancer, dermatologists treat early-stage melanoma, and gastroenterologists treat early-stage colon cancer [4]. Gynecologists may also refer patients to gynecological oncologists.

13.2.6 Physician Assistants

Physician assistants (PAs) are medically trained and licensed, and perform duties under the supervision of a physician [4]. They can diagnose and treat illness, order lab tests, prescribe medication, educate patients, and manage care plans [4]. PAs receive a generalist education and pass a national certification exam that includes content all of the major cancers [4]. Much like other professionals in this chapter, however, they receive most of their oncology knowledge through on-the-job training [4].

13.2.7 Oncology Pharmacists

Oncology pharmacists are licensed to practice pharmacy, are board certified, and have advanced knowledge and experience to work with patients with malignant disease [17]. Oncology pharmacists practice for 4 years post-license with at least half of their time devoted to oncology pharmacy activities, or they complete a residency with a focus on oncology [17]. The work of an oncology pharmacist involves an increasing number of complex therapies to prevent and treat cancer and manage adverse events [17]. This important member of the cancer care team can prepare chemotherapy dosage and safety, educate patients about side effects, or work in drug development research [18].

13.2.8 Palliative Care Professionals

Palliative care professionals work with patients and their loved ones to optimize quality of life by anticipating, preventing, and treating suffering [19]. The palliative care team can include physicians, nurses, registered dietitians, pharmacists, social workers, and other professionals who seek to address symptoms and side effects, as early as possible, to provide comfort and support to the patient [10]. These professionals address physical, intellectual, emotional, social, and spiritual needs of the patient [19]. The palliative care team can be brought into care for a cancer patient immediately following diagnosis and continue throughout treatment. They may also work with hospice professionals to assist in end-of-life care [10]. However, it is important to distinguish that patients receiving palliative care alone may still receive cancer treatment.

13.2.9 Cancer Rehabilitation Therapist

With many long-term cancer survivors, adverse effects caused by disease or treatment have led to a need for interventions to reverse or lessen the challenges facing these individuals [20]. Cancer rehabilitation therapists include physical and occupational therapists and physiatrists who work with patients and survivors to improve daily function and quality of life [21]. The field of oncology rehabilitation has evolved from supportive and palliative care to complex rehabilitation interventions [20]. Physical therapists help patients address feelings of tiredness, weakness, and challenges with balance [21]. Occupational therapists work with patients to help them complete activities of daily living such as dressing, grooming, bathing, increasing fine motor skills, saving energy, and improving memory and sight [21]. Physiatrists are physicians with training in physical medicine and rehab. They can manage medical problems experienced by many cancer patients such as fatigue, pain, and weakness [21].

13.2.10 Oncology Nurses, Nurse Practitioners, and Nurse Navigators

Nursing is defined by the American Nurses Association [22] as "the protection, promotion, and optimization, of health and abilities, prevention of illness and injury, alleviation of suffering through the diagnosis and treatment of human response, and advocacy in the care of individuals, families, communities, and populations." Nursing is a multilevel profession that includes: (1) licensed practical nurses who complete 12- to 18-month programs; (2) registered nurses who complete a 2-year associate degree program, a 3-year diploma program, or a 4-year bachelor's degree program and complete a licensure exam; (3) advanced practice registered nurses who have a master's or doctoral degree [4]. Further, nurse practitioners have a master's or doctoral degree and advanced clinical training.

Oncology nurses often specialize through on-the-job training in an oncology care setting. Many oncology nurses seek further certification to become certified in targeted areas, including the Oncology Certified Nurse, Certified Pediatric Hematology Oncology Nurse, Certified Breast Care Nurse, Blood & Marrow Transplant Certified Nurse, Advanced Oncology Certified Nurse Practitioner, Advanced Oncology Certified Clinical Nurse Specialist, Certified Pediatric Oncology Nurse, Advanced Oncology Certified Nurse, Certified General Oncology Nurse Navigator, Subspecialty (Organ Site) Certified Oncology Nurse Navigator, Certified General Patient Navigator, and others.

Nurse practitioners and clinical nurse specialists hold a master's degree in nursing yet serve two distinct roles. Clinical nurse specialists typically work in roles that are active in both clinical research and workforce and patient education. Clinical nurse specialists are frequently employed as a part of the hospital care team. Much like physician assistants, nurse practitioners work directly alongside the physician. They diagnose and treat conditions associated with the patient care experience. Both roles are integral to the comprehensive care team.

Nurse navigators are clinically licensed and focus primarily on assisting the patient and the family through many aspects of their cancer journey from understanding diagnosis through treatment and into survivorship care. They assist patients with care coordination, symptom management, emotional support, and utilize their medical, oncology, and health knowledge to provide guidance to patients [23]. Nurse navigators help patients and families understand their diagnosis and educate them about their disease [24]. Nurse navigators can be found as a part of the hospital team and also the physician office team, and they work closely with all members to ensure seamless transitions between steps of the cancer journey. They are also strong patient advocates.

13.2.11 Oncology Social Workers or Social Work Navigators

Oncology social work emerged as a subspecialty of medical social work around 1980 [25]. A professional oncology social worker is an individual with a degree in social work and a clinical license. Many social workers seek oncology social work certification (OSW-C) to demonstrate to clients and colleagues a defined and specialized skill set [26].

Oncology social workers can provide psychotherapeutic mental and behavioral health services as well as navigate patients through logistical barriers or serve as a liaison to social safety net organizations. They work with patients to address their emotional, spiritual, physical, and social health [27]. Social workers utilize a socioecological systems perspective in their work with patients. This approach allows social workers to assess micro-, meso-, and macro-level factors that influence patients' and families' experiences of cancer [28]. Social workers develop multilevel interventions that incorporate all components and institutions in a patient's life [28].

Oncology social workers typically work in a hospital, ambulatory care, or clinic setting. They may work primarily with patients in a specific phase of cancer treatment such as surgery, chemotherapy, or radiation, or they may serve patients across the treatment and care continuum. Patients are often referred to social workers by other members of the cancer care team such as the oncologist or nurse. There are also clinical social workers in private practice who specialize in treating cancer patients and their families. They often have advanced understanding of oncology, palliative care, death and dying, grief, and bereavement.

Oncology social workers and social work navigators help patients and their families with a number of issues, including accessing information to help patients understand their disease, coping with emotional reactions to a diagnosis, considering decisions about treatment options, understanding insurance coverage and other benefits, and applying for financial assistance [29]. Social workers can provide counseling to patients and their families, facilitate support groups and educational programs, refer to community counseling and social safety net programs, and consult with patients regarding their workplace or educational options.

Social workers also launched the first universal biopsychosocial screening program in the United States in the 1990s [30]. In current practice, the social worker is often responsible for administering distress screening, which is a required standard implemented by the American College of Surgeons Commission on Cancer (CoC). Psychosocial distress is defined by the CoC [31] as extending:

> "along a continuum, ranging from common normal feelings of vulnerability and sadness to problems that can be disabling, such as depression anxiety, panic, social isolation and spiritual crisis. There are a number of sources of distress that can all have negative effects from unmet psychosocial needs including poor coping skills, inadequate control of co-morbidities and financial concerns." (p. 80)

Distress screening is a process that includes the identification of "psychological, social, financial, and behavioral issues that may interfere with a patient's treatment plan and adversely affect treatment outcomes" [31] (p. 56). Social workers then work with the cancer care team as well as a network of community resources and/or nonprofit organizations to connect the patient and their loved ones with appropriate resources and services. The CoC requires that the distress screening process be implemented a minimum of one time at a pivotal medical visit; however, most oncology social workers build ongoing relationships with their patients (as well as their loved ones), consistently assessing the full range of challenges facing the patient, the strengths of the patient to overcome the challenges, the social supports of the patient, and the ability of the patient to navigate the healthcare system and work with each member of the multidisciplinary team.

Although the distress screening process is often led by social workers, the IOM [32] recommends that "all cancer care providers should ensure that every cancer patient within their practice receives care that meet the standard for psychosocial health care" (pp. 10–11). This may include all of the professionals listed in this chapter as well as psychiatrists, psychologists, pastoral counselors, and licensed professional counselors.

13.2.12 Patient Navigators

In 2012, the CoC included patient navigation as a new accreditation standard. The standard requires cancer programs to include a patient navigation process that is driven by a triennial community needs assessment [31]. The CoC [31] defines patient navigation as "specialized assistance for the community, patients, families, and caregivers to assist in overcoming barriers to receiving care and facilitating timely access to clinical services and resources (p. 54). Patient navigators help to eliminate barriers to screening, treatment, and supportive care [33].

Oncology patient navigators can be found across the full cancer continuum. Although some navigators are clinically licensed nurses or social workers as evidenced above, many are not clinically licensed but may have a related nonclinical degree such as public health or human services. Patient navigators may practice in a hospital, ambulatory care setting, or clinic. They may also be based in the community, often within a nonprofit organization or federally qualified health center. They may work with a specific population (such as breast cancer patients) or across all tumor types. Patient navigators most often work with the most underserved and vulnerable patients, such as those who are uninsured, patients living in poverty, or patients who experience disparate health outcomes such as racial and ethnic minorities. Typical patient navigator duties include, but are not limited to, addressing transportation needs to and from treatment, advocating for the patient's priorities with the medical team, navigating uninsured or underinsured patients to health insurance options, connecting patients with social service agencies, and addressing financial toxicity.

Patient navigators adhere to a set of principles that guide the profession and include adherence to a patient-centered health delivery model; integration of a fragmented healthcare system; elimination of individual and systematic barriers to timely care; adherence to boundaries and a clear scope of practice; delivery of services that are commensurate with training and skill level; provision of services that have a clear beginning and end; and delivery of services and care coordination across disconnected systems of care [34].

It is important to note the nuanced and practical differences between patient navigation and patient navigators. Patient navigation describes a process of assisting patients, families, and caregivers, while patient navigators are the professionals who specialize in implementing navigation programs and assisting patients and their loved ones. Patient navigators are key members of patient navigation processes; however, successful navigation programs rely on coordination among all members of the patient's care team.

13.2.13 Peer Navigators, Community Health Workers, and Promotores de Salud

Peer navigators, community health workers, and promotores de salud (the Spanish term for community health workers or lay health workers who work in Spanish-speaking communities [35]) may play a similar role to nonclinically licensed patient navigators. These individuals most often serve the communities from which they are from allowing for a unique level of trust, understanding, and culturally sensitive care [36]. They may work with patients who share the same cancer type (such as breast cancer), geographic location, or another identifier such as race, ethnicity, or language. These navigators focus exclusively on navigating patients to help them address logistical barriers. These individuals focus on addressing nonclinical barriers and serve as a liaison to institutions and other professionals.

Table 13.1 provides examples of the various duties of different types of navigators

Table 13.1 Patient navigator types and duties

Type of Navigator	Example of Duties[a]	Educational/Licensure Requirements
Nurse	Clinical Care Responsibilities* Care Coordination Medical Education* Symptom Management* Barrier Assessment Appointment Scheduling for Care Continuity Patient Advocacy Recommends Supportive Care Facilitates Individualized Care Encounter Documentation	Clinical License Nursing Degree
Social Worker	Clinical Mental Health Care Responsibilities* Support Group Facilitation Care Coordination Mental Health Therapy* Distress Screening Resource Referral Barrier Assessment Patient Advocacy Encounter Documentation	Clinical License Social Work Degree
Patient Navigator	Care Referral Resource Coordination Transportation Assistance Financial Assistance Communication Facilitation Insurance Assistance Education and Employment Assistance Cultural Concerns Barrier Assessment Patient Advocacy	Often holds relevant degree such as public health or human services Does not require license
Peer Navigator	Resource Referral Transportation Assistance Financial Assistance Communication Facilitation (particularly in languages other than English) Cultural Concerns Barrier Assessment Patient Advocacy	Does not require degree or license

[a]It is important to note that these duties are not an exhaustive list, and some duties may cross different types of navigators. However, due to professional boundaries, the duties that have an asterisk next to them are specific to that type of navigator.

13.3   Conclusion

The practice of oncology has become exceedingly complex, requiring the skills and expertise of a carefully orchestrated team of professionals and support staff. The purpose of this chapter was to introduce the concept of an interdisciplinary team, which is comprised of professionals working in concert with one another to seamlessly (at least to the patient) facilitate access to comprehensive, timely, afford-able healthcare services and resources. However, it is important to recognize the unique role each member of the oncology care team plays. Although no one profes-sional can provide the full range of services required to competently care for a cancer patient, it is important to understand and respect the different educational backgrounds, skill sets, professional ideologies, ethical approaches, and functional duties of each member of the healthcare team.

For the cancer care team to provide optimal care to patients, they must treat one another with respect, understand the roles of each team member, adhere to profes-sional boundaries, and refer to colleagues or external resources when appropriate. Each member of the team may serve as a leader at different points along the care continuum, whether due to the particular skill set necessary to serve the patient at a particular point in time or due to the specific caring relationship with the patient. Every patient is distinct and may look to the oncologist, nurse, social worker, patient navigator, or other members of the care team as the person guiding them through their care journey. It is important for the healthcare team to work as a cohesive unit, supporting the patient's needs, values, and preferences as they deal with one of the most challenging experiences of their life.

13.4   Case Study

The following case study illustrates the journey of a cancer patient as she interacts with a competent and integrated transdisciplinary care team that also adheres to professional boundaries and roles. This is an example of a best case scenario in which all of the team members are working within their scope, respecting one another, and utilizing their strengths and the strengths of their colleagues to best serve the patient.

Ana Maria lives in Washington, DC. She is a 42-year-old woman who immi-grated to the United States from Mexico with her mother over 30 years ago. Ana Maria and her mother were undocumented when they made their way to their new home and have neither sought nor received consistent healthcare services during their time in the United States. Ana Maria's mother, Leticia, does not speak fluent English, but Ana Maria is bilingual. Leticia worked as a housekeeper for many years and as a result suffers from various aches and pains from bending, stretching, and kneeling for long periods of time. She can no longer work, and Ana Maria takes care of them both through wages earned at her job at a restaurant. Because she is undocumented, Ana Maria does not have health insurance. Ana Maria has never been married and has no children, but she does have a long-term boyfriend named Miguel.

Several years ago, Ana Maria began feeling pain in her pelvic area, particularly during or after intercourse. She also began bleeding from her vagina, even when she was not on her period. She sometimes felt that her vagina smelled strangely and was too embarrassed to discuss these issues with anyone, including Miguel. She figured she had a yeast infection or maybe even a sexually transmitted disease and felt ashamed to seek treatment. She was also afraid that she would not be able to afford treatment and just hoped it would go away on its own.

Finally, her symptoms got so bad that Ana Maria went to the emergency room. She explained her symptoms and underwent a physical examination and screening for sexually transmitted infections. The physician assistant (PA) treating Ana Maria asked her when her last Pap smear was, and Ana Maria said that she was not sure she had ever received one. The PA collected cells from Ana Maria's cervix and told her that her results would come back in a few days. Ana Maria was extremely uncomfortable from the invasive examination and screenings. She could not remember being undressed in front of anyone other than Miguel or family members, and she hoped that this nightmare would just go away.

Ana Maria was at work the next day when the PA called her cell phone and asked her to come back to the hospital the same day. Ana Maria was worried about losing wages or getting in trouble at work, but the PA sounded concerned, so Ana Maria asked her boss for a few hours off to handle a personal matter. Her boss seemed annoyed because it was the lunch hour rush, but since Ana Maria was an excellent worker and had never requested unscheduled time off before, he allowed her to leave. When Ana Maria arrived at the hospital, she was escorted to a different area of the building where she saw the word "oncology" on the door. She was not sure what that meant, and she started to get nervous.

The PA she saw in the emergency room introduced Ana Maria to Dr. Sweeney, who was a gynecological oncologist. Dr. Sweeney told Ana Maria that she works with women who have cancer of the reproductive organs. She was sorry to tell Ana Maria that she was concerned about her Pap test results and that she wanted to do another exam and a biopsy. She told Ana Maria that her Pap smear revealed abnormal cells and that the appearance of her cervix was the cause for concern.

After the biopsy was sent for analysis, Ana Maria went home and was clearly distraught. Miguel asked her what was wrong, and she confided in him regarding her symptoms and discussion with the doctor. Miguel assured her that she would be okay and that he would go with her when she received the biopsy results. They both decided not to tell Leticia for fear that she would be too upset.

Once again, Ana Maria asked her boss for time off from work to address a personal matter. Her boss said okay but said that this better not become a regular occurrence. Ana Maria assured him it would not. Ana Maria and Miguel went to Dr. Sweeney's office, where they were told that Ana Maria appeared to have advanced cervical cancer. Dr. Sweeney explained that Ana Maria had a strain of the human papillomavirus (HPV) which caused her cancer and that it had likely been in Ana Maria's body for quite some time. Dr. Sweeney's concern was that the cancer was invasive and she needed to determine if it had spread to other organs, which was known as metastatic cancer. Dr. Sweeney needed to determine the full extent of the disease and most likely perform a surgery called a hysterectomy on Ana Maria, where her reproductive organs, including her cervix, would be removed.

Ana Maria was shocked and could not speak. She was visibly shaken and immediately feared for her life. Very quickly, however, she switched her concern to paying for treatment, taking time off from work, and ensuring that her mother would be okay. Dr. Sweeney always refers her patients to Jenna, the oncology social worker, but especially in cases of metastatic cancer. Luckily, Jenna was available and immediately came to meet Ana Maria and chat with her about her concerns. Dr. Sweeney told Ana Maria that her nurse, Stephanie, would be in touch to discuss her options and the specifics about surgery if she chose to have it. She also told her that Jenna would help answer any immediate questions.

Ana Maria started to cry, and Jenna asked her if they could walk to her office for some privacy. Jenna escorted Ana Maria and Miguel to her office and sat down with them to process the news they had just received. Jenna explained that a cancer diagnosis is almost always a shock and that the feelings Ana Maria was experiencing were completely normal. Jenna said that her job was to help assist Ana Maria with any concerns that she had, especially in terms of her feelings and emotions. She provided Ana Maria with some literature on cervical cancer and discussed it with her before giving her a chance to ask any questions she might have. She also explained that Ana Maria was not just a patient but the most important part of the healthcare team. She described the shared decision-making process and assured Ana Maria that although Dr. Sweeney and other members of the team were there to provide information or answer questions—that they also wanted Ana Maria to feel empowered to make informed decisions about her care. They wanted to understand her values and preferences so that they could work together to develop a treatment plan that was unique to her.

After their discussion, Ana Maria told Jenna that she was uninsured, and she did not know how she was going to pay for her care. Jenna told her that she might actually qualify for assistance because DC has a generous Medicaid program that covers undocumented immigrants. Jenna called her colleague Keysha, a patient navigator, to come meet Ana Maria and explain her health insurance options.

Keysha sat with Ana Maria, Miguel, and Jenna and explained that DC Medicaid would most likely insure her. Keysha would work with her to fill out her paperwork and apply for coverage. Keysha told her that she knows she is overwhelmed but that they would work together to apply for coverage so that she could schedule her surgery and take control of her treatment. Keysha asked Ana Maria a series of questions and once they were done, told her she would touch base as soon as the paperwork had been processed. She also told her that she can help connect her with charity care if she ever needs medications or treatments that are not covered by her new insurance. She told her that they would work together to help her access the care she needs. She also told her that she can help Ana Maria address her work concerns and prepare to discuss her medical condition with her boss.

Before Ana Maria and Miguel left the hospital, Jenna gave them her contact information, encouraged Ana Maria to touch base with any questions or concerns, and also told her about a support group she runs for women with gynecological cancer. She said they were meeting the next evening and encouraged Ana Maria to join. She also told her and Miguel that she ran a support group for caregivers, so if Miguel or Leticia were interested, they could join that group.

Over the next few weeks, Ana Maria worked with Keysha to obtain insurance and to talk with her boss about her impending treatment. Although she would not be paid for her missed shifts, her boss agreed to hold her position open until she returned to work. Keysha helped Ana Maria obtain government and charity assistance to pay her rent and bills, afford food, and travel to and from treatment. Ana Maria also worked with Jenna to break the news to Leticia, maintain good communication with Miguel, and process her own feelings and emotions. Keysha and Jenna worked closely together to ensure that Ana Maria was receiving the support and resources she needed.

In the meantime, Ana Maria worked with Stephanie, Dr. Sweeney's oncology nurse, to go over the surgical plan, discuss her recovery period, and answer any medical questions. Stephanie also discussed fertility options with Ana Maria since she is getting a hysterectomy. She told her that the hospital has fertility experts in case she would like to discuss next steps. Ana Maria thanked Stephanie but told her she knew she had already made a decision that she did not want to be a mother.

About a month after their initial consult, Dr. Sweeney performed a hysterectomy and confirmed that Ana Maria's cancer had spread to several other organs. She recommended that Ana Maria also undergo chemotherapy and radiation to address the spread of the cancer. Since Dr. Sweeney is a gynecological oncologist, she could perform both the surgery and administer chemotherapy. Ana Maria was worried about nausea and losing her hair. Stephanie addressed Ana Maria's physical concerns, assuring her that they would provide her with anti-nausea medication and control any physical side effects as best they could. Keysha told Ana Maria about organizations that would help her find a wig that she liked and connected her with other female patients who had lost their hair.

Dr. Sweeney introduced Ana Maria to Dr. Karimi, the radiation oncologist who would be treating her with a type of treatment called brachytherapy. Ana Maria also met Heidi, Dr. Karimi's nurse. Heidi worked with her to answer questions and schedule her treatment. Ana Maria spoke with Heidi about her concerns that she would have something radioactive placed inside of her body. Heidi discussed the safety and efficacy of the treatment and made sure that Ana Maria was completely comfortable before moving forward.

Finally, Dr. Sweeney explained to Ana Maria that she wanted her to meet with Dr. Medina, a palliative care physician, to address her quality of life and any symptoms or side effects she may experience. Dr. Medina worked closely with her physician assistant, Otis, to help Ana Maria understand the goals of palliative care and design a treatment plan that met her unique needs. They also worked with Jenna to allay Ana Maria's fears and anxieties, and address both the physical and psychosocial effects from treatment.

Throughout Ana Maria's diagnosis, treatment, and recovery, Dr. Sweeney was the primary person who coordinated her care. She was assisted by her nurse Stephanie who made sure that Ana Maria had the information necessary to make informed medical choices. Stephanie worked closely with Dr. Karimi, his nurse Heidi, and Dr. Medina and her physician assistant Otis to ensure that Ana Maria's care was coordinated. For example, they worked as a team to make appointments on the same days if possible. That way, Ana Maria would not have to make multiple trips, especially when she was not feeling well. Dr. Sweeney also relied on Jenna, the social worker, and Keysha, the patient navigator, to make sure that the full range of Ana Maria's needs were being met. This included addressing her social and emotional needs through psychotherapy and support groups but also her logistical needs. All members of the multidisciplinary care team were committed to working as a cohesive unit built on a foundation of trust and respect. They also worked under a model that put Ana Maria first. They valued her input, respected her choices, and treated her as an equal partner in the care team. This multidisciplinary team built a culture that permeated their institution. Lines of communication were open, honesty was valued, and all members of the team trusted and depended upon one another.

Although not present in this vignette, some of the challenges that are inherent to any multidisciplinary team include (1) boundary blurring, (2) role confusion, (3) hierarchical structures that are difficult to permeate, (4) competition, (5) personality conflicts, (6) reimbursement models that are not conducive to team work, and (7) preferences of the patient to work with a single provider.

References

1. Institute of Medicine. Establishing transdisciplinary professionalism for improving health outcomes. Washington, DC: National Academies Press; 2017.
2. Choi BC, Pak AW. Multidisciplinarity, interdisciplinarity, and transdisciplinarity in health research, services, education and policy: 1. Definitions, objectives, and evidence of effectiveness. Clin Invest Med. 2006;29(6):351–64.
3. McGillicuddy P, Gold K, Lowe M. Developing core competencies for interprofessional teams: a script-reading approach. In: Christ G, Messner C, Behar L, editors. Handbook of oncology social work: psychosocial care for people with cancer. New York: Oxford University Press; 2015. p. 785–91.
4. Institute of Medicine. Delivering high-quality cancer care. Washington, DC: National Academies Press; 2013.
5. Institute of Medicine. Crossing the quality chasm: a new health system for the 21st century. Washington, DC: National Academies Press; 2001.
6. National Learning Consortium. Shared decision making. 2013. www.healthit.gov/sites/default/files/nlc_shared_decision_making_fact_sheet.pdf.
7. Loscalzo M, Clark K, Bultz BD. Integrated interdisciplinary staff leadership model of patient-centered care. In: Christ G, Messner C, Behar L, editors. Handbook of oncology social work. New York: Oxford University Press; 2015. p. 595–600.
8. Smith GF, Toonen TR. Primary care of the patient with cancer. Am Fam Physician. 2007;15(75):1207–14.
9. Klabunde CN, Ambs A, Keating NL, He Y, Doucette WR, Tisnado D, Clauser S, Kahn KL. The role of primary care physicians in cancer care. J Gen Intern Med. 2009;24(9):1029–36. https://doi.org/10.1007/s11606-009-1058-x.
10. National Cancer Institute. NCI dictionary of cancer terms: medical oncologist. www.cancer.gov/publications/dictionaries/cancer-terms?cdrid=46290.
11. National Cancer Institute. Chemotherapy. 2015. www.cancer.gov/about-cancer/treatment/types/chemotherapy.
12. Bonner Millar, L. Surgical oncology. 2016. www.oncolink.org/cancer-treatment/surgery/overview/surgical-oncology-the-basics.
13. National Cancer Institute. Surgery. 2015. www.cancer.gov/about-cancer/treatment/types/surgery.

14. American College of Surgeons. Medical student FAQs. www.facs.org/education/resources/medical-students/faq.
15. American Society for Clinical Oncology. ASCO answers: radiation therapy. 2016. www.cancer.net/sites/cancer.net/files/asco_answers_radiation_therapy.pdf.
16. National Cancer Institute. Radiation therapy. 2010. www.cancer.gov/about-cancer/treatment/types/radiation-therapy/radiation-fact-sheet.
17. Board of Pharmacy Specialists. Oncology pharmacy. www.bpsweb.org/bps-specialties/oncology-pharmacy.
18. Bauer, A. Spotlight on: Oncology pharmacists—Part I, a Q&A. 2014. www.cancer.net/blog/2014-06/spotlight-oncology-pharmacists-%E2%80%93-part-i-qa.
19. National Consensus Project for Quality Palliative Care. Clinical practice guidelines for quality palliative care. 3rd ed. Author: Pittsburgh, PA; 2014.
20. Gilchrist LS, Galantino ML, Wampler M, Marchese VG, Morris GS, Ness KK. A framework for assessment in oncology rehabilitation. J Am Phys Ther Assoc. 2009;89(3):286–306.
21. The Sidney Kimmel Comprehensive Cancer Center. Cancer rehabilitation program. www.hopkinsmedicine.org/kimmel_cancer_center/centers/cancer_rehab/index.html.
22. American Nurses Association. What is nursing? www.nursingworld.org/EspeciallyForYou/What-is-Nursing.
23. Willis A, Hoffler E, Villalobos A, Pratt-Chapman M. Advancing the field of cancer patient navigation: a toolkit for comprehensive cancer control professionals. Washington, DC: The George Washington University Cancer Institute; 2016.
24. Stewart MA, Rodriguez R. Patient navigation in oncology. In: Christ G, Messner C, Behar L, editors. Handbook of oncology social work. New York: Oxford University Press; 2015. p. 659–65.
25. Messner C. Overview of oncology social work. In: Christ G, Messner C, Behar L, editors. Handbook of oncology social work. New York: Oxford University Press; 2015. p. 1.
26. Board of Oncology Social Work. Board of oncology social work. http://oswcert.org/
27. Malai, R. Oncology social workers offer many services. NASW News. 2015;60(4). www.socialworkers.org/pubs/news/2015/04/oncology-social-work.asp.
28. Zebrack B, Jones BL, Smolinksi KM. Oncology social work interventions throughout the continuum of cancer care. In: Christ G, Messner C, Behar L, editors. Handbook of oncology social work. New York: Oxford University Press; 2015. p. 35–42.
29. Association of Oncology Social Work. Oncology social workers brochure. 2015. www.aosw.org/AOSW/media/Main-Site-Files/BROCHURES%20AND%20FLYERS/OSW-BROCHURE.pdf.
30. Clark K, Loscalzo M, Bultz BD. Touch-screen technology: using a problem checklist for psychosocial oncology screening. In: Christ G, Messner C, Behar L, editors. Handbook of oncology social work. New York: Oxford University Press; 2015. p. 129–36.
31. American College of Surgeons. Cancer program standards: ensuring patient-centered care. 2016. www.facs.org/quality-programs/cancer/coc/standards.
32. Institute of Medicine. Cancer care for the whole patient: meeting psychosocial health needs. Washington, DC: The National Academies Press; 2008.
33. Harold P. Freeman Patient Navigation Institute. www.hpfreemanpni.org.
34. Freeman HP, Rodriguez RL. Principles of patient navigation. Cancer. 2011;117(15 Suppl):3539–42.
35. Centers for Disease Control and Prevention. Promotores de salud/community health workers. www.cdc.gov/minorityhealth/promotores/index.html.
36. American Public Health Association. Community health workers. www.apha.org/apha-communities/member-sections/community-health-workers.

Measuring the Impact Navigation Has on Patient Care by Supporting the Multidisciplinary Team

14

Elaine Sein, Danelle Johnston, Tricia Strusowski, and Cheryl Bellomo

14.1 Value of Measurement: Why Are Outcomes Important?

"One of the best ways for a healthcare provider to improve quality of care and reduce cost is to establish a performance improvement program with analytics, defined teams, and a focus on evidence-based practices" [1]. Research on navigation programs has not been robust for a number of reasons. Navigation programs are diverse, and the lack of standardized metrics to evaluate the impact of navigation on patient quality outcomes has made it difficult to measure programmatic success [2]. Metrics are needed to evaluate whether patient navigation can improve quality-of-care delivery, health outcomes, and overall value in healthcare during diagnosis and treatment of cancer [3]. The collection of data related to specific metrics and outcomes will be helpful to formulate program development, identify new issues/barriers, and reevaluate community needs. In its published report, *Ensuring Quality Cancer Care*, the IOM recommends that quality care is measured using a core set of metrics: "To ensure the rapid translation of research into practice, a mechanism is needed to quickly identify the results of research and quality-of-care implications and ensure that it is applied in monitoring quality" [4]. Appropriate metrics will not only define outcomes for cancer patients but may also be useful in other complex diseases, as well as in patient-centered navigation.

E. Sein, RN, BSN, CBCN (✉)
Office of Community Outreach, Fox Chase Cancer Center Partners, Philadelphia, PA, USA

D. Johnston, MSN, RN, OCN, ONN-CG
Academy of Oncology Nurse & Patient Navigators, The Lynx Group, Cranbury, NJ, USA
e-mail: djohnston@the-lynx-group.com

T. Strusowski, MS, RN
Oncology Solutions LLC, Decatur, GA, USA
e-mail: tstrusowski@oncologysolutions.com

C. Bellomo, MSN, RN, ONN-CG
Intermountain Cancer Centers, Cedar City Hospital, Cedar City, UT, USA
e-mail: cheryl.bellomo@imail.org

© Springer International Publishing AG, part of Springer Nature 2018
L. D. Shockney (ed.), *Team-Based Oncology Care: The Pivotal Role of Oncology Navigation*, https://doi.org/10.1007/978-3-319-69038-4_14

291

The development and dissemination of process and outcome measures will allow communities and researchers to evaluate the results of these programs [5]. With the standardization of metrics, navigators can be the "change agents" for their own sustainability and promote evidence-based practice (EBP) with proven outcomes. Evaluation and outcome measures, including patient-reported outcomes, for assessing the impact of navigation are essential for the success, sustainability, and future of navigation services and the navigation role [6].

To measure and, subsequently, improve the quality of cancer care, navigation programs must use standardized metrics, focusing on EBP. In 2010, the Prevention and Early Detection Workgroup of the Patient Navigation Leadership Summit established recommendations for researchers and navigation program evaluators, including: (1) clearly document key program characteristics, (2) use a set of core data elements to form the basis of reported metrics, and (3) prioritize data collection using methods with the least amount of bias [7]. Since navigation programs vary depending on the need of the institution, there is a need for evidence-based baseline metrics that can be used regardless of the structure of the navigation program.

Leaders in the field have defined EBP as the "integration of best research evidence with clinical expertise and patient values" [8]. The elements in the definition emphasize knowledge produced through rigorous and systematic inquiry, the experience of the clinician, and the values of the patient, providing an enduring and encompassing definition of EBP. This definition provides an overarching guide when choosing criteria for metric development. The science of measuring healthcare performance has made enormous progress over the last decades, and it continues to evolve, especially in the areas of patient navigation and care coordination. Measuring data represents a critical component in the national endeavor to assure all patients of high-quality care. Measures light the way, showing where systems are breaking down and where they are succeeding to help our patients. So why should we measure? Measuring drives improvement, informs consumers, and influences payment.

Since 2008, the National Priorities Partnership, a group of 48 organizations convened by the National Quality Forum, has helped galvanize healthcare's expansive and fragmented system around priorities and goals where concerted action makes the biggest difference for patients. Their initial priorities dovetail with navigation priorities with a focus on patient and family engagement, care coordination, safety, population health, overuse, and palliative and end-of-life care. As you embark on a metric selection process, it is imperative that you use rigorous scientific methods in choosing criteria of the metrics being proposed. The National Quality Forum (NQF) uses four criteria to evaluate a measure: important to measure and report, scientifically acceptable, usable and relevant, and feasible to collect, which is described in Table 14.1.

The Comprehensive Cancer Center Consortium for Quality Improvement (C4QI) is a group of administrators from NCI-designated cancer centers across the country, which began in 1997 in response to The Joint Commission focus of benchmarking quality data. The C4QI seeks to improve the quality of care for all cancer patients by identifying and promoting best practices that provide optimal clinical outcomes

Table 14.1 NQF criteria for measure development

Important to measure and report	Focus on priority areas, evidence based with highest impact
Scientifically acceptable	Implemented measure will produce reliable (consistent) and credible (valid) results
Usable and relevant	Intended users can understand results and will use for quality improvement
Feasible to collect	Data are readily available and retrievable without undue burden

National Quality Forum [9]

Table 14.2 C4QI scoring methodology

Criteria	Definitions	Score = 1	Score = 5
Meaningfulness	Measures potential impact	Less impact on quality	Highest impact on quality
Ease in Collection	Assesses level data collection difficulty	Most difficult to collect	Easiest to collect
Resource Intensity	Assesses expense/ staff time	Greatest resource intensity	Lowest resource intensity
Literature Support	Gauges degree of evidence-based practice	Less scientific evidence	Most scientific evidence
Breadth	Measures applicability	Application of the lowest percentage of patients	Applicable to the greatest number of patients

Advisory Board 2007 [10]

and patient satisfaction. One of their strategies has been to develop a comprehensive database to establish system and institutional performance on key quality and patient safety metrics that target improvement opportunities. In order to do that, they developed their criteria for metrics development using the NQF as a guideline. Table 14.2 provides a snapshot of their process presented at the annual Advisory Board Oncology Roundtable Meeting 2007 [10].

In 2015, The Academy of Oncology Nurse & Patient Navigators (AONN+) Evidence into Practice Committee formed a project team of content experts in AONN+ navigation domains, as well as metric development, to create standard metrics in the three main areas that measure success—patient experience (PE), clinical outcomes (CO), and return on investment (ROI) [2]. The AONN+ Metrics Project Team members used a blend of both sets of criteria to ensure both the integrity as well as the usefulness of the final metrics.

Another key focus for metric development is to ensure that definitions for a data dictionary are crystal clear, leaving no room for interpretation. The following outline for metric development provides the rigor needed to validate the measure being chosen.

1. Performance measure name
2. Patient population

3. Description of measure
4. Rationale for measure including literature support
5. Type—process, structure, outcome
6. Numerator statement
7. Denominator statement
8. Data collection approach
9. Data accuracy

Each metric chosen is evaluating ONE process, structure, or outcome. The definition needs to be clear and concise—using a numerator and denominator will help to make this possible. The AONN+ Metrics Project Team was cognizant that realistic data collection methods would be necessary for a nationally recognized set of core measures for navigation because the accuracy of data collected will make or break the value of the measure chosen.

Example: Metric Development
Performance Measure Name: Distress screening [11]
Patient Population: Navigated patients in your institution
Description of Measure: Number of navigated patients per month who received psychosocial distress screening at a pivotal medical visit with a validated tool

(a) Define pivotal medical visit: Period of high distress for the patient when psychosocial assessment should be completed, usually a period of transition between services.
   • Your institutions/cancer programs identified pivotal medical visit(s).
(b) Drop-down responses: Pivotal medical visit drop-down response—diagnosis, presurgical visit, postsurgical visit, first medical oncology visit to discuss chemotherapy, routine visit with radiation oncologist, post-chemotherapy follow-up, and others.
(c) Define validated tool: A validated screening questionnaire is an instrument that has been psychometrically tested for reliability (the ability of the instrument to produce consistent results), validity (the ability of the instrument to produce true results), and sensitivity (the probability of correctly identifying a patient with the condition). Source: https://manual.jointcommission.org/Manual/Questions/UserQuestionId03Sub0015.

Rationale: Commission on Cancer Standard 3.2. Each calendar year, the cancer committee develops and implements a process to integrate and monitor on-site psychosocial distress screening and referral for the provision of psychosocial care.
Definition: To address the psychosocial issues experienced by patients with cancer, the 2007 report of the IOM, "Cancer Care for the Whole Patient: Meeting Psychosocial Health Needs," emphasizes the importance of screening patients for distress and psychosocial health needs as a critical first step to providing high-quality cancer care. In addition, this report emphasizes that all patients with distress need to be referred for the appropriate provision of care and that high-quality psychosocial cancer care includes systematic follow-up and reevaluation. Cancer

programs must develop a process to incorporate the screening of distress into the standard care of oncology patients. The process will identify psychological, social, financial, and behavioral issues that may interfere with a patient's treatment plan and adversely affect treatment outcomes, and provide patients identified with distress the appropriate resources and/or referral for psychosocial need.

Type: Outcome

Numerator: Number of points given to the psychosocial screening tool

Denominator: Number of currently active navigated points

Data Collection Approach: Institutional database

Data Accuracy: Institutional quality control plan

Note: Glossary of terms is provided as appendix to chapter.

14.2   Framework for Metric Development

As evidence guides practice, it is essential for navigation programs to identify core metrics and standardize data collection in order to clearly demonstrate program outcomes. Collection of data in regard to specific outcomes can be helpful in creating a workflow for the navigator; assisting in program development, maturity, and sustainability; and providing a mechanism for resource allocation to the most needed and beneficial program pieces. Monitoring outcomes can provide valuable information on community needs, and guide future discussion of program offerings. Quality improvement and program evaluation enable navigators to provide the highest quality of care and support by anticipating and mobilizing available resources.

Metrics and quality measures as defined by the Centers for Medicare & Medicaid Services are tools to "measure or quantify healthcare processes, outcomes, patient perceptions, and organizational structure and/or systems that are associated with the ability to provide high-quality healthcare and/or that relate to one or more quality goals for healthcare" [12]. Metrics are methods used to evaluate the success of the navigator role (accurately measuring performance) in cancer programs to improve the care of patients by monitoring and measuring outcomes. Metrics for evaluating navigation programs need to include measures that assess reductions in barriers to care and improvements in the delivery of timely, effective, and equitable cancer services.

AONN+ is dedicated to improving patient care and quality of life by defining, enhancing, and promoting the role of oncology nurse and patient navigators. The objective of the metrics initiative was to develop standard metrics in the areas of patient experience, clinical outcomes, and return on investment using the domains and competencies of navigation. Ten members of AONN+, a core group of lay and clinical navigator content experts representing cancer programs/organizations across the country, were selected to participate in the project with each member being assigned a specific domain of navigation (community outreach/prevention, patient advocacy/patient empowerment, care coordination/care transitions, psychosocial assessment/support, survivorship/end of life, professional roles and responsibilities, operations management, and research/quality improvement) for the review of literature and development of metrics related to the specific domains. For a comprehensive review of the AONN+ Metrics Task Force project on Standardized Evidence-Based Oncology Navigation Metrics, please reference the following two sources:

- Strusowski P, Sein E, Johnston D, et al. Standardized Evidence-Based Oncology Navigation Metrics for All Models: A Powerful Tool in Assessing the Value and Impact of Navigation Programs. J Oncol Navig Surviv. 2017:8(5):220–237.
- Standardized Metrics Source Document: www.aonnonline.org/metrics-source-document.

The AONN+ Certification Task Force recognized that the profession of patient navigation is rapidly expanding and evolving. Therefore, AONN+ identified an opportunity to define oncology navigation areas of functional knowledge to create standardization in role definition and execution. The George Washington University Cancer Institute along with National Stakeholders developed a framework for role delineation for patient navigation. The framework includes 12 functional area domains, which were referenced to construct the AONN+ domains [13]. The task force added operations management, survivorship/end of life, and quality and performance improvement to further define functional areas for navigators. Also referenced as a source for navigation competency development was the Oncology Nursing Society Oncology Nurse Navigator Core Competencies [14]. AONN+ recognized that in order to create consistency across the profession establishing domains for functional knowledge was crucial to establish competent and skilled oncology navigation specialists.

These AONN+ navigation domains contain a comprehensive list of all areas navigators need to have functional knowledge in order to provide quality patient care and financial stability for their organizations. These domains are as follows:

AONN+ navigation role domains
Community outreach and prevention
Coordination of care/care transitions
Patient advocacy/patient empowerment
Psychosocial support services/assessment
Survivorship/end of life
Professional roles and responsibilities
Operations management/organizational development/health economics
Research/quality/performance improvement

14.2.1 Community Outreach/Prevention

Within the domain of community outreach/prevention, navigators must have core knowledge of the early signs of cancer, the current screening guidelines, as well as the available community and state resources for screening and diagnostics. Utilizing a community needs assessment, navigators can define the patient population being served, identify the needs of this population, identify gaps in resources, and determine how navigation can address these needs. Navigators are able to develop collaborative relationships and community partners, identify and provide interventions to remove barriers to care, and provide education to the community on the importance of cancer prevention and early detection for improving survival.

AONN+ competencies for the domain of community outreach/prevention are:

- Finding community resources
- Community needs assessment
- Identification of barriers to care
- Interventions to remove barriers to care
- Community education, prevention, and screening
- Population health
- Risk assessment
- Cultural competency
- Behavior modification
- Genetics

14.2.2 Coordination of Care/Care Transitions

The scope of navigation has evolved from the Freeman model of community outreach and prevention to spanning the entire continuum of care for oncology patients. Navigators help individuals overcome barriers to care and navigate through the screening/diagnostic, treatment, survivorship, and end-of-life care continuum. Navigators need to have an awareness of the healthcare system, available community resources, and act as members of the multidisciplinary team in order to address an individual's identified barriers and needs, as well as the coordination of care along the continuum. The role of the navigator along the continuum of care is bidimensional in nature with a patient-centered (empowerment with education and knowledge) and health system (multidisciplinary) orientation to deliver timely, seamless care. Within the multidisciplinary team, the navigator works as an advocate, care provider, educator, counselor, and facilitator to ensure that every patient receives comprehensive, timely, and quality healthcare services. In building collaboration among the multidisciplinary team members, coordinating execution of the treatment plan, and empowering patients, the navigator guides patients through the complicated steps along the cancer care continuum and through transitions of care, with the goal of achieving the best possible outcomes.

AONN+ competencies for the domain of coordination of care/care transitions are:

- Chronic care model (CCM)
- Identification/intervention of clinical and service barriers to care
- Patient care process/cancer care continuum (prevention, screening, risk assessment, diagnosis, clinical trials, treatment, survivorship, end-of-life care)

- Patient-/family-centered education (screening, diagnosis, treatment, side effect management, survivorship, end of life)
- Identify models of navigation
- Cultural competency
- Multidisciplinary approach to care
- Tumor board
- NCCN guidelines

14.2.3 Patient Advocacy/Patient Empowerment

A patient advocate can be defined as one who uses his or her role to promote and safeguard the well-being and the interests of patients within the community and the healthcare system by ensuring that they are aware of their rights and have access to the information they need to give informed consent and meet self-determination needs. Patient advocacy is protecting the individual's rights and autonomy, speaking up for individual and community needs, educating providers in the healthcare system on an individual's preferences of care and their needs, and ensuring that the individual's needs and preferences are integrated into the treatment and care delivery. Patient advocacy is supporting and empowering patients to make informed decisions, navigating the healthcare system, and building strong partnerships with providers while working toward system improvement to support patient-centered care. Navigators facilitate decision-making support by providing tailored, evidence-based, and culturally and health literacy appropriate education, and imparting information that can help patients achieve their goals and work in collaboration through bi-directional open communication with the patient and the healthcare team.

AONN+ competencies for the domain of patient advocacy/patient empowerment are:

- Patient problem solving
- Engagement in decision-making tools
- Relationship building/trust
- Assisting the patient with care team/communication
- Counseling: conduit between patient and providers
- Patient-/family-centered education (assess educational needs)
- Provide culturally sensitive care and education

14.2.4 Psychosocial Support Services/Assessment

The National Comprehensive Cancer Network (NCCN) defines distress as "a multifactorial unpleasant emotional experience of a psychological (cognitive, behavioral, emotional), social, and/or spiritual nature that may interfere with the ability to cope effectively with cancer, its physical symptoms, and its treatment" [15]. Distress extends along a continuum ranging from common normal feelings of vulnerability, sadness, and fear to problems that can become disabling, such as depression, anxiety, panic, social isolation, and existential and spiritual crisis. To deliver high-quality cancer care, patients' psychosocial needs must be addressed and tools/resources/support services provided to improve patient outcomes.

The NCCN Distress Thermometer was developed in 2007 as a visual analog tool for patients to indicate their distress level. The primary objective/reason for screening for psychosocial distress along the cancer continuum is to address patients' perception of quality of life (QOL). Effective psychosocial care, consisting of a multidisciplinary team approach, has been shown to positively influence patient outcomes and QOL. The NCCN Distress Thermometer has a secondary benefit of connecting patients to services that might not otherwise have been identified. Potential benefits of distress screening are that it provides patients an opportunity to partner with their healthcare team, overcomes patients' reluctance to ask for help, destigmatizes the issue and allows patients to share their vulnerabilities, and ensures timely referral to supportive services. Use of the distress thermometer tool can effectively guide and assist the nurse navigator in providing high-quality, holistic, and patient-centered care.

Navigators are instrumental in the development and implementation of a plan for psychosocial health services in their cancer program that supports patients (by providing personalized information, identifying strategies to address psychosocial needs, providing emotional support, helping patients manage their illness and health), links patients and families with psychosocial services, and coordinates psychosocial and biomedical care. Navigators can also educate patients and their families on how to use adaptive coping mechanisms, such as deep breathing mindfulness, and other self-management exercises to decrease distress. Navigators can provide a comprehensive understanding of the patient to other members of the multidisciplinary team and take the lead role in assessing the patient's needs for possible referral to a mental health specialist.

AONN+ competencies for the domain of psychosocial support services/assessment are:

- Distress screening
- Strategies for coping: disease, treatment, distress/anxiety
- Referrals to psychosocial support and resources

14.2.5 Survivorship/End of Life

Navigators have an essential role in ensuring that quality survivorship care begins at diagnosis and continues throughout the balance of patients' lives. Throughout the seasons of survival, it is imperative for healthcare providers to continually offer the components of survivorship care in the forms of prevention through health and wellness promotion, surveillance for recurrence and screening for new cancers, intervention for management of lasting physical and psychosocial effects, and coordination of care to cancer survivors. The treatment summary and survivorship care plan provides guidance for primary care physicians, the oncology team, and other healthcare providers in the coordination and continuity of care for cancer survivors.

Navigators also play an integral role in the transition of care to hospice care. Navigators should advocate the use of hospice services by recognizing seasons of survival, changes in a patient's quality of life, and understanding that patients may have end-of-life tasks to complete. Serving as the patient's advocate, navigators can help support the patient and family by providing resources for planning legally and financially for end of life, and making sure that the patient's voice is heard as to their goals for treatment and quality of life.

AONN+ competencies for the domain of survivorship/end of life are:

- Establishing goal setting, life goals
- Integrating survivor's goals/preferences into plan of care
- Providing survivorship education on late and long-term effects
- Coordinating plans of care
- Understanding of palliative and hospice care
- Understanding CoC Standard 3.3 Survivorship
- Understanding of IOM report "From Cancer Patient to Cancer Survivor: Lost in Transition"

14.2.6 Professional Roles and Responsibilities

The identification of barriers to care was a primary focus of patient navigation instituted in the 1990s by Dr. Harold Freeman to help explain delays in diagnosis, as well as incomplete care for underserved women with breast cancer [16]. This same premise was the goal of nursing utilization review in the 1970s, which evolved into utilization management, case management, and care coordination [17]. With this evolution, the process of a team approach with open communication was developed to address psychosocial distresses and financial concerns of patients, as well as coordinate care needs. Nurse navigation cultivated the bidimensional care concept—patient-centered and health system–oriented—as oncology care moved to an outpatient setting [18]. Navigation is integral to facilitate effective interprofessional collaboration and promote patient satisfaction and care quality, as well as the efficient use of healthcare resources to decrease costs across oncology patient populations and healthcare settings.

The guiding principles of navigation are to ensure that quality, confidentiality, and professionalism are threaded throughout all aspects of care and programming while demonstrating respect, compassion, and safe, culturally competent care. Common responsibilities of a navigator may include:

- Providing education and support to the patient and family
- Identifying special needs of the patient and delegating to appropriate support staff
- Enhancing understanding of treatment options available

- Facilitating patient care plan recommendations by physician
- Coordinating multidisciplinary care from time of diagnosis throughout treatment
- Improving timeliness of appointments
- Serving as a resource for the community on health issues, prevention, screening, treatment, and research

Skills such as advocacy, problem solving, time management, critical thinking, multitasking, collaboration, and communication were identified in the Oncology Nursing Society oncology nurse navigation role delineation study [19]. AONN+ also recognizes additional skills of leadership and systems management.

AONN+ competencies for the domain of professional roles and responsibilities are:

- Critical thinking
- Problem solving
- Ethics
- Team building
- Leadership
- History/evolution of navigation
- Definition of navigation and types of navigation
- Tracking workload
- Documentation

14.2.7 Operations Management/Organizational Development/ Health Economics

Operations management has been described as an area of business management concerned with designing, controlling the processes of production by managing resources efficiently, and redesigning business operations in the production of goods and services to ensure quality. While not commonly thought of, operations management is vital in the healthcare industry to ensure that processes are in place to provide safe, equitable, effective, efficient, timely, and patient-centered care.

Navigators play a key role in operations management through their daily contact with patients and their families along the continuum of care. The identification of barriers, recognizing how barriers impact patient care, and providing interventions/resources to address barriers related to flow and processes of care are at the heart of operations management. As members of the multidisciplinary team, navigators are instrumental in assessing and recognizing the patient flow process, and identifying efficient and effective ways to implement the flow process as well as determined changes.

AONN+ competencies for the domain of operations management/organizational development/health economics are:

- Healthcare reform
- Utilization of resources

- Workforce shortages
- Organizational structure, mission, and vision
- Organizational development
- Healthcare economics

14.2.8 Research, Quality, Performance Improvement

In today's healthcare environment, there are key organizations driving the focus on quality, outcomes, and evidence-based practice. The Institute of Healthcare Improvement (IHI) Triple Aim looks to improve the patient experience, improve population health, and reduce per capita cost. The Affordable Care Act of 2010 has promised quality affordable healthcare. The reports of the Institute of Medicine (IOM) have identified gaps in cancer quality care as well as the six components to quality care. The six components are engaged patients; an adequately staffed, trained, and coordinated workforce; evidence-based cancer care; a learning healthcare information technology system; translation of evidence into clinical practice, quality measurement, and performance improvement; and accessible, affordable cancer care. The 2001 Institute of Medicine report, *Crossing the Quality Chasm: A New Health System for the 21st Century,* supports the importance of research and quality improvement in its statement, "the degree in which health services (knowledge) for individuals and populations increase the likelihood of desired health outcomes and are consistent with current professional knowledge (research evidence)" [20].

Navigators can utilize research and outcomes to develop and validate the programs and services provided. The components of research and evaluation are to define the problem and establish goals, to implement strategies based on objectives and time, and to measure outcomes. The first step is to create a workgroup consisting of the cancer committee, cancer registrar, and key stakeholders to conduct a community needs assessment for determining available resources and defining the primary service area. The next step is to collect and document disparities and barriers to care in the primary community area. The data from the community needs assessment are generated and utilized to formulate the navigation process for the improvement of quality care and outcomes.

To develop implementation strategies for the identified needs, a SWOT (Strengths, Weaknesses, Opportunities, and Threats) analysis may be conducted. It is recommended that, after identifying the focus of the navigation program, SMART (Specific, Meaningful, Action Oriented, Realistic, and Timely) goals be developed [21]. Key elements of an objective are to define the time frame, criterion, target population, and action. A few criteria to consider when creating SMART goals include the following:

- What specifically do you want to achieve?
- Why is this goal important?
- What steps will be needed to achieve the goal?
- How do you know that the goal is achievable?

- When do you want to achieve the goal?
- Are the goals consistent with the policies and procedures of the organization?
- Does the initiative have enough resources?

Implementation of the plan with quality metrics and continuous process improvement are the final steps in the process. Using the PDSA (Plan, Do Study, and Act) model is recommended to implement and analyze quality studies. Continual improvement is vital, and analysis of process and data is imperative to make informed decisions in the evolving healthcare environment to improve quality of service.

AONN+ competencies for the domain of research and quality performance improvement are:

- Define Triple Aim and how this initiative drives quality.
- Define healthcare environment that is driving focus on quality and outcomes.
- Address the IOM reports that address the need for quality in healthcare and how it shapes practice and initiatives in oncology.
- Define evidence-based practice, quality, and performance improvement terminology.
- Identify regulatory agencies that mandate quality improvement.
- Identify evidence-based practice models.
- Identify key quality and performance improvement tools.
- Describe the steps to develop a quality improvement project.
- Discuss how data are used for continuous improvement.

14.3 Value of Outcome Metrics: Program Sustainability— Patient Experience, Clinical Outcomes, and Return on Investment

There have been several articles and research projects that discuss various measures that can be used to capture the impact of navigation; most of these discuss time-to-care metrics, patient satisfaction, and measures that assist with care for the underserved, but few discuss the broad range of measures that validate the role of navigation in all areas of oncology patient care. It is well known that each navigation program is developed to meet the needs of the patients and the institution where the program is being created, and those indicators to measure the success of that program need to be tailored to the navigation program. Therefore, what type of reporting is best suited to communicate patient navigator efficacy? The answer is clear: data and metrics. The challenge is that while navigation programs have existed for decades, standardized national metrics to measure programmatic success have yet to be created and standardized. After a comprehensive literature search on the topic of navigation metrics, three main categories of metrics were identified: business performance/return on investment (ROI), clinical outcomes, and patient experience. To be able to support continuation or perhaps even expansion of patient navigation services, cancer programs will need to collect quality metrics in all three of these categories.

14.3.1 Patient Experience Metrics

The "patient experience" is increasingly emerging as a more enhanced method for measuring navigation success. The 2013 Consumer Assessment of Healthcare Providers and Systems (CAHPS) cancer survey identified that patients' expectations were exceeded when they felt their healthcare provider actively listened and incorporated their personal psychosocial goals into the treatment plan. The results of this survey also confirm the importance of ensuring navigators and support staff know-how to provide the appropriate level of education, asking patients about their experience(s), and encouraging patient's active participation in their treatment discussions increased the level of understanding and satisfaction of the patient and their family. As the focus on cancer treatment broadens to include the entire continuum of care, navigators increasingly have opportunities to enhance patient experience from outreach and screening through survivorship and/or end-of-life (EOL) care. Especially as patients complete active treatments, the focus will need to shift to prevention and wellness, as well as implementing a successful surveillance plan in the outpatient setting for the balance of their life. Patient experience interventions are not difficult to create for a navigation program, but patient-centered care methodology must always be applied in order to create appropriate metrics [22].

14.3.2 Clinical Outcomes Metrics

Clinical outcome metrics are much more familiar to healthcare providers as clinicians have always measured success through patient clinical outcomes. These metrics include distress screening, pathway compliance, and timeliness of care, which identifies clinical outcome metrics related to navigation, including how to measure the metrics and corresponding benchmarks and sources [23].

14.3.3 Business Performance Metrics

Business performance metrics, unlike patient experience or clinical outcomes, are much less familiar for navigation programs. Yet, this category is becoming increasingly important as cancer program administrators question the return on investment (ROI) for navigation services. Navigators focusing on business performance metrics may require additional training or education on such measures. To fully understand the "what" and "why" of business metrics, navigators should be knowledgeable about business-related cancer topics, including in Table 14.3:

Table 14.3 Landscape for healthcare reform

• Value-based cancer care
• Federal healthcare reform and reimbursement
• The Centers for Medicare & Medicaid Services (CMS) quality measures
• Affordable care organizations (ACOs), oncology medical homes, and bundled payments
• Future reimbursement models for medical care based on quality measures rather than fee for services
• Population management and the initiation of penalties for readmission [23]

14.4   Evidence-Based Metrics for Navigation

The challenge was that although navigation programs had existed for decades, standardized national metrics to measure program success had yet to be created and standardized. The AONN+ Metrics Task Force goal was to provide a list of standardized metrics that can be used by all organizations as a baseline to prove the efficacy and sustainability of their programs. That does not mean that it will be an all-inclusive list, because there are no cookie-cutter navigation programs, and each organization will have additional metrics to capture regarding their own program. These standardized metrics will provide baseline metrics for all naviga-tion programs that are evidence based through literature support, patient prefer-ence, and clinical practice using the AONN+ domains of certification as reference points.

From the development of the 35 national evidenced-based navigation metrics collected from over 300 source documents, all navigation programs—no matter the model of navigation chosen—can utilize the same metrics to measure success and sustainability. It is imperative for navigation to continue to build a strong sustain-able business case and demonstrate that these metrics need to be measured, col-lected, and reported. The outcome metrics will be able to demonstrate with actual measurable data that navigation can impact PE, CO, and ROI.

14.4.1   Standardized Evidence-Based Oncology Navigation Metrics for All Models [24]

Community outreach, prevention		
Metric	Definition	Patient experience (PE), clinical outcomes (CO), return on investment (ROI)
Cancer screening follow-up to diagnostic workup	Number of navigated patients per quarter with abnormal screening referred for follow-up diagnostic workup *Cancer screening definition*: Screening tests can help find cancer at an early stage before symptoms will appear. When abnormal tissue or cancer is found early, it may be easier to treat or cure. By the time symptoms appear, the cancer may have grown and spread. This can make cancer harder to treat or cure	PE, CO, ROI
Cancer screening	Number of participants at cancer screening event and/or percentage increase of cancer screening	PE, CO
Completion of diagnostic workup	Number of navigated individuals with abnormal screening who completed diagnostic workup per month/quarter	CO, ROI

(continued)

(continued)

Community outreach, prevention

Metric	Definition	Patient experience (PE), clinical outcomes (CO), return on investment (ROI)
Disparate population at screening event	Number of individuals per quarter at community screening events by OMB standards	PE, CO
	Disparate population definition: The National Institute on Minority Health and Health Disparities definition is difference in the incidence, prevalence, mortality, and burden of disease and other adverse health conditions that exist among specific populations in the United States (racial and ethnic minorities, low socioeconomic status) *OMB definition*: Office of Management and Budget	

Care coordination/care transition

Metric	Definition	Patient experience (PE), clinical outcomes (CO), return on investment (ROI)
Treatment compliance	Percentage of navigated patients who adhere to institutional treatment pathways per quarter	ROI, CO
Barriers to care	Number and list of specific barriers to care identified by navigator per month	PE, CO
	Barriers to care definition: Obstacles that prevent a cancer patient from accessing care, services, resources, and/or support	
Interventions	Number of specific referrals/interventions offered to navigated patients per month	PE, CO
	Intervention definition: The act of intervening, interfering, or interceding with the intent of modifying the outcome	
Clinical trial education	Number of patients educated on clinical trials by the navigator per month	PE, CO
Clinical trial referrals	Number of navigated patients per month referred to clinical trial department	PE, CO
Patient education	Number of patient education encounters by navigator per month	PE, CO, ROI
Diagnosis to initial treatment	Number of business days from diagnosis (date pathology resulted) to initial treatment modality (date of first treatment)	PE, CO
Diagnosis to first oncology consult	Number of business days from diagnosis (date pathology resulted) to initial oncology consult (date of first appointment)	PE, CO

(continued)

Patient empowerment/patient advocacy

Metric	Definition	Patient experience (PE), clinical outcomes (CO), return on investment (ROI)
Patient goals	Percentage of analytic cases per month that patient goals identified and discussed with the navigator	PE, CO, ROI
Caregiver support	Number of caregiver needs/preferences discussed with navigator per month	CO
Identify learning style preference	Number of navigated patients per month whose preferred learning style was discussed during the intake process	PE, CO
	Learning styles:	
	• Visual (spatial): You prefer using pictures, images, and spatial understanding	
	• Aural (auditory-musical): You prefer using sound and music	
	• Verbal (linguistic): You prefer using words, both in speech and writing	
	• Physical (kinesthetic): You prefer using your body, hands, and sense of touch	
	• Logical (mathematical): You prefer using logic, reasoning, and systems	
	• Social (interpersonal): You prefer to learn in groups or with other people	
	• Solitary (intrapersonal): You prefer to work alone and use self-study	

Psychosocial support, assessment

Metric	Definition	Patient experience (PE), clinical outcomes (CO), return on investment (ROI)
Psychosocial distress screening	Number of navigated patients per month who received psychosocial distress screening at a pivotal medical visit with a validated tool	PE, CO
	Pivotal medical visit definition: Period of high distress for the patient when psychosocial assessment should be completed	
	Define various validated tools as examples: FACT, NCCN Psychosocial Distress Screening Thermometer	
Social support referrals	Number of navigated patients referred to support network per month	PE, CO, ROI

(continued)

(continued)

Survivorship and end of life

Metric	Definition	Patient experience (PE), clinical outcomes (CO), return on investment (ROI)
Survivorship care plan	Number of navigated patients (patients with curative intent) per month who received a survivorship care plan and treatment summary	PE, CO
Transition from treatment to survivorship	Percentage of navigated analytic cases per month transitioned from completed cancer treatment to survivorship	PE, CO
	Define care transitions: The movement patients make between healthcare practitioners and settings as their condition and care needs change during the course of chronic or acute illness	
Referrals to support services at the survivorship visit	Number of navigated patients per month referred to appropriate support service at the survivorship visit	PE, CO, ROI
Palliative care referral	Number of navigated patients per month referred for palliative care services	PE, CO, ROI

Professional roles and responsibilities

Metric	Definition	Patient experience (PE), clinical outcomes (CO), return on investment (ROI)
Navigation knowledge at time of orientation	Percentage of new hires who have completed institutionally developed navigator core competencies	CO
Oncology Nurse Navigator Annual Core Competencies review	Percentage of staff who have completed institutionally developed navigator core competencies annually to validate core knowledge of oncology navigation	CO

Operations management, organizational development, health economics

Metric	Definition	Patient experience (PE), clinical outcomes (CO), return on investment (ROI)
30-, 60-, 90-day readmission rate	Number of navigated patients readmitted to the hospital at 30, 60, and 90 days. Reported quarterly	ROI
Navigation operational budget	Monthly operating expenses by line item	ROI
	Definition: Operational budget is a combination of known expenses, expected future costs, and forecasted income over the course of a year	

(continued)

Operations management, organizational development, health economics

Metric	Definition	Patient experience (PE), clinical outcomes (CO), return on investment (ROI)
Navigation caseload	Number of new cases, open cases, and closed cases navigated per month	ROI
	Definitions: New cases—new patient case referred to the navigation program per month	
	Open cases: Patient case that remains open/month	
	Closed cases: Number of patient cases closed per month. Formal closing of a patient case from the navigation program	
Referrals to revenue-generating services	Number of referrals to revenue-generating services per month by navigator	ROI
No-show rate	Number of navigated patients who do not complete a scheduled appointment per month	ROI
Patient retention through navigation	Number of analytic cases per month or quarter that remained in your institution due to navigation	ROI
Emergency room utilization	Number of navigated patient visits to the emergency room per month	ROI
Emergency admissions per number of chemotherapy patients	Number of navigated patient visits per 1000 chemotherapy patients who had an emergency room visit per month	ROI

Research, quality, performance improvement

Metric	Definition	Patient experience (PE), clinical outcomes (CO), return on investment (ROI)
Patient experience/patient satisfaction with care	Patient experience or patient satisfaction survey results per month (utilize institutional specific navigation tool with internal benchmark)	PE
Navigation program validation based on community needs assessment	Monitor one major goal of current navigation program annually as defined by cancer committee	PE, CO, ROI
	Example: Population Served	

(continued)

(continued)

Research, quality, performance improvement		
Metric	Definition	Patient experience (PE), clinical outcomes (CO), return on investment (ROI)
Patient transitions from point of entry	Percentage of navigated analytic cases per month transitioned from institutional point of entry to initial treatment modality	PE, CO
	Care transitions definition: The movement patients make between healthcare practitioners and settings as their condition and care needs change during the course of chronic or acute illness	PE, CO
	Define modality: Chemotherapy, surgery, radiation therapy, endocrine therapy, and biotherapy	
Diagnostic workup to diagnosis	Number of business days from date of abnormal finding to pathology report for navigated patients	CO
	Definition for abnormal finding: Number of business days from abnormal finding diagnostic workup (date of workup) to diagnosis (date pathology resulted)	

14.5   How to Use and Report Metrics for Different Audiences

Reports and metrics are essential for program development, growth, and sustainability, yet different individuals within the cancer program, as well as patients, have diverse thoughts on quality, value, and metrics. In the Association of Community Cancer Centers (ACCC) document, *Communicating Quality in Oncology*, the forum participants agreed that defining quality in cancer care is challenging, and each stakeholder group has its own definition of quality. Given the growing number of accrediting/quality improvement organizations/standards and reporting requirements, some streamlining or consolidating of these programs would be beneficial. Patients often define quality by nonclinical parameters, such as environment of care and communication with providers. Lastly, the current reimbursement climate does not incentivize many of the approaches that improve quality and cost, and quality must be considered in tandem when determining value [25].

Clinical outcomes, patient satisfaction, and process measures are key metrics for providers and have been incorporated into present-day value-based cancer care metrics. Tracking evidence-based metrics, the Centers for Medicare & Medicaid Services (CMS) rewarded providers with monetary bonuses for reaching predetermined standards in quality care. Not only did CMS create positive incentives but it also instituted penalties for standards not met. CMS selects measures based on a wide range of factors, from patient and/or caregiver engagement to conditions that represent national public health priorities (CMS, 2013) [26].

Before work relative value units (RVUs) were used, Medicare paid for physician services using usual, customary, and reasonable reimbursement rates. Other metrics of physician value to the organization, such as accessibility, development of innovative care approaches, or team leadership and education, may gain in importance. Ethical physician incentives emphasizing those with a shared-purpose orientation can be developed without unintended harmful consequences, such as over- or under-treatment. An interesting blend of traditional productivity measures and other outcomes in the areas of quality, innovation, and education at a large integrated healthcare system has been described [27].

In the oncology setting, providers participate in metrics from Quality Oncology Practice Initiative (QOPI), Commission on Cancer (CoC), and American Society of Clinical Oncology (ASCO), just to name a few. These national databases have helped establish national oncology benchmarks, which ultimately results in improved care for the oncology patient. National standards help drive continuous quality improvement and value, and identify best practice programs that elevate cancer care on a grander scale.

The Oncology Care Model (OCM), which launched on July 1, 2016, is a program that is meant to shift reimbursement and payment to value-based quality care, and one of the six fundamental transformation processes is patient navigation [28]. The OCM is a 5-year model that combines financial incentives, including performance-based payments, to improve care coordination, appropriateness of care, and access for beneficiaries undergoing chemotherapy. It targets patients receiving chemotherapy treatment and the spectrum of care provided to a patient during a 6-month episode following the start of chemotherapy. Physician practices that furnish chemotherapy treatment may also participate in the OCM.

The OCM requires that participating physician practices meet certain practice transformation requirements to improve management and coordination of care. They include the following:

- 24/7 patient access to a clinician who has real-time access to the practice's medical records.
- Attestation and use of the Office of the National Coordinator for Health Information Technology–certified electronic medical record (EMR).
- Utilize data for continuous quality improvement.
- Provide core functions of patient navigation.
- Document care in accordance with the Health and Medicine Division (HMD; formerly Institute of Medicine) Care Management Plan.
- Treat patients with therapies consistent with nationally recognized clinical guidelines [29].

Administrators are interested in metrics that support patient- and family-centered care, financial strength of the organization, patient experience, and clinical measures. A patient who feels well taken care of and incorporated into their treatment and goals of care discussion has proven to result in a loyal long term customer. The Institute of Medicine's *Delivering High-Quality Cancer Care: Charting a New Course for a System in Crisis* revealed that the most important characteristic of their provider was when they listened to the needs of the patient. Value should always be defined around the customer, and in a well-functioning healthcare system, the creation of value for patients should determine the rewards for all other healthcare providers in the system. Since value depends on results, not inputs, value in healthcare is measured by the outcomes achieved, not the volume of services delivered, and shifting focus from volume to value is a central challenge. Nor is value measured by the process of care used; process measurement and improvement are important tactics but are no substitutes for measuring outcomes and costs.

Measuring a program with evidence-based metrics provides optimal outcomes, which translate into high-quality care and program sustainability. Navigation programs for decades were measuring different metrics; therefore no national benchmarks exist for navigation programs; thus the need to utilize standardized metrics is essential for navigation program growth and sustainability [30].

Metrics and their definitions are sometimes misinterpreted by the individuals within the cancer program, thus resulting in low-quality data, outcomes, and poor reporting. It is extremely important to have all the staff understand the definition of the metric; this may be the most important step. Metrics should be decided by the multidisciplinary team to create synergy with the metric goals for the entire cancer program. Discuss your metrics with your administrators and cancer committee; start with metrics that support the Commission on Cancer (CoC), National Accreditation Program for Breast Centers (NAPBC), or other national standards and guidelines. Many times each department, provider, or administrator will be collecting different metrics without any harmony on goals for the cancer program outcomes. When the entire team is working together on the same outcomes, the results will exceed their individual department expectations. It is also important to measure a few metrics at a time and create realistic benchmarks. Learn how to collect metrics effectively, find a model that works for your program, and create a plan to meet your metric goal and talk with your colleagues, your team, your administrators, and your physicians and their office staff.

Identifying metrics, their definitions, and how to collect them can be a daunting task; utilize experts in your program. The tumor registry, performance improvement, and information technology staff will assist with successful implementation processes as well as a sound electronic medical record (EMR) for reporting. Collecting baseline data and reports by utilizing discrete fields in your EMR is optimal. Audit and monitor until your program reaches internal goals or national benchmarks. When collecting a new metric, completing a "check-in status" is the new process to ensure your metric goal is working; if not, revise your plan. Brainstorm with your team a new process and/or identify barriers. When metric goals are reached, move on to new metrics and complete an intermittent reaudit to ensure your metric is staying on track.

Identify what needs to be reported to the administration, cancer committee, and your providers. Keep the reporting simple and understandable. Create a navigation dashboard or easily understood report for the administration, cancer committee, and your navigation staff.

The landscape of healthcare has shifted, driven by the Triple Aim to reduce cost per capita in healthcare, improve the patient experience of care, and advance health outcomes. It is essential for outcomes to be driven by standardized evidence-based metrics that can effectively be measured with the application of data analytics and implementation performance improvement initiatives. National standards for measure through CoC, NAPBC, QOPI, and value-based care are now propelling cancer programs to be accountable to measure quality of care delivery and cost. *AONN+ standardized evidence-based navigation metrics* are vital to oncology navigation programs to measure program sustainability and value focused in the domains of PE, CO, and ROI.

References

1. Brown B, Falk LH. Embarking on performance improvement. Healthc Financ Manage. 2014;68:98–103.
2. Strusowski P, Sein E, Johnston D, et al. Standardized evidence-based oncology navigation metrics for all models: a powerful tool in assessing the value and impact of navigation program. J Oncol Navig Surviv. 2017;8(5):220–37.
3. McGillicuddy P, Gold K, Lowe M. Developing core competencies for interprofessional teams: a script-reading approach. In: Christ G, Messner C, Behar L, editors. Handbook of oncology social work: psychosocial care for people with cancer. New York: Oxford University Press; 2015. p. 785–91.
4. Institute of Medicine. Delivering high-quality cancer care. Washington, DC: The National Academies Press; 2013.
5. Institute of Medicine. Crossing the quality chasm: a new health system for the 21st century. Washington, DC: The National Academies Press; 2001.
6. National Learning Consortium. Shared decision making. 2013. https://www.healthit.gov/sites/default/files/nlc_shared_decision_making_fact_sheet.pdf
7. Loscalzo M, Clark K, Bultz BD. Integrated interdisciplinary staff leadership model of patient-centered care. In: Christ G, Messner C, Behar L, editors. Handbook of oncology social work. New York: Oxford University Press; 2015. p. 595–600.
8. Stevens KR. The impact of evidence-based practice in nursing and the next big ideas. Online J Issues Nurs. www.nursingworld.org/MainMenuCategories/ANAMarketplace/ANAPeriodicals/OJIN/TableofContents/Vol-18-2013/No2-May-2013/Impact-of-Evidence-Based-Practice.html. Accessed 31 May 2017.
9. National Quality Forum. ABCs of measurement. www.qualityforum.org/Measuring_Performance/ABCs_of_Measurement.aspx. Accessed 4 May 2017.
10. National Cancer Institute. NCI dictionary of cancer terms: medical oncologist. https://www.cancer.gov/publications/dictionaries/cancer-terms?cdrid=46290
11. Standardized Metrics Source Document. www.aonnonline.org/metrics-source-document.
12. Centers for Medicare and Medicaid Services (CMS). www.cms.gov/Qualitymeasures.
13. National Cancer Institute. Surgery. 2015. https://www.cancer.gov/about-cancer/treatment/types/surgery
14. Oncology Nursing Society Oncology Nurse Navigator Core Competencies. 2013. www.ons.org/sites/default/files/ONNCompetencies_rev.pdf.
15. National Comprehensive Cancer Network. NCCN Clinical Practice Guidelines in Oncology. (NCCN Guidelines). Distress Management Version 1.2014. www.nccn.org/professionals/physician_gls/pdf/distress.pdf.
16. National Cancer Institute. Radiation therapy. 2010. https://www.cancer.gov/about-cancer/treatment/types/radiation-therapy/radiation-fact-sheet

17. Board of Pharmacy Specialists. Oncology pharmacy. https://www.bpsweb.org/bps-specialties/oncology-pharmacy/
18. Bauer, A. Spotlight on: Oncology pharmacists—Part I, a Q&A. 2014. http://www.cancer.net/blog/2014-06/spotlight-oncology-pharmacists-%E2%80%93-part-i-qa
19. National Consensus Project for Quality Palliative Care. Clinical practice guidelines for quality palliative care. 3rd ed. Author: Pittsburgh, PA; 2014.
20. Institute of Medicine. Crossing the quality chasm: a new health system for the 21st century. Washington, DC: National Academies Press; 2001.
21. Smart Goal Setting. 2010–2016. www.smart-goals-guide.com/smart-goal-setting.html.
22. Strusowski, T, Sein E, et al. Standardized metrics source document. 2017. www.aonnonline.org/metrics-source-document. Accessed 15 May 2017.
23. Strusowski T, Stabb J. Patient navigation metrics, measuring the impact of you patient navigation services. accc-cancer.org, January–February 2016.
24. Stewart MA, Rodriguez R. Patient navigation in oncology. In: Christ G, Messner C, Behar L, editors. Handbook of oncology social work. New York: Oxford University Press; 2015. p. 659–65.
25. Association of Community Cancer Centers. Communicating quality in oncology. 2014. www.accc-cancer.org/institute/pdf/2014-WhitePaper-Communicating-Quality-in-Oncology-10-3-14.pdf.
26. Gilbert E, Sherry V, et al. Health care metrics in oncology. J Adv Pract Oncol. 2015;6(1):57–61.
27. Makari-Judson G, Wrenn T, Mertens WC, et al. Using quality oncology practice initiative metrics for physician incentive compensation. J Oncol Pract. 2014;10:58–62.
28. Patel M, Patel K. The oncology care model: aligning financial incentives to improve outcomes. Oncol Pract Manage. 2016; 6. http://oncpracticemanagement.com/issue-archive/2016/december-2016-vol-6-no-12/the-oncology-care-model-aligning-financial-incentives-to-improve-outcomes. Accessed 15 Apr 2017.
29. Charland K, Zweifel R. www.ajmc.com/journals/evidence-based-oncology/2016/june-2016/quality-metrics-for-oncology-in-a-value-based-reimbursement-world-#sthash.n0mWuIQ5.dpuf.
30. Porter ME. What is value in health care? N Engl J Med. 2010;363:2477–81. https://doi.org/10.1056/NEJMp1011024.

Navigation Training, Tools, and Resources

15

Mandi Pratt-Chapman and Linda Burhansstipanov

Patient navigation has arisen quickly as a new health profession with great heterogeneity of background, training, roles, and practices [1]. However, patient navigation, at its core, aims to reduce barriers to healthcare, including access to screening, diagnosis, treatment, supportive care, and posttreatment care for those at risk for and diagnosed with cancer [2, 3]. There are a number of tools and resources available to new and experienced navigators of various types to support professional training and growth. These include core competencies, training, certificates, certification, guides, toolkits, and evaluation support.

15.1 Core Competencies

In 2015, core competencies for oncology patient navigators [4] and nurse navigators [5] were published. Core competencies are helpful in developing standardized expectations for professional knowledge, skills, and expertise in order to perform job functions. Pratt-Chapman et al. developed core competencies for navigators who work professionally, but do not have a healthcare professional license like social workers, nurses, physician assistants, or nurse practitioners. Hereafter, these professional navigators who do not have a healthcare professional license are referred to simply as "patient navigators" [4]. The resulting competencies align with the healthcare professional domains suggested by the Association of American Medical Colleges and the Accreditation Council for Graduate

M. Pratt-Chapman, MA (✉)
Institute for Patient-Centered Initiatives and Health Equity, The George Washington University Cancer Center, Washington, DC, USA
e-mail: mandi@gwu.edu

L. Burhansstipanov, MSPH, DrPH
Native American Cancer Research Corporation, Pine, CO, USA
e-mail: lindab@natamcancer.net

© Springer International Publishing AG, part of Springer Nature 2018
L. D. Shockney (ed.), *Team-Based Oncology Care: The Pivotal Role of Oncology Navigation*, https://doi.org/10.1007/978-3-319-69038-4_15

315

Medical Education [6]. These domains include patient care, knowledge for practice, practice-based learning and improvement, interpersonal and communication skills, professionalism, systems-based practice, interprofessional collaboration, and personal and professional development (see Table 15.1) [4].

In the same year, the Oncology Nurse Navigation Special Interest Group of the Oncology Nursing Society (ONS) established core competencies for oncology nurse navigators, hereafter referred to as "nurse navigators," in order to clarify the role and qualifications for navigators with a nursing license [5]. Updated in 2017, the ONS competencies emphasize the role of the nurse navigator in conducting community needs assessment, developing navigation programs, meeting patient needs, and influencing systems-based strategies. The ONS Oncology Nurse Navigator Professional Practice Framework visualizes roles that align well with the core competencies for patient navigators (see Fig. 15.1).

Differences between navigator types may be described based on licensure and scope of practice, since goals of coordination, education, communication, and facilitation of culturally sensitive care are shared by all navigators. In other words, navigators may perform different tasks, but all have common goals of getting patients to and through the healthcare they need for optimal survival and quality of life.

Core competencies are helpful in creating education and training for a profession, because clarity on what individuals in that profession need to know and do focuses professional development and certification assessment.

15.2   Certificate Programs

Training can be helpful to build navigator confidence as well as competence. Training programs are diverse, which allow navigators with different backgrounds (high school education, bachelor's degree, nursing license) the opportunity to find appropriate programs and improve their skills and expertise as patient navigators.

There are a number of training opportunities that range from undergraduate junior college associate degree programs, through bachelor degrees to adult learning-focused certificates for professionals (see Table 15.2). Curricula tend to focus on medical and cancer care basics, outreach and education, patient assessment, resource mapping, advocacy, interprofessional communication, and professional development. Trainings range from live to online formats as well as blended learning options. Emphasis ranges from foundational competencies to advanced learning or specialized skills, such as integrative or complementary care specialization.

Costs vary widely from free to nearly $5000 based on the education provider, format, and degree of customization. Programs developed using federal monies are often available at no cost. For example, The GW Cancer Center online education programs were created with Centers for Disease Control and Prevention (CDC) funding, and the Patient Navigation Training Collaborative was supported by the National Cancer Institute. However, community-based training programs created without such support typically require revenue to sustain or customize

Table 15.1 Core competencies for oncology patient navigators

Domain 1: Patient care
Facilitate patient-centered care that is compassionate, appropriate, and effective for the treatment of cancer and the promotion of health

1.1 Assist patients in accessing cancer care and navigating healthcare systems. Assess barriers to care and engage patients and families in creating potential solutions to financial, practical, and social challenges
1.2 Identify appropriate and credible resources responsive to patient needs (practical, social, physical, emotional, spiritual) taking into consideration reading level, health literacy, culture, language, and amount of information desired. For physical concerns, emotional needs, or clinical information, refer to licensed clinicians
1.3 Educate patients and caregivers on the multidisciplinary nature of cancer treatment, the roles of team members, and what to expect from the healthcare system. Provide patients and caregivers evidence-based information and refer to clinical staff to answer questions about clinical information, treatment choices, and potential outcomes
1.4 Empower patients to communicate their preferences and priorities for treatment to their healthcare team; facilitate shared decision-making in the patient's healthcare
1.5 Empower patients to participate in their wellness by providing self-management and health promotion resources and referrals
1.6 Follow up with patients to support adherence to agreed-upon treatment plan through continued non-clinical barrier assessment and referrals to supportive resources in collaboration with the clinical team

Domain 2: Knowledge for practice
Demonstrate basic understanding of cancer, healthcare systems, and how patients access care and services across the cancer continuum to support and assist patients
NOTE: This domain refers to foundational knowledge applied across other domains

2.1 Demonstrate basic knowledge of medical and cancer terminology
2.2 Demonstrate familiarity with and know how to access and reference evidence-based information regarding cancer screening, diagnosis, treatment, and survivorship
2.3 Demonstrate basic knowledge of cancer, cancer treatment, and supportive care options, including risks and benefits of clinical trials and integrative therapies
2.4 Demonstrate basic knowledge of health system operations
2.5 Identify potential physical, psychological, social, and spiritual impacts of cancer and its treatment
2.6 Demonstrate general understanding of healthcare payment structure, financing, and where to refer patients for answers regarding insurance coverage and financial assistance

Domain 3: Practice-based learning and improvement
Improve patient navigation process through continual self-evaluation and quality improvement. Promote and advance the profession

3.1 Contribute to patient navigation program development, implementation, and evaluation
3.2 Use evaluation data (barriers to care, patient encounters, resource provision, population health disparities data, and quality indicators) to collaboratively improve navigation process and participate in quality improvement
3.3 Incorporate feedback on performance to improve daily work
3.4 Use information technology to maximize efficiency of patient navigator's time
3.5 Continually identify, analyze, and use new knowledge to mitigate barriers to care
3.6 Maintain comprehensive, timely, and legible records capturing ongoing patient barriers, patient interactions, barrier resolution, and other evaluation metrics and report data to show value to administrators and funders
3.7 Promote navigation role, responsibilities, and value to patients, providers and the larger community

(continued)

Table 15.1 (continued)

Domain 4: Interpersonal and communication skills
Demonstrate interpersonal and communication skills that result in the effective exchange of information and collaboration with patients, their families, and health professionals

4.1 Assess patient capacity to self-advocate; help patients optimize time with their doctors and treatment team (e.g., prioritize questions, clarify information with treatment team)
4.2 Communicate effectively with patients, families, and the public to build trusting relationships across a broad range of socioeconomic and cultural backgrounds
4.3 Employ active listening and remain solutions-oriented in interactions with patients, families, and members of the healthcare team
4.4 Encourage active communication between patients/families and healthcare providers to optimize patient outcomes
4.5 Communicate effectively with navigator colleagues, health professionals, and health-related agencies to promote patient navigation services and leverage community resources to assist patients
4.6 Demonstrate empathy, integrity, honesty, and compassion in difficult conversations
4.7 Know and support National Standards for Culturally and Linguistically Appropriate Services (CLAS) in Health and Health Care to advance health equity, improve quality, and reduce health disparities
4.8 Apply insight and understanding about emotions and human responses to emotions to create and maintain positive interpersonal interactions

Domain 5: Professionalism
Demonstrate a commitment to carrying out professional responsibilities and an adherence to ethical principles

5.1 Apply knowledge of the difference in roles between clinically licensed and non-licensed professionals and act within professional boundaries
5.2 Build trust by being accessible, accurate, supportive, and acting within scope of practice
5.3 Use organization, time management, problem-solving, and critical thinking to assist patients efficiently and effectively
5.4 Demonstrate responsiveness to patient needs within scope of practice and professional boundaries
5.5 Know and support patient rights
5.6 Demonstrate sensitivity and responsiveness to a diverse patient population, including but not limited to diversity in gender, age, culture, race, religion, abilities, and sexual orientation
5.7 Demonstrate a commitment to ethical principles pertaining to confidentiality, informed consent, business practices, and compliance with relevant laws, policies, and regulations (e.g., HIPAA, agency abuse reporting rules, duty to warn, safety contracting)
5.8 Perform administrative duties accurately and efficiently

Domain 6: Systems-based practice
Demonstrate an awareness of and responsiveness to the larger context and system of healthcare, as well as the ability to call effectively on other resources in the system to provide optimal healthcare

6.1 Support a smooth transition of patients across screening, diagnosis, active treatment, survivorship, and/or end-of-life care, working with the patient's clinical care team
6.2 Advocate for quality patient care and optimal patient care systems
6.3 Organize and prioritize resources to optimize access to care across the cancer continuum for the most vulnerable patients

Domain 7: Interprofessional collaboration
Demonstrate ability to engage in an interprofessional team in a manner that optimizes safe, effective patient- and population-centered care

Table 15.1 (continued)

7.1 Work with other health professionals to establish and maintain a climate of mutual respect, dignity, diversity, ethical integrity, and trust

7.2 Use knowledge of one's role and the roles of other health professionals to appropriately assess and address the needs of patients and populations served to optimize health and wellness

7.3 Participate in interprofessional teams to provide patient- and population-centered care that is safe, timely, efficient, effective, and equitable

Domain 8: Personal and professional development
Demonstrate qualities required to sustain lifelong personal and professional growth

8.1 Set learning and improvement goals. Identify and perform learning activities that address one's gaps in knowledge, skills, attitudes, and abilities

8.2 Demonstrate healthy coping mechanisms to respond to stress; employ self-care strategies

8.3 Manage possible and actual conflicts between personal and professional responsibilities

8.4 Recognize that ambiguity is part of patient care, and respond by utilizing appropriate resources in dealing with uncertainty

Reprinted with permission from The GW Cancer Center [14].

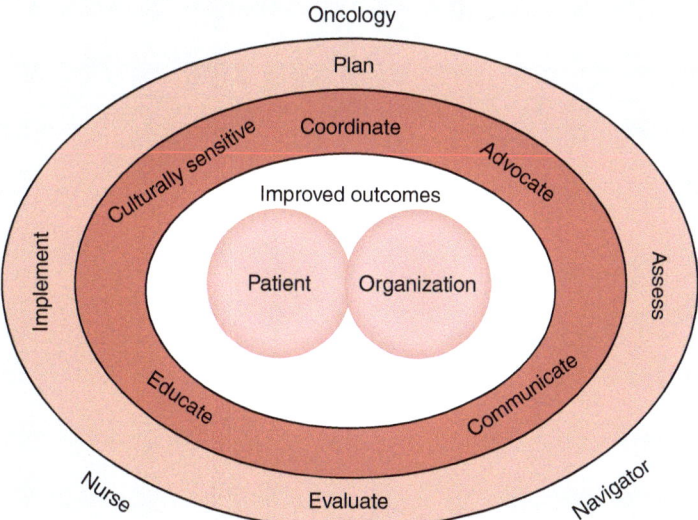

Note. From "Oncology Nurse Navigator Core Competencies," by Oncology Nursing Society, 2013. Retrieved from https://www.ons .org/sites/default/files/ONNCompetencies_rev.pdf. Copyright 2013 by Oncology Nursing Society. Reprinted with permission.

Fig. 15.1 Professional practice framework. *Note.* Reprinted with the permission from the Oncology Nursing Society (ONS). 2017 *Oncology Nurse Navigator Competencies.* www.ons.org/sites/default/files/2017ONNcompetencies.pdf. Copyright © 2017. All rights reserved [5]

Table 15.2 Professional certificate programs

Program	Website	Target audience	Cost	Course format	Curriculum
Cancer Navigator Program	cancernavigatorprogram.org	Social workers, counselors, chaplains, and other staff supporting patients, including navigators	$550	Online–21 lessons	• Cancer biology • Prevention and screening methods • Treatment options • Palliative/end-of-life care • Financial resources • Patient education • Advocacy • Resource utilization and support • Spiritual, psychosocial, and emotional support needs • Home health and hospice care • Medicare, Medicaid, and other payers
Cancer Navigator Program	cancernavigatorprogram.org	Registered nurses	$550	Online–24 lessons	• All content from general navigator program plus symptom management
The GW Cancer Center—Oncology Patient Navigator Training: The Fundamentals	bit.ly/GWCCOnlineAcademy	Any navigator	No cost	Online–20 lessons Interactive, evidence-based with case studies Comes with free online guide	• Overview of patient navigation and core competencies • Basics of healthcare • Basics of patient navigation • Enhancing communication • Professionalism • Enhancing practice
GW Cancer Center—Executive Training on Navigation and Survivorship	bit.ly/GWCCOnlineAcademy	Supervisors of navigators Program leaders	No cost	Online Interactive, evidence-based with case studies and supplemental written content and activities Comes with free online workbook	Nuts and bolts of navigation and survivorship program development, including: • Identifying Need • Planning Your Program: Models • Components, Tools, Goal Setting and more • Funding and Sustaining Your Program • Evaluating Your Program • Creating a Business Plan

	Website	Target audience	Cost	Format	Content
Harold P. Freeman Patient Navigation Institute Patient Navigation Program	www.hpfreemanpni.org	Patient navigators	$995	2 days, In-Person—10 modules including patient interaction and case studies	• Curriculum not publicly available • Focus on increased retention, diagnostic, and treatment resolution rates
Misericordia University	www.misericordia.edu/page.cfm?p=1814	Undergraduate students wishing to become navigators	Based on tuition to complete required credits	Bachelor of health science, Patient Navigation specialization Patient Navigation certificate	Helps new navigators guide patients, caregivers, and family members through a treatment plan with the goal of improving patient outcomes • Values of justice and hospitality • Physical, emotional, and social support to patients following a treatment plan • Communication and interviewing to assess barriers to care • Current healthcare trends and issues that impact the patient navigators' ability to provide care/assistance • Identify and explain health resources, including publicly funded health insurance programs and health delivery systems
Native Patient Navigator's Training	www.NatAmCancer.org	Any navigator working with indigenous peoples	$1,100	5 days In-person Learning reinforcement sessions post-training	• AI/AN history and impact on community member perceptions and healthcare • Cultural competency, goal setting and culture, navigator safety • Navigating the Healthcare Systems and the Indian Health Service (IHS) Purchased Referred Care • Outreach and education strategies • Communication • Healthcare team collaboration • Resources • Cancer continuum and tumor-specific education • Clinical trials, confidentiality, HIPAA, data collection and protocols for dissemination • Tribal IRBs and approval processes

(continued)

Table 15.2 (continued)

Program	Web site	Target audience	Cost	Course format	Curriculum
Otero	www.ojc.edu/academics/ academicprograms/ ctehealthnav.aspx	Patient navigators	Based on tuition to complete required credits	In-person	• Linking patients with services • Providing information and resources • Helping providers interact with patients • Health education and behavior change promotion
Patient Navigator Training Collaborative	patientnavigatortraining. org	Patient navigators (Level 1) Experienced patient navigators, nurses, social workers (Level 2) Administrators (Level 3)	Varies	In-person (Level 1, 2, 3) Online (Level 2) Special topic webinars	• Level 1–fundamentals: basic patient navigation skills, resources, basic health promotion, professional conduct, motivational interviewing • Level 2–for experienced navigators, nurses, or social workers: includes small group work, role-play, practice sessions, and group discussion. Real-life scenarios and examples are woven throughout each course • Level 3–supervisors of navigators, program planners, and administrators of patient navigator programs: provides a basic understanding of the patient navigator intervention model, reviews challenges facing program managers, and provides strategies for an effective program. Includes identifying evidence-based clinical guidelines, utilizing registries for identifying patients, developing standard work flows, navigator training, navigator supervision needs, and evaluation of services • E-Learning: Preventive healthcare 101, introduction to the healthcare system, introduction to chronic disease, clinical trials and patient navigation, HIV-related cancer research studies • Webinars: Poverty and self-sufficiency, 2013 CLAS standards for patient navigators, basic crisis management skills for patient navigators, managing difficult patient encounters

Shenandoah University/Inova Health System	www.su.edu/nursing/certificate-programs/care-navigator-certificate	Registered nurses	$3000	5 days in-person/blended learning 56 contact hours and a preceptorship	• Assist patients in navigating complex healthcare services across the continuum of care • Build skills in delivering care coordination services within new healthcare models and patient settings
Smith Center Patient Navigation Training in Integrative Cancer Care	smithcenter.org/institute-for-integrative-oncology-navigation	Navigators interested in integrative care	$995	Two pre-training teleconferences 5 days in-person	• Morning Yoga at Patient Navigation Training • Client Assessment • Difficult Conversations • Survivorship Issues • The Art of Healing • Spiritual Support • Nutrition • Application of Complementary Modalities • Building Trust • Planning Your Integrative Practice
University of Miami Healthcare Navigator Certificate	continue.miami.edu/en/packagedetail.aspx?p=100	Any navigator or patient advocate	$4995	Online	• Health advocacy and the role of the health advocate • Understanding the patient illness experience • Healthcare communications and professionalism • Ethical issues in healthcare • Health law • Navigating healthcare financing • Business as a healthcare advocate

Reprinted with permission from the Journal of Oncology Navigation & Survivorship [9] and the University of Michigan School of Public Health [15] training for learners. Junior colleges and universities may require students to enroll in the institution for credit. For example, Otero Junior College [7] offers an Applied Associate of Science (AAS) degree with a focus on patient navigation. Otero Junior College requires students to enroll and meet eligibility requirements prior to acceptance to the patient navigation certificate program. Credits from the AAS program can be used to help fulfill bachelor degree requirements at some 4-year colleges. Red Rocks Community College, a part of the Colorado Patient Navigator Training Collaborative, has hosted Level 1 trainings in the past with grant funding [8].

While training and certification are not currently a requirement for hire at all places of employment, documentation of training can be helpful to a navigator in a competitive job market.

15.3 Certification

Currently, there are two options for national navigation certification—breast-specific certification through the National Consortium of Breast Centers (NCBC) and certification for those who assist patients with any cancer type available through the Academy of Oncology Nurse & Patient Navigators (AONN+) (see Table 15.3). NCBC offers credentialing based on level of licensure, while AONN+ currently offers Oncology Patient Navigator–Certified Generalist (OPN-CG) and Oncology Nurse Navigator–Certified Generalist (ONN-CG) options. Some states, such as Florida, offer certification for community health workers (CHWs). Patient navigators working within Florida are encouraged to obtain the CHW certification.

Certification is different from a certificate program [9]. Certificates are granted to individuals after completing a training or program, whereas certification is granted by an external entity, usually as a result of a passing grade on a proctored examination along with other, often experiential, requirements (see Table 15.4).

To prepare for certification, NCBC provides a study guide and resources for reference. NCBC has partnered with the Harold P. Freeman Patient Navigation Institute to provide additional educational support for exam preparers. AONN+ provides online learning modules and printed learning guides. In addition, AONN+ has partnered with The GW Cancer Center to prepare test takers for the OPN-CG examination. The GW Cancer Center's Oncology Patient Navigation Training: The Fundamentals prepares navigators well for the OPN-CG examination [1].

Some state government agencies, such as the Colorado Department of Public Health and Environment, are in the process of approving programs that meet their competencies and documentation standards. Those eligible programs will be posted on the Department of Public Health and Environment website, so that patient navigators are aware of trainings that are recognized as legitimate for navigators working in Colorado.

Table 15.3 Certification options

Program	Website	Target audience	Cost	Course format	Education support
Academy of Oncology Nurse & Patient Navigators	www.aonnonline.org/certification	Patient Navigators of all cancer types *Oncology Patient Navigator–Certified Generalist* Nurse Navigators of all cancer types *Oncology Nurse Navigator–Certified Generalist*	Free with membership	Examination	AONN+ partners with the GW Cancer Center to provide educational content. See information in Table 15.2 for the GW Cancer Center training offerings AONN+ offers online learning modules to help candidates prepare for the ONN-CG certification examination Supplemental learning guides are offered through the *Journal of Oncology Navigation & Survivorship* to prepare candidates with additional resources relevant to the OPN-CG and ONN-CG examinations
National Consortium of Breast Centers	www2.bpnc.org	Any navigator *Certified Navigator–Breast (CN-B)* + individual designation based on licensure	$300 for NCBC members $450 for nonmembers at annual conference $459 at regional locations	Examination	A self-study document is emailed to applicants within 7 working days containing information about certification, resources, reference websites, and sample questions NCBC partners with the Harold P. Freeman Patient Navigation Institute to educational support to prepare for the examination. See information in Table 15.2 for Harold P. Freeman Patient Navigation Institute Patient Navigation Program

Table 15.4 Certificate versus certification

Certificate	Certification
Results from an educational process	Results from an assessment process
For both newcomers and experienced professionals	Typically requires some amount of professional experience
Awarded by educational programs and institutions	Awarded by a third-party, standard-setting organization
Indicates completion of a course with a specific focus; different from a degree-granting program	Indicates mastery or competence as measured against a defensible set of standards, usually by application or examination
May result in a document (certificate)	Typically results in a designation to use after one's name (e.g., OPN-CG)
Demonstrates knowledge of the course at the end of a determined period of time	Has ongoing requirements to show continued competence, such as continuing education units

15.4 Additional Resources

There are many resources available to assist with cancer basics, navigation knowledge, and program planning (see Table 15.5). The *GW Cancer Center Guide for Patient Navigators–A Supplement to the Oncology Patient Navigator Training: The Fundamentals* is an excellent resource to learn about the basics of healthcare and US healthcare financing, foundations of patient navigation competency, enhancing communication skills, and professional conduct as a navigator. The *Executive Training on Navigation and Survivorship: Finding Your Patient Focus–Guide for Program Development* [10] and corresponding workbook [10, 11] provide step-by-step guidance for program planning. And *Advancing the Field of Cancer Patient Navigation: A Toolkit for Comprehensive Cancer Control Professionals* [11, 12] provides tips for cancer control programs, policy strategies for navigation sustainability and resources such as sample job descriptions, group activities for navigation networks, a navigator competency self-assessment tool, and interview questions to consider when hiring a navigator. For more information, see also Chapter 4 of this book, "Building a Navigation Program."

Evaluating the impact of a navigator can be as important as the navigator developing knowledge and professional skills. Documenting value can support job retention and program sustainability. The Association of Community Cancer Centers, the Kansas Center Partnership, and the University of North Carolina provide free downloadable forms that can help navigators document the value of their services (see Table 15.6). Software can also help manage patient cases and report on navigation value metrics. There are several commercial options, including Nursenav, Cordata, and OncoNav. There is also an Excel-based case management and reporting tool called the Patient Navigation Barriers and Outcomes Tool™ (PN-BOT™) that The GW Cancer Center developed. The PN-BOT™ can be downloaded free of charge and comes with user videos and a quick-start guide. PN-BOT™ allows for case management, navigation tracking, testimonial tracking, and patient-level, case-level, and barrier-level reports (Tables 15.7 and 15.8) [13].

Table 15.5 Guides, manuals, and toolkits

Resource	Website	Target audience	Cost	Format	Content
2016 Breast Health Navigator Manual	www.educareinc.com/training_nav.php	Breast health navigators	$349.95	Online manual	Manual topics include: • Navigator role • Historical overview • Statistics and risk factors • Anatomy and physiology • Benign breast conditions • Diagnosis of breast disease • Breast pain • Breast discharge • Male breast disease • Hormones and breast disease • Understanding breast cancer • Navigator as coach • Surgical decisions • Breast reconstruction • Breast cancer treatment • Pregnancy and breast cancer • Fertility issues • Recurrent breast cancer • Sexuality after cancer • Hereditary breast cancer • Survivorship challenges • Spiritual needs • Terminal patient • Support programs • Survivorship programs • Navigation program organization • Breast center marketing • EduCare information

(continued)

Table 15.5 (continued)

Resource	Website	Target audience	Cost	Format	Content
Advancing the Field of Cancer Patient Navigation: A Toolkit for Comprehensive Cancer Control Professionals	bit.ly/PNPSEGuide	Cancer control professionals	No cost	Online toolkit	• Overview of patient navigation • Training and technical assistance options • System change and program planning • Sustaining the profession
Executive Training on Navigation and Survivorship: Finding Your Patient Focus–Guide for Program Development	bit.ly/ExecTrainGuide	Program planners	No cost	Online guide	• Program planning cycle: assess, plan, implement, evaluate • Defining your patient population • Conducting a stakeholder analysis • Program design • Questions to consider • Funding and sustainability • Evaluation • Making a business case
Boston Medical Center Patient Navigation Toolkit	sites.bu.edu/coeinwomenshealth/resources/avontoolkits	Program planners (Volume I) Navigation supervisors (Volume II) Patient navigators (Volume III)	No cost	Online toolkit	• Volume I: Provides information on program planning and design as well as relevant tools • Volume II: Building a program, hiring a navigator, supervising and training a navigator, evaluating your program • Volume III: Defining the navigator role, building skills, understanding barriers, helping patients take charge of their health, meeting your goals and self-care

(continued)

| Executive Training on Navigation and Survivorship Program Development Workbook | bit.ly/ExecTrainWorkbook | Navigators of all types Program managers Administrators | No cost | Online workbook | Provides worksheets on:
• Defining your patient population
• Determining patient flow
• Conducting an institutional analysis
• Internal and external resource mapping
• Assessing stakeholder needs
• Writing a mission and vision statement
• Developing SMART goals
• Designing your program
• Creating a logic model
• Demonstrating value
• Creating a budget
• Developing an evaluation plan
• Writing a business plan |
| Guide for Patient Navigators—A Supplement to the Oncology Patient Navigator Training: The Fundamentals | bit.ly/PNTrainingGuide | Navigators of all types | No cost | Online guide | Provides content that aligns with training
• Medical terminology
• Cancer basics
• Clinical trials
• Impact of cancer
• US healthcare system
• Healthcare payment and financing
• Role of the patient navigator
• Patient assessment
• Shared decision-making
• Identifying resources
• Communicating with patients
• Patient advocacy
• Culturally competent communication
• Scope of practice
• Ethics and patient rights
Practicing efficiently and effectively
• Healthcare team collaboration
• Program evaluation and quality improvement
• Personal and professional development |

Table 15.5 (continued)

Resource	Web site	Target audience	Cost	Format	Content
New Hampshire Colorectal Cancer Screening Program Patient Navigation Model for Increasing Colonoscopy Quality and Completion: A Replication Manual	www.cdc.gov/cancer/crccp/pdf/nhcrcsp_pn_manual.pdf	Colorectal cancer screening programs	No cost	Online manual	• Case for colorectal cancer screening, barriers to screening, and patient navigation overview • The New Hampshire Colorectal Cancer Screening Patient Navigation Model with six-topic protocol • Planning and implementing a successful intervention • Using data to maintain a quality intervention • Sample forms, letters, checklists, protocols, data metrics, and satisfaction survey
Paying for Colorectal Cancer Screening Navigation Toolkit: Strategies for Payment and Sustainability	https://nccrt.org/wp-content/uploads/v.22016_paying_pntoolkit_full_final.pdf	Colorectal cancer screening programs	No cost	Online toolkit	• Sustainability framework • Evidence base for colorectal cancer screening navigation • Examples of programs • Quality and accreditation standards • Making the business case for colorectal cancer screening navigation • Policy standards for colorectal cancer screening navigation • Evaluation of colorectal cancer screening navigation • Resources
Catholic Health Initiatives Navigation Resource Guide	https://mdpnn.files.wordpress.com/2013/04/chi-navigation-program-resource-guide-_final-012013_.pdf	Focus is on nurse navigators and supervisors Guide does include a section on community (referred to as "lay") patient navigators	Free from Internet	PDF	• Definition of Patient Navigation • Navigation Program Implementation • Navigation Program Operations • Determining Optimal Navigator Caseloads • Navigation Program Policies and Procedures • Patient Intake and Assessment Tools • Ongoing Navigation Program Evaluation and Improvement Tools and Processes • Navigation Role Clarity • Patient and Family Education • Survivorship • Emerging Trends in Navigation Appendix (includes needs assessment tools, patient acuity scales, navigator knowledge assessment tools, and several other documents)

Table 15.6 Sample forms

Resource	Website	Cost	Format	Considerations

Association of Community Cancer Centers Tool kit	www.accc-cancer.org/resources/ PatientNavigation-Tools.asp	No cost	Forms available online	• No cost
				• Paper forms for download including:
				  – Sample pre-assessment tool
				  – Sample job descriptions
				  – Sample intake forms
				  – Sample assessment forms
				  – Sample evaluation forms
				  – Sample patient satisfaction surveys

Kansas Center Partnership Toolkit	www.cancerkansas.org/download/ Cancer_Patient_Navigation_Toolkit.pdf	No cost	Forms available online	• No cost
				• Paper forms for download including:
				  – Sample position description
				  – Sample intake form and tracking tool
				  – Sample flyer
				  – Sample patient satisfaction survey
				  – Sample press release
				  – Sample cancer treatment plan and summary

UNC Cancer Network Patient Navigation Tools	unclineberger.org/unccn/patient- navigation/cancer-resource-documents	No cost	Forms available online	• No cost
				• Paper forms for download include:
				  – UNC Patient Navigation Process
				  – UNC Nurse Navigator Tracking Tool
				  – Cancer Resources
				  – Image-guided breast biopsy FAQ sheet

Table 15.7 Software for evaluating patient navigation

Resource	Website	Cost	Format	Considerations
Cordata	www.cordatahealth.com	Depends on number of users and scope of license	Software	• Tracks clinical outcomes using built-in protocols • Provides reports to document outcomes to payers • Allows patients to enter data through a patient portal • Requires financial investment

GW Cancer Center Patient Navigation Barriers and Outcomes Tool	bit.ly/AboutPNBOT	No cost	Excel database available for free download with user videos and quick-start guide	• No cost
				• Based on research-driven metrics
				• Generates preprogrammed reports including:
				  – Patient volume
				  – Patient demographic profiles
				  – Cancer treatment profiles
				  – Timeliness of cancer care
				  – Barriers to care
				  – Navigator caseload and time
				  – Navigation services provided
				  – Patient outcomes
				• Data entry only by one user at a time

Navigation Tracker	www.navigationtracker.com/Index.aspx	Monthly subscription	Software	• Requires financial investment
Nursenav	www.nursenav.com	Depends on number of users and scope of license	Secure web-based application	• Capability to invoice clients, exchange secure emails and documents, schedule and track appointments, set up shared case permissions, design and perform patient assessments, and run reports • Requires financial investment
OncoNav	www.onco-nav.com/?cid=59	Depends on number of users and scope of license	Software	• Capability to schedule appointments, customize templates, record barriers to care and track efforts, document distress screening, and generate survivorship care plans • Requires financial investment

Table 15.8 Patient Navigation Barriers and Outcomes Tool™ sections

MISCELLANEOUS SHEETS FOR NAVIGATION, USABILITY AND FUNCTIONALITY
•Home
•Set UP
•Reports List
•Reference
•Don't Delete

DATA ENTRY SHEETS FOR DATA ENTRY, MODIFICATION AND LOOKUP
•Patient Data Entry
•Case Data Entry
•Encounters Data Entry
•Testimonials Data Entry

LIST SHEETS FOR RAW DATA/DATABASE STORAGE
•Patient List
•Case List
•Encounters List
•Barriers List
•Testimonials List

REPORTS SHEETS FOR AUTOMATIC REPORT TEMPLATES
•Patient Reports
•Case Reports
•Encounter Reports
•Barriers Reports

PIVOT SHEETS FOR CUSTOM PIVOT TABLE REPORTS
•Patient Pivot
•Case Pivot
•Encounters Pivot
•Barriers Pivot

Reprinted with permission from the GW Cancer Center [13]

Native American Cancer Research Corporation (NACR), a community-based American Indian nonprofit organization, has operated and evaluated an online evaluation program [14] since 2005 that tracks patient navigation visits and activities for the full cancer continuum. The system tracks navigators' work with patients; intervals from when a screening or cancer test was recommended to when scheduled to when completed; survivorship quality of life (physical, mental-emotional, social, and spiritual); and existence of a survivorship care plan (SCP), when updated, and how patients acted upon the SCP recommendations. The system can also track pre-/posttest changes in navigator learning based on education offerings, as well as demographics and satisfaction assessments for workshop participants. The online program can tailor reports by specific navigator, span of time, or phase of cancer. This online program is being expanded and modified into a commercial tablet application that is easier to use and can load data when WiFi is not available, a common issue when working in rural areas and on Indian reservations. Based on informant interviews, this is also an attractive feature for navigators from cultures other than American Indian.

Finally, a technical assistance portal is available called Cancer Control TAP, accessible at www.cancercontroltap.org. The portal features a searchable resource repository and online academy where you can find many of the resources for patient navigation professional development mentioned here, along with resources on a variety of other topics relevant to comprehensive cancer control. For example, there are articles, fact sheets, toolkits, and webinars available from national and state-level organizations with tumor-specific information, cancer health risk information, and population-specific resources (e.g., resources targeted for specific age groups; racial, ethnic, sexual, or gender minorities; or those with low health literacy).

Conclusion

Navigators are diverse in background and skill set—and this diversity is critical to address the variety of needs that cancer patients have. This chapter provides resources to help navigators understand, become trained, and operate within their appropriate scope of practice. Available trainings, toolkits and manuals, sample protocols, and evaluation supports can optimize navigation program planning and impact as well as provide opportunities for continued learning.

References

1. Pratt-Chapman M. What does a patient navigator do?: patient navigation core competencies, training and certification. Association of Community Cancer Centers Oncology Issues. 2016.
2. Freeman HP, Rodriguez RL. History and principles of patient navigation. Cancer. 2011;117(15 Suppl):3539–42. https://doi.org/10.1002/cncr.26262.
3. Willis A, Reed E, Pratt-Chapman M, Kapp H, Hatcher E, Vaitones V, et al. Development of a framework for patient navigation: delineating roles across navigator types. J Oncol Navig Surviv. 2013;4:20–6.
4. Pratt-Chapman M, Willis A, Masselink L. Core competencies for oncology patient navigators. J Oncol Navig Surviv. 2015;6:16–21.
5. Oncology Nursing Society. 2017 Oncology Nurse Navigator Core Competencies. 2017. www.ons.org/sites/default/files/2017ONNcompetencies.pdf.
6. Englander R, Cameron T, Ballard A, Dodge J, Bull J, Aschenbrener CA. Toward a common taxonomy of competency domains for the health professions and competencies for physicians. Acad Med. 2013;88:1088–94.
7. Otero Junior College. Health navigator: Associate of Applied Science Degree & Certificate. www.ojc.edu/academics/academicprograms/ctehealthnav.aspx.
8. Center for Public Health Practice. Level I: patient navigator fundamentals. 2015. www.publichealthpractice.org/civicrm/event/info?id=62.
9. Pratt-Chapman M. Certificate or certification: what's the difference? J Oncol Navig Surviv. 2015;6:16–21.
10. The GW Cancer Center. Executive training on navigation and survivorship: finding your patient focus: guide for program development. Washington, DC: The George Washington University; 2014.
11. The GW Cancer Center. Advancing the field of patient navigation: a toolkit for comprehensive cancer control professionals. Washington, DC: The George Washington University; 2016.
12. Phillips S, Raskin S, Pratt-Chapman M. Patient navigation barriers and outcomes tool: version 1.1 quick start guide. Washington, DC: The George Washington University Cancer Center; 2016.
13. GW Cancer Center. Patient navigator competencies. 2015. http://bit.ly/PNCompReport.
14. Native American Cancer Research Corporation. Collaborative partnership in cancer prevention & control. http://natamcancer.org/nacreval/nacreval.html.
15. University of Michigan School of Public Health. Certificate v. Certification. In: Website no longer active; 2015.

Compassion Fatigue in Oncology Nurse Navigation: Identification and Prevention

16

Emily Gentry and Lillie D. Shockney

16.1 Concept of Compassion Fatigue

The concept of compassion fatigue (Exhibit 16.1) arose out of the research and observations of Charles R. Figley, PhD (1995) [1]. He defines it as a combination of burnout and secondary traumatic stress, which is stress that is caused by the emotional burden of wanting to help people who are suffering [2].

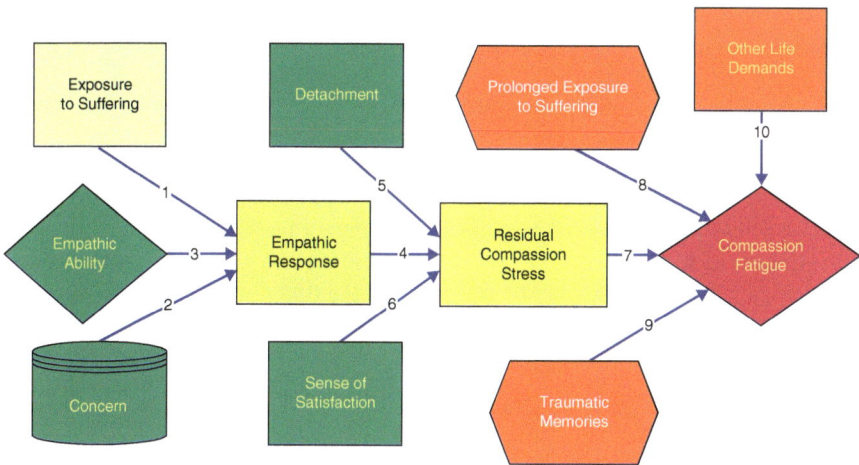

The Compassion Fatigue Process (Figley, 2001)

Exhibit 16.1 The cascade of events and emotions that can lead to compassion fatigue

E. Gentry, RN, BSN, OCN (✉)
Sarah Cannon Cancer Institute at Medical City Healthcare, Irving, TX, USA
e-mail: Emily.Gentry@MedicalCityHealth.com; Emily.Gentry@SarahCannon.com

L. D. Shockney, RN, BS, MAS, ONN-CG
Johns Hopkins University School of Medicine, Baltimore, MD, USA
e-mail: shockli@jhmi.edu

If exposure to suffering is a contributing factor to compassion fatigue, then oncology nurse navigators may be getting extra doses of suffering, given that nationally a small population of navigators is managing an ever-expanding caseload of cancer patients. This expanding caseload exacerbates the ever-present perception that there are not enough hours in the day to provide optimum care for patients. The anxiety over the lack of time creates an emotional burden that can lead to burnout and compassion fatigue. A cross-sectional study of oncology physicians examined the incidence of burnout and the connection to time pressures [3]. The study surveyed oncologists in Canada ($n = 312$). They completed questionnaires assessing burnout, compassion fatigue, workload, time pressure at work, work-family conflict, and other personal, family, and occupational characteristics. The results of the study showed that subjective time pressure at work is a key predictor of both burnout and compassion fatigue. If oncologists are burdened by time pressures, and these pressures can lead to compassion fatigue, it is just as likely that oncology nurses can experience the same results.

Many times, hospitals and health systems will create oncology navigation programs before they are operationally or administratively ready to support these programs. In a rush to answer a marketing or clinical demand, driven by national cancer care standards and patient experience literature, healthcare organizations create navigation programs without addressing broken internal business processes, ingrained physician referral practices, or inadequate medical documentation systems. The "rush to market" means that navigators have to cope with both workload stressors and work process stressors. These circumstances can also result in the navigator being pulled into administrative tasks and meetings that revolve around fixing broken processes, reducing time for care planning, and reducing the navigator's ability to apply his or her highest level of skills. These situations complicate an already stressful care environment for the navigation team members and can leave them exposed to criticism from all quarters: administrators, doctors, colleagues, patients, and families. The cumulative effect of the organizational stress, when layered with typical caregiving stress, can create job dissatisfaction and burnout, starting the compassion fatigue cascade described above.

16.2 Symptoms of Compassion Fatigue

People who have developed compassion fatigue may exhibit the following symptoms [4]:

- Slowness of thought
- Difficulty prioritizing tasks
- Difficulty initiating routine tasks
- Irritability and/or anxiety
- Preoccupation with minor issues and familiar tasks
- Indecision and lack of concentration
- Loss of initiative with fatigue
- Exhaustion and poor self-care
- Physical symptoms, such as headaches

- Substance abuse
- Loss of adaptability
- Inability to relax
- Physical symptoms (at work or when thinking of work): nausea, insomnia, heart palpitations, and other issues

Given these factors, it is easy to see how medical professionals who have developed compassion fatigue could fail to provide optimum care for patients and fail with self-care. Therefore, it is crucial for the medical industry, and individual provider entities, to understand the nexus of compassion fatigue, how to recognize it, how to prevent it, and how to effectively address the needs of practitioners who develop it. In settings where team-based care is dominant, it is also important to recognize that team members may see early indicators of compassion fatigue before managers, and they may be in a position to help a teammate or at least raise the issue for management so that aid can been offered.

16.3   The Prevalence and Impact of Compassion Fatigue

The prevalence of compassion fatigue among oncology nurses has been recorded as ranging from 8% to 38% [5]. As stated above, there is a close correlation between compassion fatigue and burnout, and research has shown that oncology nurses have a high risk for burnout because of their intense emotional involvement with patients and families and their diminished sense of accomplishment when patients perish [6].

Compassion fatigue can have a negative influence on performance at work and negatively impact the personal lives of those suffering under its influence. Given that compassion fatigue can also be a significant factor in job turnover or dropping out of oncology altogether, health administrators cannot ignore it.

16.4   Implementing Strategies to Diminish Symptoms

16.4.1 Acknowledge Emotions

To support the oncology nursing staff, the Sarah Cannon Cancer Institute at Johnston-Willis Hospital in Richmond, VA, created a bereavement committee with representatives from each oncology unit. The bereavement committee sponsored events that allowed nursing staff members to share the emotions they experienced in caregiving. One of the events was an annual service of remembrance that involved the family members of patients who have passed and any staff members who wanted to attend, even on their days off. Feedback from the nursing staff led the bereavement committee to develop a second event that was designed exclusively for the oncology nursing staff, since they had different needs than family members and didn't always feel comfortable expressing their emotions in front of the families who attended the service of remembrance. According to feedback surveys, the reflection service (created for nursing staff) provided a safe space for nursing team members to share and let go of bottled-up emotions, empowering them to face the next challenge. The unit administrators have also seen an increased sense of team-work on the units and a deeper sense of caring among the staff. All of these factors are perceived to be useful in combating compassion fatigue across the staff [7].

16.4.2 Reduce Stress

Because stress is a key factor in compassion fatigue, basic strategies for reducing the impact of stress can be effective at preventing or recovering from compassion fatigue [8]. Below are key steps to recovery and breaking the cycle of fatigue and burnout:

1. Acknowledge and identify the stressors
2. Make a commitment to self-care; involve others, i.e., colleagues and family
3. Focus on proper nutrition
4. Set up a better regimen for sleep and rest and exercise
5. Simplify your off-work schedule
6. Engage in activities that don't remind you of work, such as hobbies

At a professional level, a key to avoiding or recovering from compassion fatigue is talking about possible causes and simply acknowledging the reality of compassion fatigue. This can help managers develop strategies for recovery, such as a shift in job responsibilities.

It is often assumed that compassion fatigue is linked to the process of caring for critically ill or terminally ill patients. While this can be a factor, especially for professionals who have worked in oncology for many decades, this isn't necessarily true. Medical personnel who elect to work in oncology understand that medical interventions don't always win the battle against cancer. A certain level of mental shielding is natural and understandable for oncology personnel. This defense is not defined as compassion fatigue, and people working in oncology are no more or no less susceptible to compassion fatigue simply based on their medical specialty. Undoubtedly, the risk for compassion fatigue is high for oncology nurses, but it would also be high for nurses in critical care units.

For many oncology navigators, however, compassion fatigue can develop over time due to the sense of frustration that builds if and when they are not supported organizationally as they care for patients and families.

16.4.3 Practice Self-Care [8]

The following are basic strategies that can help combat stress and can be helpful in combating compassion fatigue:

Keep family close: Spend time or at least talk with family members regularly. Family members serve as grounding influences and provide love, encouragement, and acceptance.

Practice mindfulness: Take 5 minutes and go to a quiet spot and be "in the moment." Look at your surroundings and relate to them. Pull out of chaotic environments and try to find a quiet zone. This practice can be combined with mindful breathing. Ideally, the hospital or healthcare organization will dedicate space for quiet reflection for staff members.

Find ways to improve operational efficiency at work, especially if inefficiencies add stress to your workday: Identify activities that result in wasted time at work and objectively try to help the organization improve processes and practices that elevate work frustration.

Stay current on medical research that promotes a positive impact on cancer treatments: Review information about promising cancer therapies to help balance the reality of daily struggles with patients who face difficult outcomes.

Eat healthy: Try to eat healthy meals and healthy snacks. Hydrate frequently.

Change your mode of travel if traveling to work adds more stress: Consider public transportation or carpooling, especially if the additional human interaction is helpful.

Massage: Get a massage once or twice a month or create a spa environment at home if possible. Try soft lights, soft music, scented candles, and scented oils.

Keep a journal: Write thoughts about your workday each night. It may just be a few words that sum up the day. Expand on the topic if it was something positive, and record these positive thoughts in red so they are easy to find. Review them occasionally. Also add thoughts on being grateful about some aspect of work or life outside of work.

Laugh more: Go online and watch funny videos. Laughter is one of the best stress relievers known.

Tap into employee assistance programs: Take advantage of any employee assistance programs that are designed to provide confidential and professional support during difficult times. Psychologists and psychotherapists can be very helpful in giving perspective and advice and serving as sounding boards.

Add music to your day: Create a positive environment by adding music to each day.

Focus on what is possible, not on what is impossible: Manage expectations. Just as nurses want patients to focus on what they can still do, and less on what they are no longer able to do, so should nursing professionals. Focus on the glass half full and not the glass half empty.

Get a pet [9]: Adopt a pet. Studies show that people with pets are generally happier and have lower stress levels, primarily because pets offer love and affection and force a measure of structure to each day, which can help lower stress.

16.5   Recognizing Compassion Fatigue Across Multidisciplinary Teams

It is often assumed that people working in multidisciplinary teams have built-in support networks that reduce the risk of compassion fatigue. No studies support or explicitly refute this theory. At day's end, each individual caregiver has his or her set of internal and external pressures that create incremental weight to job duties. The compilation of these pressures can create the environment for compassion fatigue, even with the natural release valve that team relationships may provide.

Identifying individuals within a team structure who are at risk for compassion fatigue is probably of greater importance than with staff members who are not involved in team structures. While identifying signs of compassion fatigue in any employee is critical, when a team member goes down, he or she will impact their own performance and hinder the effectiveness of the overall team. Like most industries, healthcare is team-driven, so understanding team health is critical for managers.

Leadership Strategies for Managing Compassion Fatigue in Team Environments

1. *Provide regular opportunities for team members to discuss stressors that contribute to development of compassion fatigue, both individually and as a team.*
2. *Facilitate forums to combat stress, i.e., add self-care topics to team meeting agendas, include guest speakers to equip colleagues with new self-care skills.*
3. *Ask employees to complete regular self-assessments.*
4. *Implement an annual staff retreat, emphasizing team/relationship building and self-care activities, and concurrently implement these types of activities in regular team meetings.*
5. *Celebrate employee milestones, i.e., birthdays, employee anniversaries, career accomplishments.*
6. *Share patient appreciation/employee recognition with the team.*
7. *Listen to your team to implement efficiencies in work processes.*
8. *Provide time for those navigators working alone to share their patient experiences with bereavement; connect those navigators working in isolation with oncology nursing teams, pastoral care, and social work.*
9. *Refer employees at risk to employee assistance programs, behavioral health resources, or wellness programs.*

16.6   Prevention Strategies

16.6.1 Mentorship

Significant research has shown that mentorship not only improves job satisfaction but also improves productivity, facilitates personal growth, and can rekindle our passion while lessening the risk of compassion fatigue [10]. One could assume that having a mentor adds an additional layer of checks and balances that could help staff cope with the pressures and emotions that might lead to compassion fatigue. Implementing a mentorship program, with voluntary participation, might be one strategy to address compassion fatigue prevention.

16.6.2 Perform a Self-Assessment

It is often very difficult for caregivers who are experiencing compassion fatigue to admit it to themselves or others. After all, caregivers are supposed to care. They are naturally caring empathetic people, which is why they entered the healthcare profession, so it often doesn't make sense initially that they are experiencing compassion fatigue. They may simply tell themselves they are angry about various work issues, or they may lack energy or enthusiasm about work. They may feel more comfortable working in isolation, rather than relating at a normal level with colleagues.

All of these tendencies can be associated with compassion fatigue. Because it is so difficult to self-identify compassion fatigue, a useful strategy for management to deploy in support of personnel is to offer a mandatory self-assessment tool that can be completed annually by staff.

By offering the tool and making it mandatory, it becomes possible for managers to review baseline scores and address any negative trends that are observed.

Having staff members complete scheduled self-assessments might provide data that can be used to request resources to implement interventions to stave off compassion fatigue.

Compassion Fatigue Self-Assessment Tools
www.avenidas.org/assets/pdf/Fatigue.pdf
www.valueoptions.com/providers/Education_Center/Training_Workshops/
   Handouts/032106/032106_Compassion_Fatigue_Test_from_ACE.pdf

16.7   Conclusion

The medical industry is wrestling with numerous issues that impact patient care—medical errors, inefficient information systems, increasing regulatory burdens, reimbursement challenges, nursing and physician shortages, etc. Compassion fatigue is an issue that can be added to this important list of topics. Compassion fatigue concretely impacts medical personnel and, therefore, patient care. People who enter nursing, especially oncology nursing, may or may not understand their risk for developing compassion fatigue. It is the obligation of every healthcare organization and every manager to observe and intervene if and when signs of compassion fatigue begin to arise. Without early intervention, the individual's ability to recover could be significantly eroded, which might place patients at risk and push the individual out of the nursing profession. Both of these outcomes are harmful to healthcare. Fortunately, effective tools and strategies exist to prevent and treat compassion fatigue among oncology nursing staff.

Beating compassion fatigue once is no guarantee that an individual will consistently win this battle. Given that many of the pressures in health care that act as catalysts for compassion fatigue will not be going away, there is an ongoing need for empirical resource into the subject. The research should evaluate the effectiveness, feasibility, and nurses' experiences of interventions. Because of the global increase in the number of patients being diagnosed and living with cancer, oncology nurses must be equipped to be able to recognize and manage compassion fatigue. Recent research has shown that no single intervention is completely effective and an integrated approach is likely best [11]. The key to defeating compassion fatigue is preventing it before it starts and using the strategies outlined herein. Equally important would be efforts to diminish the stress or at least the effects of stress that can lead to job dissatisfaction and eventually to burnout. Identifying the stressors and feelings of stress is a first step in reducing the incidences of burnout among healthcare workers. With a growing oncology patient population, healthcare leaders must accept the challenge of addressing compassion fatigue among oncology nurses, even as it competes for attention with so many other important issues in health care.

16.8   Case Study

16.8.1 Case Study

Janet is an experienced nurse, having worked for nearly 15 years in oncology settings, so she assumed her new job as an oncology nurse navigator would match her skill set. The role sounded well defined when she first accepted the position, but each week she found new responsibilities and expectations being added, sometimes without her input or checking to see if the tasks were appropriate for the nurse navigator. The oncology director and the COO, both new to their own roles, had established aggressive plans for marketing and growing the oncology program at the hospital.

Soon Janet found it difficult to keep up with her patient volume. She started calling patients from her home in the evening after work. Janet also couldn't stop thinking about the patients she was caring for, wondering: "How are they doing?" "Will she be there when I call?" "Is she still alive?" Janet carried these concerns and emotions regarding her patients into her personal time away from work. Eventually, she began to outwardly display frustration at work, specifically complaining about the new leaders, who had lofty program goals, but little understanding of how navigation fit into the big picture.

One day, Janet responded to a suggestion about a new job task by lashing out verbally to a peer. As a result, her supervisor set up a coaching meeting with Janet to review her communication shortcomings. Feeling guilty about her lapse in professional behavior, Janet withdrew from her colleagues for a period and took a long weekend away. During the next month, Janet continued to feel burdened by what happened at work. Meanwhile, the opening of the new lung cancer center increased Janet's patient load further. The new responsibilities stretched Janet physically and mentally, and left her little time to relax and recharge. Each day, Janet felt less and less excited about going to work or helping patients.

As a result of her work stress, Janet sought comfort in food, eating late at night. The natural consequence of the food regimen was a 30-pound weight gain over the proceeding months. The weight gain brought new emotional stress for Janet, creating embarrassment that caused her to retreat from her family and friends. The weight gain also made sleep difficult, which impacted Janet's decision-making ability and caused irritability. Her expanded workdays frustrated her children and husband, who urged her to quit.

After a particularly frustrating day where she had a tearful outburst about a work issue, Janet's supervisor recommended she seek help through the hospital's employee assistance program. After an initial counseling session, it was quickly determined that Janet exhibited the classic signs of compassion fatigue.

With a clearer picture of her problem, Janet revisited with her supervisor all of the additional tasks Janet felt had been dumped on her. They worked to create a clearer job description and educated others on the team about Janet's actual roles and responsibilities as a navigator: barrier assessment, providing disease site pathway support, coordination of care activities, serving as an advocate and educator for the patient and caregiver, accompanying patients on the emotional journey of cancer from diagnosis through survivorship, palliative care and bereavement, and identifying hospital and community resources to support patients. Janet and her manager also identified operational barriers that needed to be removed to fix frustrating inefficiencies in the patient care flow.

A nursing colleague also informed Janet of an informal coffee that several nurses attended weekly in a location near the hospital. The coffee gathering served as a place where nurses could speak their mind without judgment or retribution. One of the other attendees who also struggled with obesity agreed to join Janet in a weight loss program and hold each other accountable. The friendships that Janet established in the group helped her to recover a sense of normalcy and empathy, especially as she listened to others share about their own daily struggles with work and family issues.

Appendix: Best Practice Model

Sarah Cannon Cancer Institute
Medical City Healthcare

The Sarah Cannon Cancer Institute Medical City Healthcare navigation team maintains its perspective on compassion fatigue by implementation of surveys and employee self-assessments, and regularly focuses on the subject during team meetings. The team participates in self-care modules and holds an annual team retreat where the topic is discussed.

Surveys

The team is asked to participate in the Professional Quality of Life (ProQOL) Scale (Exhibit 16.2) survey twice a year (June/December). The scale measures levels of compassion satisfaction, burnout, and secondary traumatic stress. The results are combined with data gleaned from the self-care modules and an annual navigator retreat survey, which identifies the navigation team's biggest stressors, their preferred frequency of participation in self-care modules, and how they would prefer those events be structured. The larger goal with these surveys is to ensure that a high level of quality of life is maintained within the team and to ensure that the management team is meeting the needs of the navigation team members, where possible.

The ProQOL Scale survey was first initiated for the Medical City Healthcare navigation team in the spring of 2016. The team has exhibited a high level for compassion satisfaction and low levels of burnout and secondary trauma. The results would indicate the typical team member represents a person who receives positive reinforcement from their work. The typical team member carries no significant concerns about being "bogged down" or the inability to be efficacious in their work—either as an individual or within their organization. The navigator does not suffer any noteworthy fears resulting from their work. He or she may benefit from engagement, opportunities for continuing education, and other opportunities to grow in their career. He or she is likely a good influence on colleagues and the organization. The individual is probably liked by the patients who seek out assistance.

The following information depicts the manager's report for the Sarah Cannon oncology navigation team ProQOL survey from the summer of 2017.

ProQOL Scale Results: Summer 2017

Compassion Satisfaction—Compassion satisfaction is characterized by feeling satisfied by one's job and from helping. It is characterized by people feeling invigorated by work they like to do. They feel they can keep up with new technology and protocols. They experience happy thoughts, feel successful, are happy with the work they do, want to continue to do it, and believe they can make a difference.

- *Raw score summer 2017*: 43
- *Level of compassion satisfaction*: HIGH
- *Raw score fall 2016*: 45
- *Level of compassion satisfaction*: HIGH
- *Raw score spring 2016*: 43
- *Level of compassion satisfaction*: HIGH

Burnout—Burnout is part of compassion fatigue that is characterized by feelings of unhappiness, disconnectedness, and insensitivity to the work environment. Symptoms can include exhaustion, feeling overwhelmed or bogged down, and being "out-of-touch" with the person he or she wants to be, while having no sustaining beliefs.

- *Raw score summer 2017*: 18
- *Level of burnout*: LOW
- *Raw score fall 2016*: 20

- *Level of burnout*: LOW
- *Raw score spring 2016*: 19
- *Level of burnout*: LOW

Professional Quality of Life Scale (ProQOL)

Compassion Satisfaction and Compassion Fatigue
(ProQOL) Version 5 (2009)

When you *[help]* people you have direct contact with their lives. As you may have found, your compassion for those you *[help]* can affect you in positive and negative ways. Below are some questions about your experiences, both positive and negative, as a *[helper]*. Consider each of the following questions about you and your current work situation. Select the number that honestly reflects how frequently you experienced these things in the *last 30 days*.

1=Never	2=Rarely	3=Sometimes	4=Often	5=Very Often

_____ 1.   I am happy.
_____ 2.   I am preoccupied with more than one person I *[help]*.
_____ 3.   I get satisfaction from being able to *[help]* people.
_____ 4.   I feel connected to others.
_____ 5.   I jump or am startled by unexpected sounds.
_____ 6.   I feel invigorated after working with those I *[help]*.
_____ 7.   I find it difficult to separate my personal life from my life as a *[helper]*.
_____ 8.   I am not as productive at work because I am losing sleep over traumatic experiences of a person I *[help]*.
_____ 9.   I think that I might have been affected by the traumatic stress of those I *[help]*.
_____ 10. I feel trapped by my job as a *[helper]*.
_____ 11. Because of my *[helping]*, I have felt "on edge" about various things.
_____ 12. I like my work as a *[helper]*.
_____ 13. I feel depressed because of the traumatic experiences of the people I *[help]*.
_____ 14. I feel as though I am experiencing the trauma of someone I have *[helped]*.
_____ 15. I have beliefs that sustain me.
_____ 16. I am pleased with how I am able to keep up with *[helping]* techniques and protocols.
_____ 17. I am the person I always wanted to be.
_____ 18. My work makes me feel satisfied.
_____ 19. I feel worn out because of my work as a *[helper]*.
_____ 20. I have happy thoughts and feelings about those I *[help]* and how I could help them.
_____ 21. I feel overwhelmed because my case [work] load seems endless.
_____ 22. I believe I can make a difference through my work.
_____ 23. I avoid certain activities or situations because they remind me of frightening experiences of the people I *[help]*.
_____ 24. I am proud of what I can do to *[help]*.
_____ 25. As a result of my *[helping]*, I have intrusive, frightening thoughts.
_____ 26. I feel "bogged down" by the system.
_____ 27. I have thoughts that I am a "success" as a *[helper]*.
_____ 28. I can't recall important parts of my work with trauma victims.
_____ 29. I am a very caring person.
_____ 30. I am happy that I chose to do this work.

Exhibit 16.2   The compassion fatigue process

Secondary Traumatic Stress—Secondary traumatic stress is an element of compassion fatigue that is characterized by being preoccupied with thoughts of people one has helped. Caregivers report feeling trapped, on edge, exhausted, overwhelmed, and infected by others' trauma. Characteristics include an inability to sleep, sometimes forgetting important things, and an inability to separate one's private life and his or her life as a helper and experiencing the trauma of someone you have helped, even to the extent of avoiding activities that are reminders of the trauma. It is important to note that developing problems as a result of secondary traumatic stress is rare, but it does happen.

- *Raw score summer 2017*: 18
- *Level of secondary traumatic stress*: LOW
- *Raw score fall 2016*: 18
- *Level of secondary traumatic stress*: LOW
- *Raw score spring 2016*: 18
- *Level of secondary traumatic stress*: LOW

Meetings and Retreats

Giving team members regularly scheduled opportunities to discuss the subject of compassion fatigue and burnout is also considered crucial to creating a healthy workplace environment. The 19-member Sarah Cannon Cancer Institute Medical City Healthcare navigation team, which is responsible for oncology patients in 10 hospitals, engages in monthly meetings that offer opportunities to discuss compassion fatigue and stressors, as well as twice-yearly retreats that include compassion fatigue as part of the agenda.

- **Self-Care Modules**—Monthly, hour-long sessions that focus on self-care, reflection, and team bonding. Opportunities have included an open discussion/support group, a yoga instructor teaching chair yoga, journaling instruction, and community partners who have shared resources regarding how their services can support the navigation team.
- **Navigator Retreats**—Twice yearly, in the summer and winter, the team participates in retreats that focus on team bonding. Activities have included a team lunch with a presentation about self-care by a psychologist, an afternoon of bowling and games, holiday parties, and professional education offerings.

Internal surveys of these navigation team members following these gatherings revealed a variety of perspectives related to stressors and compassion fatigue strategies. The surveys help the team supervisor specifically understand the challenges team members face and how they wish to see those challenges addressed, if possible.

Self-Care Module and Navigator Retreat Survey Results: Summer 2017

Navigator Stressors/Challenges

- *The largest stressors/challenges in working with patients*:
    - Not having enough information to do my job or spending a lot of time finding it.
    - Brevity of life. Although this is an area that I do extremely well with, it is just hard. One day last week I was calling patients, and I discovered that eight had died. That doesn't happen every week. It is just hard when it does.
    - Getting the referral early enough in the patient's diagnosis to help them at maximum capacity.
    - Repetitive documentation and spreadsheet work, even though it is getting a little better.
    - Cooperation from doctors and staff.
    - Volume of load is heavy at intervals.
    - Due to the number of patients in the *documentation system*, I can't keep up with all my patients in a timely manner.
    - Not feeling like I am able to do enough for my patients, limited resources, limited transportation, etc.
    - The biggest is resources; sometimes you are not able to assist where they really need it; a lot of services are tightening their services.
    - Nothing.
- *The largest daily stressor/challenge*:
    - Time.
    - Completing survivorship care plans. It takes approximately 1 hour 15 minutes to complete just one.
    - Data.
    - Having many leaders to report to within the hospital setting and leadership not being aware of my role as a navigator.
    - Due to the number of patients I navigate, I can't keep up with all my patients in a timely manner.
    - Not enough time in the day to get everything I want done.
    - Is trying to stay in contact regularly with my patients. Very high volume.
    - Balancing work and home life.

Self-Care Modules

- *Ideal frequency*:
    - Monthly, 20%
    - Every other month, 20%
    - Quarterly, 50%
    - Yearly, 10%
- *Ideal topics*:
    - Delivering a cancer diagnosis, 10%
    - Communication techniques, 20%
    - Compassion fatigue/burnout, 20%

- – Workplace stress, 10%
- – Balancing work/home life, 30%
- – Other, 10%
  All of the above
- *Ideal format of time*:
  - – Speakers, 90%
  - – Support group/group sharing, 40%
  - – Handouts, 0%
  - – Reflection/growth activities, 50%
  - – Quiet/reflection time, 10%
  - – Guided meditation, 20%
  - – Other, 10%
    Sometimes I just need more time for me.

Navigator Retreats

- *Ideal frequency*:
  - – Yearly, 30%
  - – Every 6 months, 60%
  - – Every quarter, 10%
- *Ideal format of time*:
  - – Fun icebreaker activities to get to know each other, 30%
  - – Open activities (bowling, pool, etc.), 60%
  - – No activities (open time to sit and talk), 20%
  - – Social hour, 30%
  - – Formal, guided team building, 10%
  - – Other, 10%
    Just some extra time to rest and relax
- *Other ideas for a team retreat*:
  - – Team recreational activities such as golf, painting

Summary

The Self-Care and Navigator Retreat Survey provides further insight into the barriers facing the navigation team. Most of the issues are not easily amended (which is the reason for annual distribution vs twice a year), such as the amount of data entry required, lack of time for tasks, and the inherent nature of physicians/staff (willingness to collaborate, communicate, etc.). The navigators did identify the need for access to new community resources, which the team is are attempting to meet with new online applications. The team seemed comfortable with the frequency of both the self-care modules and the navigator retreats, and offered easy-to-implement suggestions for future team health events.

References

1. Figley CR. Renewing spirits: lessons from thirty years of trauma work, invited keynote address to the William Wendt Center for Loss and Health Conference on Illness, Grief & Trauma, Washington, DC, October 6, 2001.
2. Beaton RD, Murphy SA. Working with people in crisis: research implications. In: Figley CR, editor. Compassion fatigue: Coping with secondary traumatic stress disorder in those who treat the traumatized. New York: Brunner/Mazel; 1995. p. 51–81.
3. Kleiner S, Wallace JE. Oncologist burnout and compassion fatigue: investigating time pressure at work as a predictor and the mediating role of work-family conflict. BMC Health Services Research. Published online, September 11, 2017.
4. The American Institute of Stress. Online resource. www.stress.org/military/for-practitionersleaders/compassion-fatigue.
5. Potter P, Deshields T, Divanbeigi J, Berger J, Cipriano D, Norris L, Olsen S. Compassion fatigue and burnout: prevalence among oncology nurses. Clin J Oncol Nurs. 2010;14(5):E56–62.
6. Aycock N, Boyle D. Interventions to manage compassion fatigue in oncology nursing. Clin J Oncol Nurs. 2009;13:183.
7. Collins J. Normalizing feelings of grief & loss in oncology nurses. Oncol Issues. 2017;July–August:26–31.
8. Shockney LD. Preventing burnout and compassion fatigue among providers caring for patients with metastatic cancer. In: Fulfilling hope: supporting the needs of patients with advanced cancers. Nova Science Pub; 2014. p. 143–51.
9. Allen KM, Blascovich J, Tomaka J, Kelsey RM. Presence of human friends and pet dogs as moderators of autonomic responses to stress in women. J Pers Soc Psychol. 1991;61(4):582–9.
10. Cooke KJ, Patt DA, Prabhu RS. The road of mentorship. American Society of Clinical Oncology Meeting Presentation. 2017.
11. Wentzel D. Integrative review of facility interventions to manage compassion fatigue. Oncol Nurs Forum Online Article; 2017 May.

Lillie D. Shockney

17.1 Determining One's Chosen Career Path

It also can be difficult to determine what career path someone wishes to take until they have explored and understood a bit more about themselves. It is not unusual that someone believes they want to become a manager and then, having achieved that promotion, learns that they actually don't like supervising people and prefer more patient contact, which now they miss. A nurse navigator may actually have not chosen to even become a nurse navigator, but due to structural changes within their organization, their position was converted into an ONN without clear guidance or even a job description. Therefore the first step for a navigator is to take a closer look at the work they currently are doing and identify what aspects they enjoy the most versus like the least. Are the ones that are enjoyed the least due to the task itself or due to the people that one needs to work with in order to get the task done? This requires stepping back and assessing the job piece by piece. For example, a nurse navigator may be spending time standing at a fax machine sending documents to insurance companies when this could likely be performed by a clerical person. The task is unpleasant because it is a clerical task that lacks any mental challenges that require nursing skills and training. On the other hand, a navigator may dislike providing patient education to cancer patients about their upcoming surgeries, because she finds it too repetitive or doesn't feel so many questions should be coming up during the educational sessions. This is an issue that focuses more on not enjoying patient contact as it relates to patient education, and could mean that the navigator isn't in the best role within their multidisciplinary team. She enjoys more case preparation for tumor board discussion. In the first scenario with the fax machine, the

L. D. Shockney, RN, BS, MAS, ONN-CG
Johns Hopkins University School of Medicine, Baltimore, MD, USA
e-mail: shockli@jhmi.edu

© Springer International Publishing AG, part of Springer Nature 2018
L. D. Shockney (ed.), *Team-Based Oncology Care: The Pivotal Role of Oncology Navigation*, https://doi.org/10.1007/978-3-319-69038-4_17

ONN doesn't feel productive standing idly faxing papers, and would prefer to spend more time directly with her patients. In the second scenario, the ONN is not a real "people person" and prefers to apply her nursing knowledge by creating the case presentations for the multidisciplinary tumor board that meets weekly to discuss new cases and determine the optimal treatment plans for each patient presented.

Many ONNs prior to becoming navigators were medical oncology nurses working in infusion centers. During that time, nurses saw patients cyclically when due for their next IV treatment. Due to patient volume, it would be unusual today for a medical oncology nurse to have time to sit and get to know her patients. With an ONN, however, the patient is usually navigated beginning at the point of diagnosis (or even sooner) across their continuum of care into survivorship or end of life. This results in ONNs getting to know their patients very well, along with the patient's family members and friends. This is a relationship that is formed, and with it, ONNs are more personally involved in the lives of the patients they are navigating and supporting. They know their finances, their concerns, and their clinical situation, including if they are going to live or die. It's a much more intimate role than before, and for some it is the driving force why someone wants to become and remain a navigator. For others, it is too personal, and an ONN may choose to return to the infusion center or another nursing specialty within the cancer center so that they are happier with their professional choices. Bottom line, navigation isn't for everyone. Clearly defining and writing down what elements of the navigation roles and responsibilities are enjoyed the most and enjoyed the least provides a framework for determining what may be the next and most logical career step. Even an ONN in their current navigation position needs to have a comprehensive skill set.

17.2   The Need for a Comprehensive Skill Set

Without good communication skills, writing skills, problem-solving skills, and the ability to do critical thinking, it may be difficult for someone to climb a career ladder in the direction of one's choosing. Below is a list of skills that are valuable to have, whether planning to remain in the current navigation role or pursue a career change up the ladder, or even for prepare to make a lateral move:

17.2.1 Critical Thinking

Critical thinking is a deliberative thought process. During this process, an individual uses a set of critical thinking skills to consider a specific issue. At the end of these thought processes, the individual makes a judgment about what to believe or a decision about what to do.

1. There are a number of critical thinking skills. A core set includes the following [1]:
   Suspending judgment to check the validity of a proposition or action

Taking into consideration multiple perspectives
Examining implications and consequences of a belief or action
Using reason and evidence to resolve disagreements
Reevaluating a point of view in light of new information
2. There is a specific method called the "infusion method" [1] that can explicitly teach critical thinking skills.
3. Some questions used to stimulate critical thinking within the infusion method are:
What is your point of view?
What are your reasons for supporting this point of view?
Why do you think that?
Are there different perspectives on the issue?

17.2.2 Problem-Solving

Problem-solving is a process—an ongoing activity in which someone takes what they know to figure out and learn what they currently don't know. It involves overcoming obstacles by generating hypotheses, testing those predictions, and arriving at satisfactory solutions. It actually could be considered a basic element of the navigation process. Barriers to care require problem-solving. There is a strategy to problem-solving, however, that may go beyond providing a patient's resources to address their barriers to care [2].

1. Problem-solving involves three basic functions:
Seeking information
Creating new knowledge
Making decisions based on this new and prior information
Navigators need to be able to take personal action to solve problems, resolve conflicts, and discuss alternatives/options. It provides the ability to have new opportunities to use their newly acquired knowledge in meaningful, real-life activities, and assists them in working at higher levels of thinking.

It's vitally important to assess one's own problem-solving skills and solutions. The process of self-assessment is not simple. It involves risk-taking, self-assurance, and a certain level of independence. The following questions should be asked of oneself:

"How do you feel about your progress so far?"
"Are you satisfied with the results you obtained?"
"Why do you believe this is an appropriate response to the problem?"

There are always learning opportunities when performing problem-solving. It can be difficult to be objective, too, especially if the issue involves patient care needs. Others may not be able to hear valid solutions however from a navigator if they are said with too much passion or emotion. It is important to keep that in check. Recording the process that was taken and how the solution was derived, as well as later documenting if the solution worked, is all part of developing and applying effective problem-solving skills.

17.3 Team Building

By definition, a team is a group of people who are dependent upon one another to accomplish specific goals, who share in the outcomes for those goals, who are viewed as one entity by others, and who manage relationship building across organizational boundaries. While teams are made up of groups of people, not all groups of people are teams. A group of engineers, for example, working in the same unit are not considered a team, because their work is not dependent upon one another nor do they share in each other's outcomes [3].

17.3.1 Effective Teams Follow a Specific Method for Building Teams [3]

1. Purpose—In order for teams to be successful, the team members have to know why the team was created in the first place. Organizations build teams to help solve specific problems, such as reducing costs, improving productivity, and improving quality. A multidisciplinary oncology team is designed to diagnose and treat cancer patients in a cost-effective way while delivering the highest quality of care, with the goal to save lives and preserve the patients' life goals as well as preserve their quality of life during and after cancer treatment. A navigation team may have been created to navigate all newly diagnosed cancer patients across the continuum of care, identifying and eliminating barriers to care, empowering patients so they can participate in the decision-making about their treatments, and serving as patient advocates while providing cross coverage for one another so no patient goes without navigation.
2. Participation—Team members are more effective when they feel they have something of specific value to contribute rather than when they feel required to participate. Every team must have their own team spirit. This means that team members' contributions need to be acknowledged and valued. It is common today that members of a multidisciplinary oncology team are not familiar nor understand the roles and responsibilities of a navigator who has been added to the team without any explanation of their role. This can make it difficult to effectively participate, because team members either don't feel a need for adding new members, team members feel insulted that a new member was added, perhaps believing someone finds them to be failing at their role, or the navigator herself does a poor job of understanding where she fits into the overarching goals of the team. This is a critical step to team buy-in, and when it doesn't happen, months or even years can be spent without the team working cohesively with the addition of a navigation professional. Worst-case scenario, the navigator remains alienated from the group and finds herself working in a vacuum. This can result in

duplication of effort, rework, and loss of efficiency and effectiveness not to mention low morale. The individual who is charged with recruitment for a navigator and who adds the navigator to the team needs to be held accountable for getting buy-in, having all team members understand where the navigator's role fits within the team and that the purpose goes well beyond that of "trying to meet any Commission on Cancer navigation standard."

3. Communication—In an age where people are connected 24/7 through cell phones, the Internet, and social media, it should be relatively easy to communicate with one another. In order to be successful, team members need to agree on how often they will communicate and the methods they will use to communicate with one another. Team members should be able to challenge others' ideas while being respectful at the same time. The navigator needs to know what strategies her team practices to ensure they are communicating at all times. This may be via the electronic patient record, tumor board meetings, inpatient rounds every morning, texting, sign-offs at end of shifts, and other methods. Technology is amazing for communication; however it also results in losing face-to-face contact. This needs to be kept in mind.

4. Strengths—Individual team members should be selected based upon their strengths and skill set. Therefore the navigator needs to know her strengths, confirm this with the team members and whomever added her to the team that these are her strengths, and how these strengths complement those of other members.

5. Group dynamics—Small teams, those between two and nine members, have advantages of being able to interact easily, communicate or share information, stay motivated, and see the importance of their individual contribution to the overall team. Large teams, those consisting of ten or more members, have advantages as well. They often have the experience, skills, knowledge, and resources to accomplish goals more quickly. Large groups are able to split up the work more easily, whereas this task is difficult to manage in smaller groups due to a lack of (or limited) resources. A disadvantage of large groups is their inability to communicate or coordinate functions as they tend to get bogged down in processes [3].

6. Agreement—Team members will stick to rules they create. How much time will each member be allowed to discuss a point on the agenda? Who will be the scribe for the team (or how will this activity be rotated among team members)? What is the role of the scribe? By establishing rules upfront, it will be easier to point out when someone ignores the rules. With a multidisciplinary oncology team, there is a built-in hierarchy usually with a physician (surgeon or medical oncologist) at the helm. This can mean that not all of the rules appear to apply to all members in the same way. This means once again understanding the group dynamics and the onco-politics of the team members.

7. Team effectiveness—A team's effectiveness is measured by performance, outcomes, and attitudes. A team that meets its goals is based on clinical and financial outcomes. This requires effective ways to measure performance. Quality metrics for navigators is one of the best ways to measure performance and contribution to the team's overarching goals. A total of 35 metrics have been

developed by the Evidence into Practice Subcommittee and are available for use (see Chapter 11 for more information).

8. Oftentimes, management will create teams that work well. Occasionally, no matter how hard they try, teams are ineffective or truly a nightmare. In those cases, management needs to identify the source of the problem quickly. If the wrong person is on the team, they need to be replaced immediately. This, however, is very difficult to do within a healthcare system. A physician may be identified as not being a team player; however, he has the largest volume of cancer patients, which fulfills the financial outcomes required of the team. This is also part of the onco-politics of the team. This, too, is an example of the strength of that one team member toward fulfilling the overall goals of the team, understanding where everyone fits and what needs to be understood by everyone. This is definitely not simple.

17.4 Professional Development

On an annual basis, it is important to step back and look at what has been accomplished in the past year; was it in keeping with professional development goals created last year and deciding what new professional development goals are desired to fulfill this coming year? To do this, a navigator needs to answer some questions for herself. If someone doesn't know where they are along their trajectory of learning and growing, then it will be difficult to establish meaningful, measurable goals going forward. This list of questions is recorded below [4]:

1. Identify your strengths. What are a few of your core strengths?
2. Identify areas for development.
   Where does feedback over the past year's performance suggest you have some opportunities for improvement and growth?
   What opportunities do you see in your area/department, or elsewhere, that you'd like to contribute to in new ways?
3. Prioritize your strengths and skill sets that need further development.
   Which strengths are most important in contributing to your continued success and enjoyment in your role?
   Which areas of development to improve your skill set will be most critical in your current and/or future role?
   How motivated are you to develop your skill set in these areas?
4. Create a professional development goal. Effective development goals are those that are important to you and those to which you can commit to accomplishing. It also must be explicitly measurable.
5. What type of learning opportunities or activities would you like to participate in as part of your development plan, beyond conferences and classrooms?

Another option for determining what appropriate and useful professional goals to develop can be determined by answering instead this set of questions. Both sets of questions have proved to be useful in developing these goals and creating a strategy to achieve them. These questions are [5]:

1. What types of tasks or activities motivate you to do your best work?
2. What skills, talent, or knowledge do you possess that could be used more fully?
3. What are two ways you have contributed to your area/department?
4. What is happening in your area/department that could provide you with a developmental opportunity?
5. What types of tasks or activities would you like to do in the next 6 months?

17.5 Creating SMART Goals [6]

SMART goals provide a concrete way to measure one's success. When a goal is too loosely worded, it can make it difficult to measure. A SMART goal is defined as one that is specific, measurable, achievable, results-focused, and time bound. Below is the formula to use for creating SMART goals:

SMART goals are:

Specific—What exactly would you like to accomplish? What is your desired outcome?

Measurable—How will you measure progress? How will you know when you have successfully reached your goal?

Achievable—Do you have the ability and motivation to successfully accomplish this goal? Is the goal achievable given needed resources and support?

Relevant—Does the goal support your work and reflect your priorities as well as those of your department/group? Why is this important to you at this time?

Timely—What is the time frame for achieving the goal? Is the time frame realistic?

17.6 Mentorship Skills: Finding a Mentor or Serving as a Mentor

Mentoring has been regarded for decades, and perhaps centuries, as one of the key components of research training and faculty development. For most individuals just starting to build their navigation careers, they need to have a mentor rather than serve as a mentor. There is a mentorship section on the AONN+ website to help AONN+ members find a mentor within the organization or even serve as a mentor if they meet the criteria for fulfilling such an important educational and supportive role.

Good navigation mentors are experienced, knowledgeable navigation professionals who are experts in their own fields, whether it be patient navigation, nurse navigation, or administratively and managerially. By being such, it enables mentors to provide guidance in navigating organizational structures, serve as advocates for their mentee at various levels, and provide mentees with opportunities to network crucial to their professional socialization. Some individuals perceive themselves to be good mentors when in fact they are not. Being experienced in the field of interest isn't sufficient knowledge and training to necessarily become a mentor.

17.6.1 Key Characteristics of an Effective Mentor

An effective mentor is motivated, committed, genuinely interested, and passionate about developing their mentee. Mentors are compassionate and sensitive of cultural differences, just as they are when navigating a cancer patient. By being available and responsive to the evolving needs of their mentees, demonstrating nonjudgmental listening and a belief in the mentee's abilities, a mentor brings out the best in the mentee and allows them to reach their desired potential. By creating a sense of safety, the mentor becomes a coach, a confidant, a sounding board, and an educator, challenging the mentee to achieve full potential. A good mentor is willing to be challenged. A good mentor is secure in their position, demonstrates self-awareness, is mature, and is self-confident; by manifesting these characteristics, the mentor is then able to celebrate the mentee's success rather than feeling threatened, vying with the mentee for credit, or potentially pushing forth a personal agenda [7, 8].

17.7 Assessing One's Own Motivations and Leadership Styles

We all possess strengths and weaknesses. Although we may assume we know what they are, there is value in learning more about ourselves and how we think. There is an online evaluation tool that can aid in learning these strengths and weaknesses. Go to www.viacharacter.org, offered free by the VIA Institute on Character. Character strengths are present in every aspect of our lives. Strengths are where our energy is. We need for everyone, mentor and mentee, to focus on their most significant strengths—which focus on a positive presence—practice mindfulness, and be empathetic, warm, calm, zestful, fun, and courageous, as these all facilitate growth. Active mindfulness focuses a great deal on listening. (Note: the letters in the word "listen" spell "silent" when rearranged. Most people don't listen with the intent to understand; they listen with the intent to reply.) Mentoring is about fostering the mentee's autonomy competence.

17.8 Determining If Someone Is Ready to Become a Mentor

Mentoring is not an easy task and requires investment of time and sacrifice. Mentors not only need training to equip themselves as well as develop their own mentoring skills but also benefit from receiving mentoring themselves. Sam Davies has provided a useful acronym that demonstrates the key components of mentoring. The MENTOR acronym: manage needs, effective communicator and feedback provider, nonjudgmental and confronting and challenging when appropriate, trustworthy and empathetic, offer strategies to promote self-reflection and development, and role modeling and respect [9–11].

17.8.1 Roles of the Mentor [12]

A mentor wears many hats and performs many roles in her mentorship responsibilities to the mentee. Some roles of a mentor are described as follows.

1. Coach

    A mentor ensures optimal performance of a mentee by inspiring the attainment of one's best potential, affirming the strengths and talents of the mentee, and empowering the mentee with skills to attain greater achievement in personal and professional growth. During challenging situations, a mentor encourages perseverance and determination, supports the mentee to overcome obstacles encountered, and focuses mentees on the goal ahead. The mentor does not take over the project or initiative on behalf of the mentee, however. The mentor needs to leverage their own strengths and that of the mentee, as well.

2. Educator

    The mentor creates a calm, blame-free environment for the mentee to develop knowledge and skills. Much of the training that mentors provide take the form of role modeling where mentors showcase professional and moral values and behavior in clinical and academic practice.

3. Sponsor and advocate

    The mentor assists mentees in career planning, providing networking opportunities and acting as advocates for mentees to advance their careers and research opportunities or in the face of challenges that may arise. Maximizing strengths can lead to greater productivity and happiness. We need three positive emotions to offset one negative emotion. Positive emotions are 50% genetic, 10% external, and 40% actions and thoughts.

4. Confidant and advisor

    A positive affirming relationship allows mentors to facilitate reflective practice and helps the mentee overcome blind spots while providing constructive feedback and facilitating mentee-led problem-solving.

17.9 Characteristics of a Good Mentee [13, 14]

17.9.1 Goal Setting

The mentoring relationship should be centered on a mentee's goals and motivated by the initiatives of the mentee. A mentee should be able to evaluate their needs, state their mentoring goals, and be responsible for working toward these goals with their mentor's guidance.

17.10 Characteristics of a Mentee

A teachable, motivated, engaging spirit is crucial to being an effective mentee, as is being flexible, humble, and appreciative. Mentees should be open, honest, and reflective so as to facilitate open communication.

17.11 Advice to Mentees

A suitable mentor can be challenging to find; selecting the right mentor is crucial. It is suggested that mentees identify their own educational and developmental needs and seek out mentors based on these. A single mentee may consider having multiple mentors at different points of one's career due to diverse needs and as one's professional and personal journey evolves. There must be one mentor at a time however. External controlled motivation is weak and will not result in you achieving your goals. Internal autonomous motivation is strong—Why do you want to do this goal? How will you make it happen? Visualize achieving it. Feel emotional control of your experience.

17.12 Benefits to Mentee

The ways in which mentoring contributes to career progression and personal growth is described below:

1. Research and academia [15, 16]

   Mentees who receive mentoring in research and academia have been shown to have increased research output and increased success in obtaining grants, promotions, higher levels of job satisfaction, and happiness.

2. Ensuring sustainability [17, 18]

   Mentoring ensures sustainability and has been shown to improve job satisfaction and reduce staff turnover. Mentors provide valuable guidance in time management and prioritization of work, thus allowing mentees to achieve better work–life balance. This in turn can decrease compassion fatigue and burnout. Mentees also gain increased sense of self-efficacy and self-confidence through a mentor's support and guidance. The support that a mentor provides enables the mentee to have increased psychological and behavioral competence.

3. Learn to think outside the box

A good mentor inspires the mentee to want to learn more and inspires a mentee to think outside the box and will serve as a catalyst for developing intellectual curiosity. They also instill in the mentee a sense of history and belonging to the profession, helping the mentee to develop a strong professional identity.

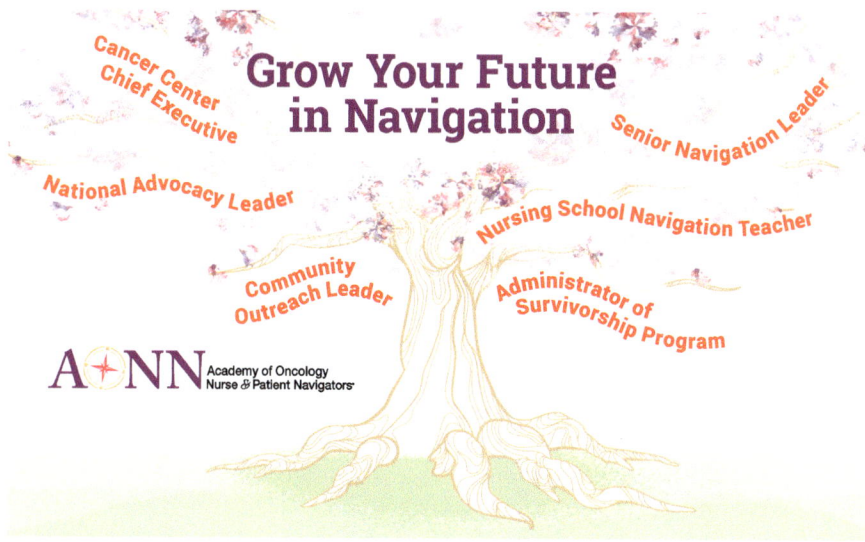

Fig. 17.1

17.13   The Need for Different Mentorship Over One's Career Pathway

More than likely AONN+ has what is needed for navigation mentors. Some individuals who are currently navigators may have aspirations to become navigation managers and cancer center administrators or take some other career path that leads them somewhat away from the day-to-day operations that nurse navigators perform. This means that when looking at the career path decision tree, decisions need to be made about what type of mentorship support will be needed to climb up the trunk of the tree and out onto a new unfamiliar branch to achieve the career goals that one has established for themselves (Fig. 17.1). Before deciding definitely what branch to take, a navigator should consider spending time with and shadowing a professional who has achieved the next level of their career path. Getting a candid look into that world helps in confirming it is the path of interest or realizing that this type of professional role was not what it was perceived to be. If this career pathway is a branch on the tree that deviates quite a bit from the day-to-day functions performed as a nurse navigator, consider finding a way to do some volunteer hours with someone in this role currently. This is something, too, that can be added to one's CV and enables additional opportunities to oftentimes unfold for the volunteer while learning new skills along the way.

17.14   The Value of Certification for Oncology Nurse Navigators and Patient Navigators

One of the ways that a professional group can demonstrate their competence, knowledge, and skill set is by getting formally certified in the profession they represent. It has taken time to develop and implement a certification program for oncology nurse navigators, as well as for patient (lay) navigators; however, such certification programs were developed and implemented several years ago by AONN+. By becoming certified, the navigator demonstrates their knowledge along with elevating their professional category personally and nationally. Certification is not something that can be achieved by just anyone who chooses to take the test(s). It represents considerable experience in the field along with knowledge of the profession, manifesting the core competencies, and demonstrating their ability to apply domains of navigation effectively. Certification elevates the profession locally, regionally, and nationally. It also helps ensure that those who are in navigation positions, and certified, are performing their navigation functions in a consistent way, based on having the same baseline principles of navigation. Once an oncology nurse navigator has achieved her general oncology nurse navigation certification (ONN-CG), she is eligible to consider getting certified in a subspecialty that focuses on specific organ site navigation certification. AONN+ has been developing organ-specific certification programs and will continue to do so, providing the opportunity for nurse navigators who specialize in specific types of cancer patients to be further recognized for their knowledge and experience. Maintaining certification once it is achieved is important. It requires accruing a specific number of CEUs annually to ensure that the navigator remains up to date on navigation principles, as well as healthcare economics, operations management, performance improvement, coordination of care, genetics and genomics, community outreach, survivorship care, end-of-life care, Commission on Cancer standards, and other key elements that encompass the navigation profession.

17.15   National Organizations for Navigation Professionals

Today, the only national organization solely devoted to the profession of navigation for nurse navigators as well as patient navigators is the Academy of Oncology Nurse & Patient Navigators (AONN+). This organization is continuously striving to have navigators recognized as valuable members of an oncology multidisciplinary team. What the membership's goals and needs are is what the organization works to provide on a continuous basis. It provides mentorship for those navigators needing support as they expand their knowledge and experiences, and educates and keeps its membership abreast of the newest information and quality improvement results and on research outcomes focused on navigation. It also provides education about changes in treatment modalities for different types of cancer, updates on clinical standards as they occur, the ability to measure one's own performance through the use of evidence-based quality metrics, and opportunities to network with others so no one tries to reinvent the wheel.

17.16 Case Study: Climbing the Career Ladder as an ONN

17.16.1 Objectives of This Case Study

Learn the value of having a qualified mentor to educate and train an ONN for professional advancement opportunities

Recognize the importance of developing personal and professional goals and reassess them at least annually

17.16.2 Introduction

There are vast opportunities for those currently in a navigator position to achieve professional advancement. It requires having professional goals, as well as personal goals, to help keep the navigator on point. Professional advancement takes time and should not be rushed, or there is risk of failure. Knowing one's strengths and weaknesses must be identified. Recruiting a good mentor and being a good mentee are part of the ingredients for professional success.

17.16.3 Background Situation

Susan, a 41-year-old oncology nurse, had transferred from her former position as an infusion nurse into an oncology nurse navigator position 3 years ago. She has aspirations to become a manager who would have oversight of the oncology navigation program at her cancer center. Currently, she worked within the breast center, did not know what other cancer patient populations within the cancer center had navigators, and reported to a breast surgeon. She joined AONN+ and also became certified through this professional organization. She networked with other AONN+ members to identify individuals who were in management roles overseeing their broader navigation programs at their cancer centers. She learned a great deal about the various structures and processes used within cancer centers to create consistent methods of performing navigation, measuring navigation processes, tracking of barriers and resolutions, and also the ratio of navigators to patient volumes based on the severity of illness and intensity of services, along with the type of cancers and where navigation begins and ends.

17.16.4 Challenges

Susan took this information and began gathering data at her cancer center by meeting with the tumor registrar to obtain statistics and then met the CAO of the cancer center. She presented her concept of having one navigation program that served all cancer patients from the moment of diagnosis through completion of treatment/end of life. The CAO was intrigued with this idea but knew little about navigation in general and was not interested in or able to consider adding another full-time employee to the cancer center budget.

The breast surgeon she reported to was annoyed that she had been spending time looking at statistics "beyond the breast center patient population."

Her idea died, and she remained in her current navigator role, feeling that there was no opportunity to grow in her chosen nursing field.

17.16.5 Opportunities

There is value in becoming formally certified as an ONN as it elevates the individual within the nursing profession one has chosen to specialize in. More education and experience is needed, however, to consider professionally advancing further into a managerial role. Taking courses on operations management, team building, and course work associated with an MBA education can be very valuable in preparation for a managerial role. Knowing one's strengths and weaknesses must take place with a focus on converting the weaknesses into future strengths.

In Susan's case, she would have benefited from first learning more within her own doors what already exists from a navigation perspective. This can be accomplished by networking within her own cancer center and learning if there are patient navigators and/or nurse navigators supporting patients who have different types of cancers other than breast cancer, offering to bring these individuals together monthly for networking purposes and promoting the concept of a navigation team. She should not imply she is their leader but instead a fellow colleague who can serve as the catalyst for exchanging ideas. This can grow into developing and implementing initiatives that everyone agrees are worthy to take on together. These can be created through identification of similar barriers and what are all of the solutions available internally and within the community to resolve such barriers. From there, navigators can exchange job descriptions, sources of funding of navigation positions, and identify group goals.

During this time, Susan is taking advantage of in-house offered courses on team building, team leadership, effective communication, and also taking college courses on operations management.

If Susan has good communication and team-leading skills, she will be able, over a multi-year period, to be able to document these shared goals, create a document that outlines the navigation program that is currently in place within this cancer center, and be in a better position to present these findings to the central cancer committee. At this point the other navigators should see Susan as their informal leader. Susan could offer volunteer time to continue to work on these shared goals, with the Cancer Committee's blessing. She has now planted the seed within the cancer center leadership that she has worked on this endeavor because of her passion about navigation. She will return to report to the cancer center committee at least semiannually. This can lead into a more formal discussion of the value of having central oversight of a formalized navigation program, with Susan being the ideal person to lead that charge.

17.16.6 Implications for Stakeholders

Susan was placing herself in a situation that was going to cause her disappointment. She needed to gather more information, including statistics, but also learn more about the organizational structure of the cancer center, identify where other navigators may be and how those positions came about, and understand what drove the implementation of navigation within the institution (CoC standards? Patient satisfaction feedback? Philanthropic support?), including her own navigation position. She needed to present herself as not being a threat but a coworker to other navigators she identified within the organization. She also needed to keep her boss, the breast surgeon, informed of her volunteer work to bring together other navigation professionals for networking purposes.

The final outcome can be improved usage of resources for undoing barriers to care, and development of more consistent methods of performing navigation functions across the cancer center and across the continuing of care. The cancer center committee benefits by having a clearer understanding of what navigation functions and processes are in place, how effective they are currently working, and where help is needed to improve and finally having statistical information that reflects the volume of patients being navigated, what barriers aggregately persist, which barriers have solutions, and where help in creating additional solutions to barriers is needed. Bottom line—improvements in patient care.

Conclusion

Oftentimes, where someone professionally begins is far from where they professionally end. Determining one's strengths and weaknesses is a learning process. Identifying what portions of one's job they like and dislike is very much a learning process, too. People are limited by how they view their own capabilities and not necessarily by those constraints placed on them by others.

Oncology nurse navigation is an evolving role for nurses today. Although still misunderstood in some clinical settings, those who serve in navigation roles need to help ensure that the tasks and functions performed impact the clinical and financial outcomes for the institution where they are employed.

Before embarking on a career change, whether it be a lateral move or a promotional move, there is value in having a mentor who can candidly provide insight as well as help train someone for such a professional change. Mentors can be utilized for a short period of time or for those seeking to climb the career ladder relatively high, for a longer period of time. Not everyone who is in a professional position that a navigator is interested in exploring is a good mentor, however.

Getting involved in professional organizations, like AONN+, is a great way to have access to a large volume of individuals who professionally serve as navigators, administrators, team leaders, etc. Some may be ideal mentors, too. Providing opportunities for professional growth is part of the foundation of AONN+ and why it exists.

References

1. http://thinkeracademy.com/critical-thinking-skills.
2. www.teachervision.com/problem-solving/problem-solving.
3. www.lifecoachhub.com/coaching-articles/7-strategies-for-effective-team-building.
4. http://hrweb.mit.edu/system/files/all/other/pd_goal_templates.pdf.
5. http://web.mnstate.edu/gracyk/courses/phil%20115/Four_Basic_principles.htm.
6. www.hr.virginia.edu/uploads/documents/media/Writing_SMART_Goals.pdf.
7. Chandrashekhar Y, Narula J. Mentees, mentors, and the mentorship…. JACC Cardiovasc Imaging. 2014;7(4):434–7. https://doi.org/10.1016/j.jcmg.2014.03.003.
8. Zhang YY, Qian Y, Wu J, Wen F, Zhang Y. The effectiveness and implementation of mentoring program for newly graduated nurses: a systematic review. Nurse Educ Today. 2016;37:136–44. https://doi.org/10.1016/j.nedt.2015.11.027.
9. www.viacharacter.org.
10. McBride AB, Campbell J, Woods NF, Manson SM. Building a mentoring network. Nurs Outlook. 2017;65(3):305–14. https://doi.org/10.1016/j.outlook.2016.12.001. pii: S0029-6554(16)30196-8.
11. Davies S, Gibbs T. Mentoring in general practice: a real activity or a theoretical possibility? Educ Prim Care. 2011;22(4):210–5.
12. Maxwell JC. Mentoring 101: what every leader needs to know.
13. McBurney EI. Strategic mentoring: growth for mentor and mentee. Clin Dermatol. 2015;33(2):257–60. https://doi.org/10.1016/j.clindermatol.2014.12.019.
14. Singla MB. How to take advantage of mentorship. ACG Case Rep J. 2015;2(3):124. https://doi.org/10.14309/crj.2015.26.
15. Barkun A. Maximizing the relationship with a mentor. Gastrointest Endosc. 2006;64(6):4–6. https://doi.org/10.1016/j.gie.2006.11.006.
16. Tolloczko TS. The mentor and the trainee in academic clinical medicine. Sci Eng Ethics. 2006;12(1):95–102.
17. Thoms L, Parmar K, Williamson T. A symbiotic approach to mentoring future academics. Clin Teach. 2013;10(5):337–8. https://doi.org/10.1111/tct.12042.
18. Smith J, Halloway A. Coaching and mentoring for success: supporting learners in the workplace. 2011.

Glossary

Criterion An accepted standard, principle, or rule used to make a decision or to inform an evaluator's judgment.

Denominator The lower part of a fraction used to calculate a rate, proportion, or ratio. It can be the same as the initial population or a subset of the initial population to further constrain the population for the purpose of the measure. Continuous variable measures do not have a denominator but instead define a measure population.

Denominator statement A statement that describes the population evaluated by the performance measure.

Feasibility criteria Extent to which the specifications, including measure logic, require data that are readily available or that could be captured without undue burden and can be implemented for performance measurement.

Grey literature Unpublished or not commercially indexed material that can include any documentary materials issued by government, academia, business, and industry such as technical reports, working papers, and conference proceedings. For example, contributors to the New York Academy of Medicine Grey Literature website include the AHRQ, NQF, CDC, HHS, The Joint Commission, National Academy of Sciences, RAND, and RTI International.

Measure (performance measure or quality measure) A mechanism to assign a quantity to an attribute by comparison to a criterion [228]. A measure may stand alone or belong to a composite, subset, set, and/or collection of measures. A healthcare performance measure is a way to calculate whether and how often the healthcare system does what it should. Measures are based on scientific evidence about processes, outcomes, perceptions, or systems that relate to high-quality care.

Measure steward Also called measure owner, this is an individual or organization that owns a measure and is responsible for maintaining the measure. Measure stewards are often the same as measure developers, but not always. Measure stewards are also the ongoing point of contact for people interested in a given measure.

Numerator The upper portion of a fraction used to calculate a rate, proportion, or ratio. Also called the measure focus, it is the target process, condition, event, or outcome. Numerator criteria are the processes or outcomes expected for each

L. D. Shockney (ed.), *Team-Based Oncology Care: The Pivotal Role of Oncology Navigation*, https://doi.org/10.1007/978-3-319-69038-4

patient, procedure, or other unit of measurement defined in the denominator. A numerator statement describes the clinical action that satisfies the conditions of the performance measure.

Outcome measure   A measure that assesses the results of healthcare that are experienced by patients: clinical events, recovery and health status, experiences in the health system, and efficiency/cost.

Population   The total group of people of interest for a quality measure, sometimes called the initial population. The measure population is a defined subset appropriate to the measure set who are not excluded from the individual measure.

Process measure   A measure that focuses on steps that should be followed to provide good care. There should be a scientific basis for believing that the process, when executed well, will increase the probability of achieving a desired outcome.

Reliability (part of scientific acceptability)   Reflects that the measure is well defined and precisely specified so it can be implemented consistently within and across organizations and that it distinguishes differences in performance.

Scientific acceptability of the measure properties   Extent to which the measure, as specified, produces consistent (reliable) and credible (valid) results about the quality of care when implemented.

Structural measure   A structural measure is one that assesses features of a healthcare organization or clinician relevant to its capacity to provide healthcare.

Systematic literature review   A review of a clearly formulated question that uses systematic and explicit methods to identify, select, and critically appraise relevant research. A systematic review also collects and analyzes data from studies that are included in the review. Two sources of systematic literature reviews are the AHRQ Evidence-Based Clinical Information Reports and the Cochrane Library.

Usability criteria   Extent to which intended audiences (e.g., consumers, purchasers, providers, policy makers) can understand the measure's results and find them useful for quality improvement and decision making. Usability criteria ask if the measure is strong enough to be used for various types of measurement programs, including public reporting, whether it leads to actual improvement for patients and whether the benefits of the measure outweigh any potential harms.

Validity (scientific acceptability of measure properties subcriterion)   Measure validity

The measure accurately represents the concept being evaluated and achieves the purpose for which it is intended (to measure quality). For example, the measure:

Clearly identifies the concept being evaluated (face validity); includes all necessary data elements, codes, and tables to detect a positive occurrence when one exists (construct validity); includes all necessary data sources to detect a positive occurrence when one exists (construct validity) (CMS Blueprint for measure development. www.cms.gov/Medicare/Quality-Initiatives-Patient-Assessment-Instruments/MMS/MMS-Blueprint.html. Accessed June 2017).